2009
YEAR BOOK OF
VASCULAR SURGERY®

The 2009 Year Book Series

Year Book of Anesthesiology and Pain Management™: Drs Chestnut, Abram, Black, Gravlee, Lee, Mathru, and Roizen

Year Book of Cardiology®: Drs Gersh, Cheitlin, Elliott, Graham, Sundt, and Waldo

Year Book of Critical Care Medicine®: Drs Dellinger, Parrillo, Balk, Bekes, Dorman, and Dries

Year Book of Dermatology and Dermatologic Surgery™: Drs Thiers and Lang

Year Book of Diagnostic Radiology®: Drs Osborn, Abbara, Birdwell, Elster, Levy, Manaster, Oestreich, Offiah, Rosado de Christenson, and Walker

Year Book of Emergency Medicine®: Drs Hamilton, Bruno, Handly, Quintana, and Werner

Year Book of Endocrinology®: Drs Mazzaferri, Bessesen, Clarke, Howard, Kennedy, Leahy, Meikle, Molitch, Rogol, and Schteingart

Year Book of Gastroenterology™: Drs Lichtenstein, Dempsey, Drebin, Jaffe, Katzka, Kochman, Makar, Morris, Osterman, Rombeau, and Shah

Year Book of Hand and Upper Limb Surgery®: Drs Yao and Steinmann

Year Book of Medicine®: Drs Barkin, Berney, Frishman, Garrick, Khardori, Loehrer, and Phillips

Year Book of Neonatal and Perinatal Medicine®: Drs Fanaroff, Ehrenkranz, and Stevenson

Year Book of Neurology and Neurosurgery®: Drs Klimo and Rabinstein

Year Book of Obstetrics, Gynecology, and Women's Health®: Drs Dungan and Shulman

Year Book of Oncology®: Drs Loehrer, Arceci, Glatstein, Gordon, Hanna, Morrow, and Thigpen

Year Book of Ophthalmology®: Drs Rapuano, Cohen, Eagle, Flanders, Hammersmith, Myers, Nelson, Penne, Sergott, Shields, Tipperman, and Vander

Year Book of Orthopedics®: Drs Morrey, Beauchamp, Huddleston, Swiontkowski, and Trigg

Year Book of Otolaryngology-Head and Neck Surgery®: Drs Sindwani, Balough, Franco, Gapany, and Mitchell

Year Book of Pathology and Laboratory Medicine®: Drs Raab, Parwani, Bejarano, and Bissell

Year Book of Pediatrics®: Dr Stockman

Year Book of Plastic and Aesthetic Surgery™: Drs Miller, Bartlett, Garner, McKinney, Ruberg, Salisbury, and Smith

2009

The Year Book of
VASCULAR
SURGERY®

Editor-in-Chief
Gregory L. Moneta, MD
Professor and Chief of Vascular Surgery, Oregon Health and Science
University; and Chief of Vascular Surgery, Oregon Health and Science
University Hospital and Portland VA Hospital, Portland, Oregon

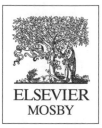

ELSEVIER
MOSBY

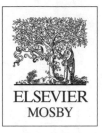

Vice President, Continuity: John A. Schrefer
Editor: Ruth Malwitz
Production Supervisor: Donna M. Skelton
Electronic Article Manager: Travis L. Ross
Illustrations and Permissions Coordinator: Dawn Vohsen

2009 EDITION

Printed in the United States of America
Composition by TNQ Books and Journals Pvt Ltd, India
Printing/binding by Sheridan Books, Inc.

Editorial Office:
Elsevier
Suite 1800
1600 John F. Kennedy Blvd.
Philadelphia, PA 19103-2899

International Standard Serial Number: 0749-4041
International Standard Book Number: 978-1-4160-5730-7

Associate Editors

David L. Gillespie, MD, RVT
Professor of Surgery, Division of Vascular Surgery; University of Rochester School of Medicine and Dentistry, Rochester, New York

Benjamin W. Starnes, MD
Associate Professor and Chief, Vascular Surgery, University of Washington, Seattle, Washington

Michael T. Watkins, MD
Associate Professor of Surgery, Harvard Medical School; and Director, Vascular Surgery Research Laboratory, Massachusetts General Hospital, Boston, Massachusetts

Contributor

Marc A. Passman, MD
Associate Professor of Surgery, Section of Vascular Surgery and Endovascular Therapy, University of Alabama at Birmingham, Birmingham, Alabama

Table of Contents

JOURNALS REPRESENTED xi

1. Basic Considerations 1
2. Coronary Disease 29
3. Epidemiology 37
4. Vascular Lab and Imaging............................. 51
5. Perioperative Considerations........................... 73
6. Grafts and Graft Complications 93
7. Aortic Aneurysm 97
8. Abdominal Aortic Endografting 117
9. Visceral and Renal Artery Disease...................... 129
10. Thoracic Aorta...................................... 141
11. Leg Ischemia.. 157
12. Upper Extremity and Dialysis Access 199
13. Carotid and Cerebrovascular Disease 215
14. Vascular Trauma..................................... 249
15. Nonatherosclerotic Conditions 259
16. Venous Thrombosis and Pulmonary Embolism 269
17. Chronic Venous and Lymphatic Disease.................. 289
18. Technical Notes 303
19. Miscellaneous 319

ARTICLE INDEX 323

AUTHOR INDEX 333

Journals Represented

Journals represented in this YEAR BOOK are listed below.

Acta Orthopaedica
American Heart Journal
American Journal of Cardiology
American Journal of Kidney Diseases
American Journal of Medicine
American Journal of Neuroradiology
Annals of Internal Medicine
Annals of Surgery
Annals of Thoracic Surgery
Annals of Vascular Surgery
BMJ
British Journal of Surgery
Canadian Medical Association Journal
Chest
Circulation
Dermatologic Surgery
European Heart Journal
European Journal of Internal Medicine
European Journal of Nuclear Medicine and Molecular Imaging
European Journal of Obstetrics & Gynecology and Reproductive Biology
European Journal of Radiology
European Journal of Vascular and Endovascular Surgery
Hypertension
Journal of Diabetes and its Complications
Journal of Clinical Epidemiology
Journal of Hand Surgery
Journal of Pediatric Surgery
Journal of the American College of Cardiology
Journal of the American College of Surgeons
Journal of the American Geriatrics Society
Journal of the American Medical Association
Journal of the American Society of Nephrology
Journal of the Neurological Sciences
Journal of Thoracic and Cardiovascular Surgery
Journal of Ultrasound in Medicine
Journal of Vascular Surgery
Lancet
Nature
New England Journal of Medicine
Pharmacotherapy
Radiology
Stroke
Surgery
Thrombosis Research

STANDARD ABBREVIATIONS

The following terms are abbreviated in this edition: acquired immunodeficiency syndrome (AIDS), cardiopulmonary resuscitation (CPR), central nervous system (CNS), cerebrospinal fluid (CSF), computed tomography (CT), deoxyribonucleic acid (DNA), electrocardiography (ECG), health maintenance organization (HMO), human immunodeficiency virus (HIV), intensive care unit (ICU), intramuscular (IM), intravenous (IV), magnetic resonance (MR) imaging (MRI), ribonucleic acid (RNA), and ultrasound (US).

NOTE

The YEAR BOOK OF VASCULAR SURGERY® is a literature survey service providing abstracts of articles published in the professional literature. Every effort is made to assure the accuracy of the information presented in these pages. Neither the editors nor the publisher of the YEAR BOOK OF VASCULAR SURGERY®can be responsible for errors in the original materials. The editors' comments are their own opinions. Mention of specific products within this publication does not constitute endorsement.

To facilitate the use of the YEAR BOOK OF VASCULAR SURGERY® as a reference tool, all illustrations and tables included in this publication are now identified as they appear in the original article. This change is meant to help the reader recognize that any illustration or table appearing in the YEAR BOOK OF VASCULAR SURGERY®may be only one of many in the original article. For this reason, figure and table numbers will often appear to be out of sequence within the YEAR BOOK OF VASCULAR SURGERY®.

1 Basic Considerations

Rosuvastatin to Prevent Vascular Events in Men and Women with Elevated C-Reactive Protein
Ridker PM, for the JUPITER Study Group (Brigham and Women's Hosp, Harvard Med School, Boston, MA)
N Engl J Med 359:2195-2207, 2008

Background.—Increased levels of the inflammatory biomarker high-sensitivity C-reactive protein predict cardiovascular events. Since statins lower levels of high-sensitivity C-reactive protein as well as cholesterol, we hypothesized that people with elevated high-sensitivity C-reactive protein levels but without hyperlipidemia might benefit from statin treatment.

Methods.—We randomly assigned 17,802 apparently healthy men and women with low-density lipoprotein (LDL) cholesterol levels of less than 130 mg per deciliter (3.4 mmol per liter) and high-sensitivity C-reactive protein levels of 2.0 mg per liter or higher to rosuvastatin, 20 mg daily, or placebo and followed them for the occurrence of the combined primary end point of myocardial infarction, stroke, arterial revascularization, hospitalization for unstable angina, or death from cardiovascular causes.

Results.—The trial was stopped after a median follow-up of 1.9 years (maximum, 5.0). Rosuvastatin reduced LDL cholesterol levels by 50% and high-sensitivity C-reactive protein levels by 37%. The rates of the primary end point were 0.77 and 1.36 per 100 person-years of follow-up in the rosuvastatin and placebo groups, respectively (hazard ratio for rosuvastatin, 0.56; 95% confidence interval [CI], 0.46 to 0.69; P<0.00001), with corresponding rates of 0.17 and 0.37 for myocardial infarction (hazard ratio, 0.46; 95% CI, 0.30 to 0.70; P=0.0002), 0.18 and 0.34 for stroke (hazard ratio, 0.52; 95% CI, 0.34 to 0.79; P=0.002), 0.41 and 0.77 for revascularization or unstable angina (hazard ratio, 0.53; 95% CI, 0.40 to 0.70; P<0.00001), 0.45 and 0.85 for the combined end point of myocardial infarction, stroke, or death from cardiovascular causes (hazard ratio, 0.53; 95% CI, 0.40 to 0.69; P<0.00001), and 1.00 and 1.25 for death from any cause (hazard ratio, 0.80; 95% CI, 0.67 to 0.97; P=0.02). Consistent effects were observed in all subgroups evaluated. The rosuvastatin group did not have a significant increase in myopathy or cancer but did have a higher incidence of physician-reported diabetes.

Conclusions.—In this trial of apparently healthy persons without hyperlipidemia but with elevated high-sensitivity C-reactive protein levels, rosuvastatin significantly reduced the incidence of major cardiovascular events. (ClinicalTrials.gov number, NCT00239681.) (Fig 1).

▶ This article generated a great deal of media attention and is, in fact, likely to have huge impact. It demonstrates for the first time the potential for lowering cardiovascular events with statin therapy (Fig 1) in patients targeted for therapy by the presence of an elevated level of C-reactive protein (CRP), but with LDL cholesterol levels generally considered to be below levels recommended for treatment. The findings are compatible with the now well-accepted postulate that inflammation contributes and is essential to the atherosclerotic process. The end points were all clinical in this study and there were no objective measurements of the presence, absence, or progression of atherosclerotic

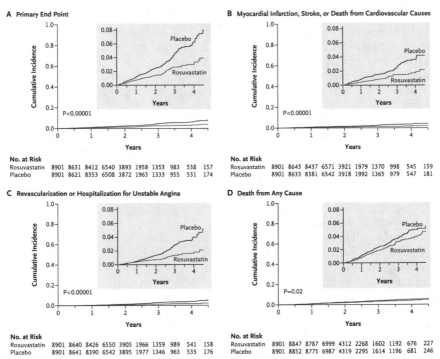

FIGURE 1.—Cumulative incidence of cardiovascular events according to study group. Panel A shows the cumulative incidence of the primary end point (nonfatal myocardial infarction, nonfatal stroke, arterial revascularization, hospitalization for unstable angina, or confirmed death from cardiovascular causes). The hazard ratio for rosuvastatin, as compared with placebo, was 0.56 (95% confidence interval [CI], 0.46 to 0.69; P<0.00001). Panel B shows the cumulative incidence of nonfatal myocardial infarction, nonfatal stroke, or death from cardiovascular causes, for which the hazard ratio in the rosuvastatin group was 0.53 (95% CI, 0.40 to 0.69; P<0.00001). Panel C shows the cumulative incidence of arterial revascularization or hospitalization for unstable angina, for which the hazard ratio in the rosuvastatin group was 0.53 (95% CI, 0.40 to 0.70; P<0.00001). Panel D shows the cumulative incidence of death from any cause, for which the hazard ratio in the rosuvastatin group was 0.80 (95% CI, 0.67 to 0.97; P=0.02). In each panel, the inset shows the same data on an enlarged y axis and on a condensed x axis. (Reprinted from Ridker PM, for the JUPITER Study Group. Rosuvastatin to prevent vascular events in men and women with elevated C-reactive protein. *N Engl J Med.* 2008;359:2195-2207. Copyright © 2008, Massachusetts Medical Society. All rights reserved.)

plaque. Because the study was stopped relatively soon after its inception raises the possibility that the events that occurred may be independent of the usual mechanisms of progression of atherosclerotic plaque. It does seem unusual that patients with relatively favorable LDL cholesterol levels would have marked progression of atherosclerosis in such a short time period. The results may therefore indicate more of a plaque stabilization effect of lowering CRP levels than an inhibition of bulky progression of existing plaque. It is important to examine this article in the context of another article that also appeared in the *New England Journal of Medicine*,[1] which suggested treatment of CRP alone is unlikely to be of benefit. The 2 articles are not incompatible, in that it is certainly reasonable to postulate that to derive benefit from treatment of elevated CRP it is also necessary to drive the LDL cholesterol level down as well. It seems it will eventually be required to do trials with agents that can lower elevated levels of CRP and not affect cholesterol levels to tease out the mechanism of benefit of rosuvastatin therapy in patients with otherwise "acceptable" LDL cholesterol levels and elevated CRP.

G. L. Moneta, MD

Reference

1. Zacho J, Tybjaerg-Hansen A, Jensen JS, et al. Genetically elevated C-reactive protein and ischemic vascular disease. *N Engl J Med.* 2008;359:1897-1908.

Genetically Elevated C-Reactive Protein and Ischemic Vascular Disease
Zacho J, Tybjærg-Hansen A, Jensen JS, et al (Copenhagen Univ Hosp, Univ of Copenhagen, Herlev, Denmark; et al)
N Engl J Med 359:1897-1908, 2008

Background.—Elevated levels of C-reactive protein (CRP) are associated with increased risks of ischemic heart disease and ischemic cerebrovascular disease. We tested whether this is a causal association.

Methods.—We studied 10,276 persons from a general population cohort, including 1786 in whom ischemic heart disease developed and 741 in whom ischemic cerebrovascular disease developed. We examined another 31,992 persons from a cross-sectional general population study, of whom 2521 had ischemic heart disease and 1483 had ischemic cerebrovascular disease. Finally, we compared 2238 patients with ischemic heart disease with 4474 control subjects and 612 patients with ischemic cerebrovascular disease with 1224 control subjects. We measured levels of high-sensitivity CRP and conducted genotyping for four CRP polymorphisms and two apolipoprotein E polymorphisms.

Results.—The risk of ischemic heart disease and ischemic cerebrovascular disease was increased by a factor of 1.6 and 1.3, respectively, in persons who had CRP levels above 3 mg per liter, as compared with persons who had CRP levels below 1 mg per liter. Genotype combinations of the four CRP polymorphisms were associated with an increase in CRP levels of up to 64%, resulting in a theoretically predicted increased risk of up to 32% for ischemic heart disease and up to 25% for ischemic cerebrovascular disease. However, these genotype combinations were not associated with an increased risk of ischemic vascular disease. In contrast, apolipoprotein E genotypes were associated with both elevated cholesterol levels and an increased risk of ischemic heart disease.

Conclusions.—Polymorphisms in the CRP gene are associated with marked increases in CRP levels and thus with a theoretically predicted increase in the risk of ischemic vascular disease. However, these polymorphisms are not in themselves associated with an increased risk of ischemic vascular disease.

▶ It is well known that the elevated plasma levels of C-reactive protein (CRP) are associated with increased risk of ischemic cerebrovascular and ischemic cardiac disease. What is unknown is whether CRP levels themselves contribute to causation of ischemic cerebrovascular or cardiac disease, or are merely markers of the existence of ischemic cerebrovascular or cardiovascular disease. The authors use the fact that there are genetic variations of the gene for CRP. These variants increase levels of CRP to different degrees and therefore could theoretically be used to assess the consequences of lifelong high CRP levels independent of additional risk factors. Sorting out the precise role of CRP in atherosclerosis is potentially commercially important also. There are drugs being developed to specifically target lowering CRP levels.[1] The ultimate goal would be to lower CRP levels and, if CRP is associated with causing atherosclerosis, ultimately prevent the development of vascular disease. This study suggests that such a strategy is likely to be barking up the wrong tree. Although epidemiologic studies have observed increased risk of ischemic vascular disease associated with higher plasma CRP levels, the current data indicate that increased CRP levels are perhaps more a marker for atherosclerosis than a cause of atherosclerosis. Please also see the abstract for a related article[2] for a different perspective on the possibility of targeting CRP levels for intervention to decrease cardiovascular disease.

G. L. Moneta, MD

References

1. Lowe GD, Pepys MB. C-reactive protein and cardiovascular disease: weighing the evidence. *Curr Atheroscler Rep.* 2006;8:421-428.
2. Ridker PM, Danielson E, Fonseca FA, et al. Rosuvastatin to prevent vascular events in men and women with elevated C-reactive protein. *N Engl J Med.* 2008;359:2195-2207.

Glucose Control and Vascular Complications in Veterans with Type 2 Diabetes

Duckworth W, Abraira C, Moritz T, et al (Phoenix Veterans Affairs (VA) Health Care Ctr, AZ; Miami VA Med Ctr, FL; Hines VA Cooperative Studies Program Coordinating Ctr, IL; et al)
N Engl J Med 360:129-139, 2009

Background.—The effects of intensive glucose control on cardiovascular events in patients with long-standing type 2 diabetes mellitus remain uncertain.

Methods.—We randomly assigned 1791 military veterans (mean age, 60.4 years) who had a suboptimal response to therapy for type 2 diabetes to receive either intensive or standard glucose control. Other cardiovascular risk factors were treated uniformly. The mean number of years since the diagnosis of diabetes was 11.5, and 40% of the patients had already had a cardiovascular event. The goal in the intensive-therapy group was an absolute reduction of 1.5 percentage points in the glycated hemoglobin level, as compared with the standard-therapy group. The primary outcome was the time from randomization to the first occurrence of a major cardiovascular event, a composite of myocardial infarction, stroke, death from cardiovascular causes, congestive heart failure, surgery for vascular disease, inoperable coronary disease, and amputation for ischemic gangrene.

Results.—The median follow-up was 5.6 years. Median glycated hemoglobin levels were 8.4% in the standard-therapy group and 6.9% in the intensive-therapy group. The primary outcome occurred in 264 patients in the standard-therapy group and 235 patients in the intensive-therapy group (hazard ratio in the intensive-therapy group, 0.88; 95% confidence interval [CI], 0.74 to 1.05; P = 0.14). There was no significant difference between the two groups in any component of the primary outcome or in the rate of death from any cause (hazard ratio, 1.07; 95% CI, 0.81 to 1.42; P = 0.62). No differences between the two groups were observed for microvascular complications. The rates of adverse events, predominantly hypoglycemia, were 17.6% in the standard-therapy group and 24.1% in the intensive-therapy group.

Conclusions.—Intensive glucose control in patients with poorly controlled type 2 diabetes had no significant effect on the rates of major cardiovascular events, death, or microvascular complications. (ClinicalTrials.gov number, NCT00032487.)

▶ There are many interventions that can affect prognosis in patients with type 2 diabetes. These include lifestyle changes, control of blood pressure and lipids, and use of antiplatelet agents. It appears that blood pressure control has better benefit than glucose control.[1] Previously there had been mixed results as to whether glucose control can independently reduce cardiovascular complications in patients with advanced type 2 diabetes. The UK Prospective Diabetes Study,[1] the ADVANCE Trial,[2] and the ACCORD Trial[3] all studied the effects of intensive glucose control in patients with diabetes. None of these studies, and now this study, provided significant evidence for favorable effects of intensive glucose control in controlling cardiovascular events in patients with diabetes. Some, in fact, even suggested harm from this approach. At this point we can say that intensive glucose control early in the course of patients with diabetes may be of benefit; however, in patients with well-established diabetes it appears that management of other cardiovascular risk factors such as hypertension and increased lipids is a more effective approach to prevent cardiovascular morbidity and mortality than tight glucose control.

G. L. Moneta, MD

References

1. Tight blood pressure control and risk of macrovascular and microvascular complications in type 2 diabetes: UKPDS 38. UK Prospective Diabetes Study Group. *BMJ*. 1998;317:703-713.
2. Patel A, MacMahon S, Chalmers J, et al. ADVANCE Collaborative Group. Intensive blood glucose control and vascular outcomes in patients with type 2 diabetes. *N Engl J Med*. 2008;358:2560-2572.
3. Gernstein HC, Miller ME, Byington RP, et al. Action to Control Cardiovascular Risk in Diabetes Study Group. Effects of intensive glucose lowering in type 2 diabetes. *N Engl J Med*. 2008;358:2545-2559.

Low-Dose Aspirin for Primary Prevention of Atherosclerotic Events in Patients With Type 2 Diabetes: A Randomized Controlled Trial
Ogawa H, for the Japanese Primary Prevention of Atherosclerosis With Aspirin for Diabetes (JPAD) Trial Investigators (Kumamoto Univ, Kumamoto City, Japan; et al)
JAMA 300:2134-2141, 2008

Context.—Previous trials have investigated the effects of low-dose aspirin on primary prevention of cardiovascular events, but not in patients with type 2 diabetes.

Objective.—To examine the efficacy of low-dose aspirin for the primary prevention of atherosclerotic events in patients with type 2 diabetes.

Design, Setting, and Participants.—Multicenter, prospective, randomized, openlabel, blinded, end-point trial conducted from December 2002 through April 2008 at 163 institutions throughout Japan, which enrolled 2539 patients with type 2 diabetes without a history of atherosclerotic disease and had a median follow-up of 4.37 years.

Interventions.—Patients were assigned to the low-dose aspirin group (81 or 100 mg per day) or the nonaspirin group.

Main Outcome Measures.—Primary end points were atherosclerotic events, including fatal or nonfatal ischemic heart disease, fatal or nonfatal stroke, and peripheral arterial disease. Secondary end points included each primary end point and combinations of primary end points as well as death from any cause.

Results.—A total of 154 atherosclerotic events occurred: 68 in the aspirin group (13.6 per 1000 person-years) and 86 in the nonaspirin group (17.0 per 1000 person-years) (hazard ratio [HR], 0.80; 95% confidence interval [CI], 0.58-1.10; log-rank test, $P = .16$). The combined end point of fatal coronary events and fatal cerebrovascular events occurred in 1 patient (stroke) in the aspirin group and 10 patients (5 fatal myocardial infarctions and 5 fatal strokes) in the nonaspirin group (HR, 0.10; 95% CI, 0.01-0.79; $P = .0037$). A total of 34 patients in the aspirin group and 38 patients in the nonaspirin group died from any cause (HR, 0.90; 95% CI, 0.57-1.14; log-rank test, $P = .67$). The composite of hemorrhagic stroke and significant gastrointestinal bleeding was not significantly different between the aspirin and nonaspirin groups.

Conclusion.—In this study of patients with type 2 diabetes, low-dose aspirin as primary prevention did not reduce the risk of cardiovascular events.

Trial Registration.—clinicaltrials.gov Identifier: NCT00110448.

▶ In patients with previous cardiovascular events, aspirin therapy can serve as a secondary prevention strategy. In addition, clinical guidelines recommend patients with risk factors for coronary heart disease should take aspirin for primary prevention. The American Diabetes Association recommends aspirin as a primary prevention strategy in patients with diabetes who are at increased cardiovascular risk, such as those > 40 years of age who have additional risk factors such as family history of coronary disease, hypertension, smoking, albuminuria, or dyslipidemia.[1] However, subgroup analyses of large trials of aspirin for primary prevention have not demonstrated significant effects in patients with diabetes. Because these analyses were subgroup analyses, it is possible they were underpowered to demonstrate primary prevention of cardiovascular events with aspirin in patients with diabetes, hence the motivation for this study. Unfortunately, although this study had a relatively large sample size, it also had a relatively low event rate (Fig 2 in the original article). The low event rate, perhaps, makes the study underpowered for demonstrating that aspirin may have a significant effect on reducing total atherosclerotic events.

It is clearly becoming frustrating to demonstrate any means of decreasing atherosclerotic events in patients with diabetes. Recent trials have suggested strictly controlling plasma glucose levels is also ineffective in reducing cardiovascular events in patients with type 2 diabetes.

Because of the low event rate in this trial, and the fact that it was conducted on an entirely Japanese population, it is probably too early to conclude that aspirin is ineffective as primary preventative therapy in patients with type 2 diabetes.

G. L. Moneta, MD

Reference

1. Colwell JA. Aspirin therapy in diabetes. *Diabetes Care*. 2003;26:S87-S88.

The prevention of progression of arterial disease and diabetes (POPADAD) trial: factorial randomised placebo controlled trial of aspirin and antioxidants in patients with diabetes and asymptomatic peripheral arterial disease

Belch J, MacCuish A, Campbell I, et al (Univ of Dundee, UK; Glasgow Royal Infirmary, UK; Royal Victoria Hosp, Kirkcaldy, UK; et al)
BMJ 337:a1840, 2008

Objective.—To determine whether aspirin and antioxidant therapy, combined or alone, are more effective than placebo in reducing the development of cardiovascular events in patients with diabetes mellitus and asymptomatic peripheral arterial disease.

Design.—Multicentre, randomised, double blind, 2×2 factorial, placebo controlled trial.

Setting.—16 hospital centres in Scotland, supported by 188 primary care groups.

Participants.—1276 adults aged 40 or more with type 1 or type 2 diabetes and an ankle brachial pressure index of 0.99 or less but no symptomatic cardiovascular disease.

Interventions.—Daily, 100 mg aspirin tablet plus antioxidant capsule (n=320), aspirin tablet plus placebo capsule (n=318), placebo tablet plus antioxidant capsule (n=320), or placebo tablet plus placebo capsule (n=318).

Main Outcome Measures.—Two hierarchical composite primary end points of death from coronary heart disease or stroke, non-fatal myocardial infarction or stroke, or amputation above the ankle for critical limb ischaemia; and death from coronary heart disease or stroke.

Results.—No evidence was found of any interaction between aspirin and antioxidant. Overall, 116 of 638 primary events occurred in the aspirin groups compared with 117 of 638 in the no aspirin groups (18.2% *v* 18.3%): hazard ratio 0.98 (95% confidence interval 0.76 to 1.26). Forty three deaths from coronary heart disease or stroke occurred in the aspirin groups compared with 35 in the no aspirin groups (6.7% *v* 5.5%): 1.23 (0.79 to 1.93). Among the antioxidant groups 117 of 640 (18.3%) primary events occurred compared with 116 of 636 (18.2%) in the no antioxidant groups (1.03, 0.79 to 1.33). Forty two (6.6%) deaths from coronary heart disease or stroke occurred in the antioxidant groups compared with 36 (5.7%) in the no antioxidant groups (1.21, 0.78 to 1.89).

Conclusion.—This trial does not provide evidence to support the use of aspirin or antioxidants in primary prevention of cardiovascular events and mortality in the population with diabetes studied.

Trial Registration.—Current Controlled Trials ISRCTN53295293.

▶ Patients with asymptomatic peripheral arterial disease (PAD) are at increased risk of myocardial infarction and stroke. They are 6 times more likely to die from cardiovascular disease within 10 years than patients without PAD.[1] Aspirin as a secondary preventative measure in patients with diabetes and cardiovascular disease is well established. This has led to recommendations for use of aspirin as primary preventative therapy as well. However, a meta-analysis has demonstrated no efficacy for aspirin as primary preventative therapy in patients with diabetes.[2] There is also some evidence that there is an increase in oxidative stress in patients with diabetes with free radicals increasing platelet aggregation and antioxidants decreasing platelet aggregation. Based on the strength of the data for secondary prevention of cardiovascular events with aspirin therapy, the lack of data investigating aspirin as primary preventative therapy, and potential effects of antioxidants in patients with diabetes, the authors sought to study these agents in a group of patients with diabetes and asymptomatic PAD. The objective was to determine whether aspirin and antioxidant therapy, combined or alone, was more effective than placebo in reducing cardiovascular events in patients with diabetes and asymptomatic peripheral arterial disease. However, once again, aspirin fails as a primary preventative therapy in patients with diabetes, this time in diabetic patients with asymptomatic PAD (see Fig 2 in the original article). This should not be construed as justification for failure to use aspirin as secondary preventative therapy in patients with cardiovascular disease and diabetes. Aspirin may be a so-called wonder drug, but it doesn't seem to be good for everything.

G. L. Moneta, MD

References

1. Criqui MH, Langer RD, Fronek A, et al. Mortality over a period of 10 years in patients with peripheral arterial disease. *N Engl J Med.* 1992;326:381-386.
2. Antithrombotic Trialists' Collaboration. Collaborative meta-analysis of randomised trials of antiplatelet therapy for prevention of death, myocardial infarction, and stroke in high risk patients. *BMJ.* 2002;324:71-86.

Effect of Statins Alone Versus Statins Plus Ezetimibe on Carotid Atherosclerosis in Type 2 Diabetes: The SANDS (Stop Atherosclerosis in Native Diabetics Study) Trial

Fleg JL, Mete M, Howard BV, et al (National Heart, Lung, and Blood Inst, Bethesda, MD; MedStar Research Inst, Hyattsville, MD; et al)
J Am Coll Cardiol 52:2198-2205, 2008

Objectives.—This secondary analysis from the SANDS (Stop Atherosclerosis in Native Diabetics Study) trial examines the effects of lowering low-density lipoprotein cholesterol (LDL-C) with statins alone versus statins plus ezetimibe on common carotid artery intima-media thickness (CIMT) in patients with type 2 diabetes and no prior cardiovascular event.

Background.—It is unknown whether the addition of ezetimibe to statin therapy affects subclinical atherosclerosis.

Methods.—Within an aggressive group (target LDL-C ≤70 mg/dl; non-high-density lipoprotein cholesterol ≤100 mg/dl; systolic blood pressure ≤115 mm Hg), change in CIMT over 36 months was compared in diabetic individuals >40 years of age receiving statins plus ezetimibe versus statins alone. The CIMT changes in both aggressive subgroups were compared with changes in the standard subgroups (target LDL-C ≤100 mg/dl; non-high-density lipoprotein cholesterol ≤130 mg/dl; systolic blood pressure ≤130 mm Hg).

Results.—Mean (95% confidence intervals) LDL-C was reduced by 31 (23 to 37) mg/dl and 32 (27 to 38) mg/dl in the aggressive group receiving statins plus ezetimibe and statins alone, respectively, compared with changes of 1 (−3 to 6) mg/dl in the standard group (p < 0.0001) versus both aggressive subgroups. Within the aggressive group, mean CIMT at 36 months regressed from baseline similarly in the ezetimibe (−0.025 [−0.05 to 0.003] mm) and nonezetimibe subgroups (−0.012 [−0.03 to 0.008] mm) but progressed in the standard treatment arm (0.039 [0.02 to 0.06] mm), intergroup p < 0.0001.

Conclusions.—Reducing LDL-C to aggressive targets resulted in similar regression of CIMT in patients who attained equivalent LDL-C reductions from a statin alone or statin plus ezetimibe. Common carotid artery IMT increased in those achieving standard targets. (Stop Atherosclerosis in Native Diabetics Study [SANDS]; NCT00047424).

▶ Ezetimibe is an anti-hyperlipidemic medication used to lower cholesterol levels. It acts by decreasing cholesterol absorption in the intestine. It can be used alone or with other cholesterol lowering medications. It may be combined with a statin medication (eg, ezetimibe/simvastatin is marketed as Vytorin). It is generally indicated for use when cholesterol levels are unable to be controlled with statins alone.

Implicit in the use of ezetimibe to lower low-density lipoprotein cholesterol (LDL-C) is the idea this should translate into a reduction in clinical atherosclerotic events similar to that observed with statins. Carotid artery intima-media thickness (CIMT) is considered as a marker of future cardiovascular risk and thus can serve as a short-term surrogate for potential long-term cardiovascular events. The current trial has, therefore, 2 potential significant implications. The first is that ezetimibe does not provide any advantage over a statin alone in reducing long-term cardiovascular risk. The results would therefore seem to confirm the Enhanced Trial[1] of 720 patients with familial hypercholesterolemia where there was no statistically significant difference in the primary end-point of mean increase in CIMT over 24 months in the patients treated with statins alone versus statin plus ezetimibe. The implication is that it matters how you lower cholesterol, and not just how much you lower cholesterol and the pleotropic effects of statins may be more important, as is suspected by many, than the cholesterol-lowering effects of statins.

The second point is that it does appear possible to actually reduce surrogate markers of future atherosclerosis by aggressively lowering cholesterol beyond standard target levels. In its early stages, atherosclerosis may be a reversible disease.

G. L. Moneta, MD

Reference

1. Kastelein JJ, Akdim F, Stroes ES, et al. Simvastatin with or without ezetimibe in familial hypercholesterolemia. *N Engl J Med.* 2008;358:1431-1433.

Plasma Levels of Soluble Tie2 and Vascular Endothelial Growth Factor Distinguish Critical Limb Ischemia From Intermittent Claudication in Patients With Peripheral Arterial Disease

Findley CM, Mitchell RG, Duscha BD, et al (Duke Univ Med Ctr, Durham, NC; et al)

J Am Coll Cardiol 52:387-393, 2008

Objectives.—Our purpose was to determine whether factors that regulate angiogenesis are altered in peripheral arterial disease (PAD) and whether these factors are associated with the severity of PAD.

Background.—Alterations in angiogenic growth factors occur in cardiovascular disease (CVD), but whether these factors are altered in PAD or correlate with disease severity is unknown.

Methods.—Plasma was collected from patients with PAD (n = 46) and healthy control subjects (n = 23). Peripheral arterial disease patients included those with intermittent claudication (IC) (n = 23) and critical limb ischemia (CLI) (n = 23). Plasma angiopoietin-2 (Ang2), soluble Tie2 (sTie2), vascular endothelial growth factor (VEGF), soluble VEGF receptor 1 (sVEGFR-1), and placenta growth factor (PlGF) were measured by enzyme-linked immunoadsorbent assay. In vitro, endothelial cells (ECs) were treated with recombinant VEGF to investigate effects on sTie2 production.

Results.—Plasma concentrations of sTie2 (p < 0.01), Ang2 (p < 0.001), and VEGF (p < 0.01), but not PlGF or sVEGFR-1, were significantly greater in PAD patients compared with control subjects. Plasma Ang2 was significantly increased in both IC and CLI compared with control subjects (p < 0.0001), but there was no difference between IC and CLI. Plasma VEGF and sTie2 were similar in control subjects and IC but were significantly increased in CLI (p < 0.001 vs. control or IC). Increased sTie2 and VEGF were independent of CVD risk factors or the ankle-brachial index, and VEGF treatment of ECs in vitro significantly increased sTie2 shedding.

Conclusions.—Levels of VEGF and sTie2 are significantly increased in CLI, and sTie2 production is induced by VEGF. These proteins may provide novel biomarkers for CLI, and sTie2 may be both a marker and a cause of CLI.

▶ Patients with peripheral arterial disease (PAD) are at increased risk for cardiovascular mortality. Risk is higher for those patients with critical limb ischemia (CLI) versus those with intermittent claudication (IC). The diagnosis of IC versus CLI is, however, purely clinical. In addition, although a lower ankle-brachial index (ABI) is also a marker for increased cardiovascular mortality, ABI in itself does not distinguish between CLI and IC. A potential biomarker that can distinguish between patients with CLI and IC may, therefore, be useful in risk stratification in patients with PAD.

The authors are experts in fields of angiogenesis and it is known that alterations in angiogenic growth factors occur in patients with vascular disease. It is, however, unknown whether these growth factors are altered in the subset of cardiovascular disease patients with PAD or whether these potential alterations in growth factors can correlate with the disease severity.

Based on the data presented, it is a bit of a stretch to suggest at this time that vascular endothelial growth factor (VEGF) and soluble Tie2 (sTie2) have any use as biomarkers for the large cohort of patients with CLI. If, however, these biomarkers could be used as a predictor of amputation risk in patients with CLI, adjusted for wound size and ABI, that would be useful. The only real conclusion that can come from this study is that plasma levels of sTie2 and VEGF are increased in patients with PAD, and are different in those with a clinical diagnosis of CLI versus those with IC. What we really need in the group of patients with CLI is a predictor of short-term amputation risk, and the data here are not sufficient for that degree of risk stratification.

G. L. Moneta, MD

Long-term clinical outcome after intramuscular implantation of bone marrow mononuclear cells (Therapeutic Angiogenesis by Cell Transplantation [TACT] trial) in patients with chronic limb ischemia

Matoba S, TACT Follow-up Study Investigators (Kyoto Prefectural Univ of Medicine, Japan)

Am Heart J 156:1010-1018, 2008

Background.—Angiogenic cell therapy by intramuscular injection of autologous bone marrow mononuclear cells was first attempted in patients with peripheral artery disease (PAD) with critical limb ischemia, and the feasibility was shown by a randomized controlled Therapeutic Angiogenesis by Cell Transplantation (TACT) study.

Methods and Results.—The present study was designed to assess the 3-year safety and clinical outcomes of this angiogenic cell therapy by investigating the mortality and leg amputation-free interval as primary end points. The median follow-up time for surviving patients was 25.3 months (range, 0.8-69.0 months), and 3-year overall survival rates were 80% (95% CI 68-91) in patients with atherosclerotic peripheral arterial disease (11 died in 74 patients) and 100% (no death) in 41 patients with thromboangiitis obliterans (TAO; Buerger's disease). Three-year amputation-free rate was 60% (95% CI 46-74) in PAD and 91% (95% CI 82-100) in patients with TAO. The multivariate analysis revealed that the severity of rest pain and repeated experience of bypass surgery were the prognostic factors negatively affecting amputation-free interval. The significant improvement in the leg pain scale, ulcer size, and pain-free walking distance was maintained during at least 2 years after the therapy, although the ankle brachial index and transcutaneous oxygen pressure value did not significantly change.

Conclusions.—The angiogenic cell therapy using bone marrow mononuclear cells can induce a long-term improvement in limb ischemia, leading to extension of amputation-free interval. The safety and efficacy are not inferior to the conventional revascularization therapies.

▶ Methods of inducing angiogenesis as a treatment for chronic limb ischemia are under active investigation. These authors published an earlier clinical trial of therapeutic angiogenesis using bone marrow mononuclear cells (BMMCs) in patients with chronic limb ischemia secondary to peripheral arterial disease (PAD) or thromboangiitis obliterans (TAO).[1] In that trial, intramuscular implantation of autologous BMMCs resulted in improvement in transcutaneous oxygen pressure, rest pain, ankle-brachial index, and pain-free walking time.

BMMCs contain cell fractions that include endothelial progenitor cells (EPC) and that also release various antigenic factors. Incorporation of EPCs in newly formed vessels and angiogenesis/arteriogenesis by angiogenic factors released from injected cells may contribute to increased blood flow in the treated patients. The stimulus for this study was the occasional sudden death after intramuscular injection of BMMCs.[2] Thus, this study was essentially a safety analysis of the patients treated under previously approved protocols. There were no prospectively identified control subjects, and therefore, the authors' conclusion that "the safety and efficacy are not inferior to the conventional revascularization therapies" is not really valid. Angiogenesis, however, remains an intriguing potential therapy for chronic limb ischemia. Overall, the data thus far are fairly underwhelming. Studies like this, however, with some hints of improvement in clinically relevant end points, will serve to sustain interest in angiogenesis. Some approach – probably not one of the current approaches – using angiogenesis, at least as an adjunct in the treatment of chronic limb ischemia, ought to prove beneficial someday.

G. L. Moneta, MD

References

1. Tateishi-Yuyama E, Matsubara H, Murohara T, et al. Therapeutic angiogenesis for patients with limb ischaemia by autologous transplantation of bone-marrow cells: a pilot study and a randomised controlled trial. *Lancet.* 2002;360:427-435.
2. Miyamoto K, Nishigami K, Nagaya N, et al. Unblinded pilot study of autologous transplantation of bone marrow mononuclear cells in patients with thromboangiitis obliterans. *Circulation.* 2006;114:2679-2684.

Hepatocyte Growth Factor, but not Vascular Endothelial Growth Factor, Attenuates Angiotensin II-Induced Endothelial Progenitor Cell Senescence
Sanada F, Taniyama Y, Azuma J, et al (Osaka Univ Graduate School of Medicine; et al)
Hypertension 53:77-82, 2009

Although both hepatocyte growth factor (HGF) and vascular endothelial growth factor (VEGF) are potent angiogenic growth factors in animal models of ischemia, their characteristics are not the same in animal experiments and clinical trials. To elucidate the discrepancy between HGF and VEGF, we compared the effects of HGF and VEGF on endothelial progenitor cells under angiotensin II stimulation, which is a well-known risk factor for atherosclerosis. Here, we demonstrated that HGF, but not VEGF, attenuated angiotensin II–induced senescence of endothelial progenitor cells through a reduction of oxidative stress by inhibition of the phosphatidylinositol-3,4,5-triphosphate/rac1 pathway. Potent induction of neovascularization of endothelial progenitor cells by HGF, but not VEGF, under angiotensin II was also confirmed by in vivo experiments using several models, including HGF transgenic mice (Fig 5).

▶ These investigators used a sophisticated combination of in vivo and in vitro experiments to demonstrate that hepatocyte growth factor (HGF) but not vascular endothelial cell growth factor (VEGF) markedly decreased angiotensin II induced oxidative stress in human endothelial progenitor cells (EPC). Furthermore, they showed the hepatocyte growth factor selectively increased human EPC neovascularization in murine model of hind limb ischemia, even in the setting of extrinsic stress mediated by angiotensin II (Fig 5). These elegant, well-thought-out experiments provide a major rationale for ongoing clinical trials into the use of HGF, but not VEGF for limb ischemia in humans. These experiments have extensive clinical importance because human EPC are sensitive to oxidative stress and can become senescent, limiting their ability to contribute to proangiogenic processes in vivo.

M. T. Watkins, MD

FIGURE 5.—Effect of transplanted ex vivo expanded human EPCs on neovascularization in the ischemic hindlimb model of athymic nude mice. A, Representative micoscopic photographs of double fluorescence in ischemic hindlimb on day 7. Transplanted human DiI-labeled EPC was identified as red. Host mouse vasculature was identified as green. Bar = 100 μm. B, Quantitative analysis of incorporated DiI-labeled EPC (red) and host endothelial cells (green) in tissue sections retrieved from ischemic adductor muscles. n = 4. *$P<0.01$ vs nonischemic, #$P<0.01$ vs Ang II or VEGF + Ang II. (Reprinted from Sanada F, Taniyama Y, Azuma J, et al. Hepatocyte growth factor, but not vascular endothelial growth factor, attenuates angiotensin II-induced endothelial progenitor cell senescence. *Hypertension* 2009;53:77-82.)

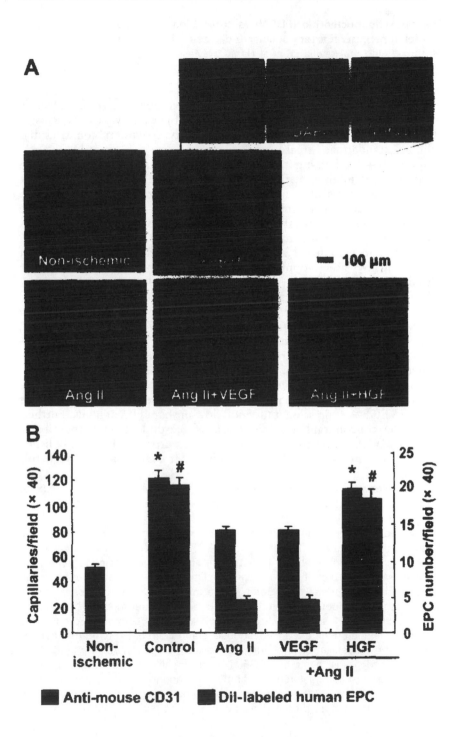

A

Non-ischemic

100 μm

Ang II   Ang II+VEGF   Ang II+HGF

B

Anti-mouse CD31   Dil-labeled human EPC

Polydeoxyribonucleotide (PDRN) restores blood flow in an experimental model of peripheral artery occlusive disease
Bitto A, Polito F, Altavilla D, et al (Univ of Messina, Italy)
J Vasc Surg 48:1292-1300, 2008

Objective.—This study investigated whether polydeoxyribonucleotide (PDRN) may be efficacious in the treatment of peripheral artery occlusive diseases, which are a major cause of morbidity in Western countries and still lack standardized treatment.

Methods.—We investigated the effects of PDRN, a mixture of deoxyribonucleotides, in an experimental model of hind limb ischemia (HLI) in rats to stimulate vascular endothelial growth factor (VEGF)-A production and to avoid critical ischemia. The femoral artery was excised to induce HLI. Sham-operated on rats (sham HLI) were used as controls. Animals were treated daily with intraperitoneal PDRN (8 mg/kg) or its vehicle. Animals were euthanized at day 7, 14, and 21 after the evaluation of blood flow by laser Doppler. Dissected muscles were used to measure VEGF-A messenger RNA (mRNA) and protein expression, to evaluate edema, and to assess histologic damage.

Results.—Administration of PDRN dramatically increased VEGF mRNA throughout the study (day 14: HLI, 7 ± 2.2 n-fold/β-actin; HLI + PDRN, 13.3 ± 3.8 n-fold/β-actin; $P < .0001$) and protein expression (HLI, 11 ± 3.4 integrated intensity; HLI + PDRN, 16 ± 3.8 integrated intensity; $P < .0001$). The compound stimulated revascularization, as confirmed by blood flow restoration ($P < .005$ vs HLI + vehicle), and blunted the histologic damage and the degree of edema. PDRN did not modify VEGF-A expression and blood flow in sham HLI animals. Furthermore, the concomitant administration of 3,7-dimethyl-1-propargilxanthine (DMPX), a selective adenosine A_{2A} receptor antagonist, abolished the positive effects of PDRN, confirming that PDRN acts through this receptor.

Conclusion.—These results led us to hypothesize a role for PDRN in treating peripheral artery occlusive diseases.

▶ Polydeoxyribonucleotide (PDRN) is a compound known to stimulate Vascular Endothelial Cell Growth Factor (VEGF) production in ischemic models of thermal injury and diabetes through the action of adenosine receptors. In Italy, these compounds have been used clinically to facilitate wound repair for a number of medical conditions. These investigators sought to determine whether these compounds limited ischemic injury in a rat model of acute limb ischemia. Using a clinically relevant post ischemic treatment protocol, the investigators demonstrate a dose response relationship between PDRN administration and decreased tissue injury, increased perfusion, capillary infiltration, and increased tissue levels of VEGF. To confirm the specificity of this drug, the investigators administered an inhibitor of adenosine receptors in select experiments, which abolished the improvement in tissue perfusion and decreased inflammatory profile. These encouraging results must be viewed in context of the fact that the experiments were performed in young healthy rodents. Tissue repair and components of the angiogenic response in humans are known to be dependent in part on circulating stem cells whose populations are depleted with age and associated vascular comorbidities. It would be helpful to know whether these agents mediate the inflammation and necrosis in ischemic skeletal muscle in the setting of hypercholesterolemia and/or hyperglycemia.

M. T. Watkins, MD

Gene expression analysis of a porcine native abdominal aortic aneurysm model
Sadek M, Hynecek RL, Goldenberg S, et al (New York Univ School of Medicine; Columbia Univ College of Physicians and Surgeons; NY; Mount Sinai School of Medicine, NY)
Surgery 144:252-258, 2008

Introduction.—We sought to characterize the gene expression patterns occurring during the development of aneurysms in the native porcine aorta.

Methods.—In Yorkshire swine, the infrarenal aorta was balloon dilated and infused with a solution of type I collagenase/pancreatic porcine elastase (16,000 U/1,000 U). Aneurysmal and control aortic samples were obtained at 1 (n = 3), 2 (n = 6), and 4 (n = 5) weeks following aneurysm induction. RNA was isolated, converted to biotin-modified antisense RNA and hybridized to porcine genome arrays. Aneurysmal and control gene intensities were compared using the 2-sample-for-means z-test. $P < .01$ was considered statistically significant.

Results.—Extracellular matrix remodeling genes that were upregulated in aneurysmal compared with control tissue included matrix metalloproteinase-1, -2, -3, and -9; MT-MMP; cathepsin-D, -H, -K, and -S; tissue inhibitor of metalloproteinase-1; and collagen I-α1 chain ($P < .01$). Elastin exhibited temporally downregulated gene expression ($P < .01$). Inflammatory genes that were upregulated included intercellular adhesion molecule-2, tumor necrosis factor-α, interleukin (IL)-1β, IL-10, chemokine receptor-4, and tissue plasminogen activator ($P < .01$). Atherosclerosis and cancer genes that were upregulated included apolipoprotein E, acyl-CoA binding protein, friend leukemia virus integration-1, and E26 transformation-specific sequence ($P < .01$).

Conclusion.—The porcine model replicates the gene expression patterns that are observed during the development of aneurysms in human studies as well as in rodent models. The porcine model thereby represents a novel method to study the impact of endovascular, cell-based, and other therapeutic interventions on AAA pathophysiology.

▶ Investigators are always seeking relevant animal models to human disease. Relevant animal models are obviously important in basic research and have contributed greatly to the understanding of many biologic processes affecting the vascular system. There are rodent models for abdominal aortic aneurysms (AAA) where gene expressions more or less mimic those of the human condition. Rodents, however, are too small to test endovascular devices. In this study, the authors have demonstrated broad similarities between gene expressions that exist in the porcine model of AAA previously described well with rodent models and the human condition of AAA. Although the similarities are not exact, and there may be differences in temporal expressions of RNA, it is likely this model will prove useful in investigations of abdominal aortic aneurysms, and in particular, in the use of endoluminal devices to treat abdominal aortic aneurysms.

G. L. Moneta, MD

Intra-abdominal fat and metabolic syndrome are associated with larger infrarenal aortic diameters in patients with clinically evident arterial disease

Gorter PM, Visseren FLJ, Moll FL, et al (Univ Med Ctr Utrecht, The Netherlands)
J Vasc Surg 48:114-120, 2008

Objective.—Abdominal obesity and its associated metabolic consequences are major determinants for the development of vascular disease. Fat tissue close to arteries may also directly affect atherogenesis. The study examined whether intra-abdominal fat accumulation is an independent determinant of infrarenal aortic diameter in patients with clinically evident arterial disease. The relationship between metabolic syndrome and infrarenal aortic diameter was also assessed in this patient group.

Methods.—Cross-sectional study was done of 2726 patients with clinically evident arterial disease enrolled in the Second Manifestations of ARTerial Disease (SMART) study. Intra-abdominal fat was measured with ultrasonography and by measuring waist circumference. Metabolic syndrome was defined according to the Adult Treatment Panel III. The maximal anteroposterior diameter of the infrarenal aorta was measured using ultrasonography. The relation between intra-abdominal fat, metabolic syndrome, and infrarenal aortic diameter was determined with linear regression analyses and adjusted for age, sex, height, and smoking.

Results.—Infrarenal aortic diameters (mm) increased across quartiles of intra-abdominal fat derived by ultrasonography (quartile 4, 19 ± 7 mm vs quartile 1, 17 ± 5 mm; adjusted beta, 1.34; 95% confidence interval [CI], 0.73-1.94) and across quartiles of waist circumference (quartile 4, 19 ± 7 mm vs quartile 1, 17 ± 5 mm; adjusted β, 1.43; 95% CI, 0.82-2.04). Patients with metabolic syndrome had slightly larger infrarenal aortic diameters (18 ± 7 mm vs 17 ± 6 mm; adjusted beta, 0.70; 95% CI, 0.27-1.13) compared with those without metabolic syndrome.

Conclusions.—Intra-abdominal fat accumulation and metabolic syndrome are associated with larger infrarenal aortic diameters in patients with clinically evident arterial disease. These data may indicate a role for intra-abdominal fat in the development of larger aortic diameters.

▶ If you are overweight, where you deposit your fat seems to matter. There is evidence that intra-abdominal fat results in some sort of altered adipocyte function with increased levels of interlukin-6 free fatty acids and low plasma concentrations of adiponectin. These changes and others result in increased insulin resistance and may contribute to accelerated atherosclerosis. This study found an association between the accumulation of intra-abdominal fat and larger aortic diameters. Obviously, no cause and effect mechanism can be inferred from the type of data presented here. I suppose at some point a measurement of intra-abdominal fat may be useful in classifying patients at risk for aortic expansion and development of aneurysm. However, at this point, a connection between intra-abdominal fat and aortic aneurysm development is only speculative. The study will have no immediate clinical impact. It is, however, interesting that obesity, and particularly patterns of obesity may contribute to potential aortic enlargement.

G. L. Moneta, MD

Biomechanical properties of abdominal aortic aneurysms assessed by simultaneously measured pressure and volume changes in humans
van 't Veer M, Buth J, Merkx M, et al (Catharina Hosp, Eindhoven, The Netherlands; Univ of Technology, Eindhoven, The Netherlands)
J Vasc Surg 48:1401-1407, 2008

Background.—Abdominal aortic aneurysms (AAA) are at risk of rupture when the internal load (blood pressure) exceeds the aneurysm wall strength. Generally, the maximal diameter of the aneurysm is used as a predictor of rupture; however, biomechanical properties may be a better predictor than the maximal diameter. Compliance and distensibility are two biomechanical properties that can be determined from the pressure-volume relationship of the aneurysm. This study determined the compliance and distensibility of the AAA by simultaneous instantaneous pressure and volume measurements; as a secondary goal, the influence of direct and indirect pressure measurements was compared.

Methods.—Ten men (aged 73.6 ± 6.4 years) with an infrarenal AAA were studied. Three-dimensional balanced turbo field echo (3D B-TFE) images were acquired with noncontrast-enhanced magnetic resonance imaging (MRI) for the aortic region proximal to the renal arteries until just beyond the bifurcation. Volume changes were extracted from the electrocardiogram-triggered 3D B-TFE MRI images using dedicated prototype software. Pressure was measured simultaneously within the AAA using a fluid-filled pigtail catheter. Noninvasive brachial cuff measurements were also acquired before and after the imaging sequence simultaneously with the invasive pressure measurement to investigate agreement between the techniques. Compliance was calculated as the slope of the best linear fit through the pressure volume data points. Distensibility was calculated by dividing the compliance by the diastolic aneurysmal volume. Young's moduli were estimated from the compliance data.

Results.—The AAA maximal diameter was 5.8 ± 0.6 cm. A strong linear relation between the pressure and volume data was found. Distensibility was 1.8 ± 0.7 × 10^{-3} kPa^{-1}. Average compliance was 0.31 ± 0.15 mL/kPa with accompanying estimates for Young's moduli of 9.0 ± 2.5 MPa. Brachial cuff measurements demonstrated an underestimation of 5% for systolic ($P < .001$) and an overestimation of 12% for diastolic blood pressure ($P < .001$) compared with the pressure measured within the aneurysm.

Conclusion.—Distensibility and compliance of the wall of the aneurysm were determined in humans by simultaneous intra-aneurysmal pressure and volume measurements. A strong linear relationship existed between the intra-aneurysmal pressure and the volume change of the AAA. Brachial cuff measurements were significantly different compared with invasive intra-aneurysmal measurements. Consequently, no absolute distensibility values can be determined noninvasively. However, because of a constant and predictable difference between directly and indirectly derived blood pressures, MRI-based monitoring of aneurysmal distensibility may serve the online rupture risk during follow-up of aneurysms.

▶ This unique study for the first time measured compliance and distensibility of the aortic aneurysm wall in humans. The goal, of course, is to find a better predictor of rupture of abdominal aortic aneurysms (AAAs). Currently, based on the results of the ADAM Study[1] and the UK Small Aneurysm Trial,[2] it is recommended that aortic aneurysms not be repaired until they exceed 5.5 cm in diameter. Small aneurysms, however, do on occasion rupture, and while they may comprise 5% to 10% of all series of aortic aneurysm ruptures, the percentage of small aneurysms that rupture is likely much smaller. The question, therefore, becomes whether it is more effective to eventually try to predict AAA rupture in patients with small AAAs, or try to predict which patients with large AAAs will not have the aneurysms rupture!

The authors' approach to determine aneurysm rupture is sophisticated science but is clinically impracticle. One is not going to relegate a patient with a small AAA with a minimal likelihood of rupture to the sophisticated combination of MR studies and invasive pressure measurements used in this article. However, this approach may be of use in the patient with a large AAA who is a marginal candidate for either endovascular or open repair. In such patients, determination of the biomechanical properties of AAA might influence the clinician one way or the other when considering whether or not to recommend repair. I have no doubt that in 10 to 15 years we will be using some sort of measure of the biomechanical properties of the aortic wall to help stratify aneurysm risk of rupture. Whether it is an MRI-based measurement of aneurysm distensibility or something else is unknown, but it will be something.

G. L. Moneta, MD

References

1. Lederle FA, Wilson SE, Johnson GR, et al. Immediate repair compared with surveillance of small abdominal aortic aneurysms. *N Engl J Med.* 2002;346: 1437-1444.
2. Mortality results for randomised controlled trial of early elective surgery or ultra-sonographic surveillance for small abdominal aortic aneurysms. The UK Small Aneurysm Trial Participants. *Lancet.* 1998;352:1649-1655.

Genomewide Association Studies of Stroke

Ikram MA, Seshadri S, Bis JC, et al (Erasmus MC Univ Med Ctr, Rotterdam, The Netherlands; Boston Univ School of Medicine, MA; Univ of Washington; et al)
N Engl J Med 360:1718-1728, 2009

Background.—The genes underlying the risk of stroke in the general population remain undetermined.

Methods.—We carried out an analysis of genomewide association data generated from four large cohorts composing the Cohorts for Heart and Aging Research in Genomic Epidemiology consortium, including 19,602 white persons (mean [±SD] age, 63 ± 8 years) in whom 1544 incident strokes (1164 ischemic strokes) developed over an average follow-up of 11 years. We tested the markers most strongly associated with stroke in a replication cohort of 2430 black persons with 215 incident strokes (191 ischemic strokes), another cohort of 574 black persons with 85 incident strokes (68 ischemic strokes), and 652 Dutch persons with ischemic stroke and 3613 unaffected persons.

Results.—Two intergenic single-nucleotide polymorphisms on chromosome 12p13 and within 11 kb of the gene *NINJ2* were associated with stroke ($P < 5 \times 10^{-8}$). *NINJ2* encodes an adhesion molecule expressed in glia and shows increased expression after nerve injury. Direct genotyping showed that rs12425791 was associated with an increased risk of total (i.e., all types) and ischemic stroke, with hazard ratios of 1.30 (95% confidence interval [CI], 1.19 to 1.42) and 1.33 (95% CI, 1.21 to 1.47), respectively, yielding population attributable risks of 11% and 12% in the discovery cohorts. Corresponding hazard ratios were 1.35 (95% CI, 1.01 to 1.79; P = 0.04) and 1.42 (95% CI, 1.06 to 1.91; P = 0.02) in the large cohort of black persons and 1.17 (95% CI, 1.01 to 1.37; P = 0.03) and 1.19 (95% CI, 1.01 to 1.41; P = 0.04) in the Dutch sample; the results of an underpowered analysis of the smaller black cohort were nonsignificant.

Conclusions.—A genetic locus on chromosome 12p13 is associated with an increased risk of stroke (Fig 1).

▶ Through analysis of stroke patterns within families and twin studies, it has been determined that stroke has a significant genetic component.[1,2] There have been 2 previous genome-wide association studies of stroke. These studies were smaller and limited by case-controlled design and, therefore, more

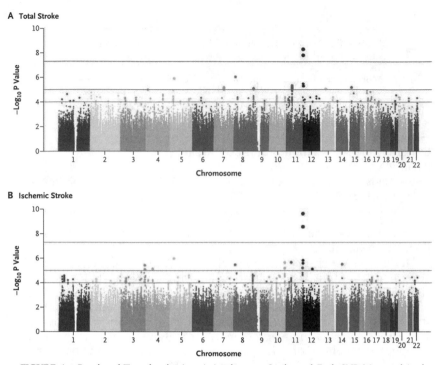

FIGURE 1.—Results of Tests for the Association between Stroke and Each SNP Measured in the Genomewide Association Study. P values (based on the fixed-effects model) are shown in signal-intensity (Manhattan) plots relative to their genomic position for total stroke (Panel A) and ischemic stroke (Panel B). Within each chromosome, the results are plotted left to right from the p-terminal end. The top horizontal line indicates the chosen threshold for genomewide significance, $P = 5 \times 10^{-8}$; the middle line indicates the threshold for $P = 10^{-5}$; and the bottom line indicates the threshold for $P = 10^{-4}$. (Reprinted from Ikram MA, Seshadri S, Bis JC, et al. Genomewide association studies of stroke. *N Engl J Med.* 2009;360:1718-1728, with permission from Massachusetts Medical Society. All rights reserved.)

susceptible to selection bias. In this study the authors carried out an analysis of genome-wide association data generated from 4 large prospective population-based cohorts. The study indicates that 2 previously unsuspected common single-nucleotide polymorphisms (SNPs) on chromosome 12p13 (Fig 1) are associated with total and ischemic stroke, and particularly athero-embolic stroke in white patients. The data was duplicated in an additional cohort of Dutch white patients, and also in an independent sample of North American black persons. The intergenic SNPs are probably not the causal variants of stroke, but more likely they reflect linkage disequilibrium with the causal variants. Clarification of this point will require more detailed genotyping and translational studies.

G. L. Moneta, MD

References

1. Bak S, Gaist D, Sindrup SH, Skytthe A, Christensen K. Genetic liability in stroke: a long-term follow-up study of Danish twins. *Stroke.* 2002;33:769-774.
2. Jousilahti P, Rastenyte D, Tuomilehto J, Sarti C, Vartiainen E. Parental history of cardiovascular disease and risk of stroke. A prospective follow-up of 14371 middle-aged men and women in Finland. *Stoke.* 1997;28:1361-1366.

Local Delivery of Gene Vectors From Bare-Metal Stents by Use of a Biodegradable Synthetic Complex Inhibits In-Stent Restenosis in Rat Carotid Arteries

Fishbein I, Alferiev I, Bakay M, et al (Children's Hosp of Philadelphia, PA)
Circulation 117:2096-2103, 2008

Background.—Local drug delivery from polymer-coated stents has demonstrated efficacy for preventing in-stent restenosis; however, both the inflammatory effects of polymer coatings and concerns about late outcomes of drug-eluting stent use indicate the need to investigate innovative approaches, such as combining localized gene therapy with stent angioplasty. Thus, we investigated the hypothesis that adenoviral vectors (Ad) could be delivered from the bare-metal surfaces of stents with a synthetic complex for reversible vector binding.

Methods and Results.—We synthesized the 3 components of a gene vector binding complex: (1) A polyallylamine bisphosphonate with latent thiol groups (PABT), (2) a polyethyleneimine (PEI) with pyridyldithio groups for amplification of attachment sites [PEI(PDT)], and (3) a bifunctional (amine- and thiol-reactive) cross-linker with a labile ester bond (HL). HL-modified Ad attached to PABT/PEI(PDT)-treated steel surfaces demonstrated both sustained release in vitro over 30 days and localized green fluorescent protein expression in rat arterial smooth muscle cell cultures, which were not sensitive to either inhibition by neutralizing anti-Ad antibodies or inactivation after storage at 37°C. In rat carotid studies, deployment of steel stents configured with PABT/PEI(PDT)/HL-tethered adenoviral vectors demonstrated both site-specific arterial Ad(GFP) expression and adenovirus-luciferase transgene activity per optical imaging. Rat carotid stent delivery of adenovirus encoding inducible nitric oxide synthase resulted in significant inhibition of restenosis.

Conclusions.—Reversible immobilization of adenovirus vectors on the bare-metal surfaces of endovascular stents via a synthetic complex represents an efficient, tunable method for sustained release of gene vectors to the vasculature.

▶ Polymer-coated stents facilitate local drug delivery to the vasculature and have proven efficacious in preventing in-stent restenosis in the coronary circulation. There are, however, concerns about the inflammatory effects of polymer coatings and late outcomes of drug-eluting stents. This study investigated local delivery of gene therapy from bare-metal stent surfaces using reversible chemical attachment of vectors to the bare-metal stents. Adenovirus vectors on the surfaces of the stents demonstrated greater than 1-month release kinetics and site-specific transduction of target cell types in-vitro and in-vivo in the rat model used. Deployment of stents configured with 10^9 adenovirus vectors that were encoded for inducible nitric oxide synthase resulted in significant reduction of in-stent restenosis. It appears that the concept of gene-eluting stents is valid and may provide a mechanism of local and systemic delivery of gene products via the vasculature.

G. L. Moneta, MD

Adventitial delivery of platelet-derived endothelial cell growth factor gene prevented intimal hyperplasia of vein graft

Handa M, Li W, Morioka K, et al (Univ of Fukui, Japan)
J Vasc Surg 48:1566-1574, 2008

Background.—Platelet-derived endothelial cell growth factor (PD-ECGF), also known as thymidine phosphorylase (TP) reportedly inhibits vascular smooth muscle cells (VSMCs) migration and proliferation. We hypothesized that adventitial administration of the *PD-ECGF/TP* gene will suppress intimal hyperplasia and prevent vein graft failure.

Methods.—The study used 68 female rabbits. Rabbit jugular vein was autogenously transplanted into carotid artery with a cuff anastomotic technique. To define vascular wall gene transfer efficiency, poloxamer hydrogel (20%) containing plasmid vector encoding the *LacZ* gene and different concentrations of trypsin (0%, 0.1%, 0.25%, and 0.5%, n = 5 for each group) was applied to the adventitia of the vein graft. Gene transfer efficiency was evaluated 7 days later by X-gal staining. An additional 48 rabbits received poloxamer hydrogel (20%) containing 0.25% trypsin and the human *PD-ECGF/TP* gene, *LacZ* gene, or saline. Intima thickness was evaluated at 2 and 8 weeks after grafting (n = 8 for each group at each time point). Transgene expression was examined by reverse transcriptase-polymerase chain reaction, immunoblotting assay, and immunohistochemical staining. Immunohistochemical staining was also used to determine VSMC proliferation, heme oxygenase-1 expression, and macrophage infiltration.

Results.—Incorporation of trypsin into the poloxamer hydrogel significantly increased vessel wall gene transfer. Trypsin at 0.25% and 0.5% resulted in higher gene transfer at the same level without effecting intimal hyperplasia and inflammation; thus, trypsin at 0.25% concentration was used for subsequent experiments. Compared with the *LacZ* and saline groups, grafts receiving the *PD-ECGF/TP* gene significantly reduced intimal thickness at 2 and 8 weeks after treatment. The ratio of proliferative VSMC was lower in *PD-ECGF/TP* treated grafts. Histologic examination of the *PD-ECGF/TP* transgene grafts demonstrated high expression of heme oxygenase-1, which has been reported to inhibit VSMC proliferation, suggesting that heme oxygenase-1 may be important in the inhibition effect of PD-ECGF/TP on VSMC. No neoplastic or morphologic changes were found in the remote organs.

Conclusions.—A safe and highly efficient gene transfer method was developed by using poloxamer hydrogel and a low concentration of trypsin. Neointimal hyperplasia was significantly reduced by adventitial application of the *PD-ECGF/TP* gene to the vein graft. Our data suggest that adventitial delivery of the *PD-ECGF/TP* gene after grafting may be promising method for preventing vein graft failure.

▶ This novel article describes a useful experimental technique using poloxamer gel to achieve gene delivery to arterialized vein grafts using a rabbit model. The target gene delivered to vein graft *PD-ECGF/TP* has been known to promote angiogenesis in vivo by stimulating chemotaxis of endothelial cells. The rationale for these experiments was based on in vitro studies where this gene has been shown to conclusively inhibit smooth muscle cell proliferation and migration. The experimental results clearly demonstrate the efficacy of gene transfection and the ability of the *PD-ECGF/TP* gene to ameliorate intimal hyperplasia. The article falls short of providing conclusive mechanistic insight into how this happens, largely because the authors focus on expression of heme oxygenase-1 in transfected tissue. No experiments are performed with an in vivo inhibitor of heme oxygenase-1 to conclusively demonstrate its role in vein graft intimal hyperplasia.

M. T. Watkins, MD

Metalloproteinase expression in venous aneurysms
Irwin C, Synn A, Kraiss L, et al (Univ of Texas Medical Branch, Galveston)
J Vasc Surg 48:1278-1285, 2008

Introduction.—Although recognized with increasing frequency, the pathogenesis of venous aneurysms (VA) remains poorly understood. We evaluated 8 patients with 10 VA for the presence, localization and activity of metalloproteinases (MMPs).

Methods.—Tissue specimens from VA (n = 8), normal saphenous vein (NSV n = 7) and varicose veins (VV n = 7 were compared by histology and immunohistochemistry (IHC). Histologic sections were stained with H&E, Movats pentachrome and toluidine blue, and IHC specimens with antibodies to CD68, MMP2, MMP9, and MMP13. Protein expression and enzyme activity were determined by Western immunoblotting and zymography.

Results.—Three of 4 patients with popliteal VA presented with edema and leg pain and the remaining patient with deep venous thrombosis (DVT) and pulmonary embolism (PE). The 5 popliteal VA were treated by; excision and reanastomosis (n = 2) lateral venorrhaphy (n = 2) and spiral saphenous vein graft (n = 1). The 3 patients with 4 upper extremity VA had discomfort over a compressible mass. Two of the VA were excised

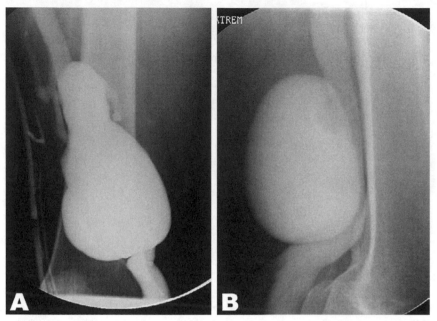

FIGURE 2.—Phlebography showing lobulated (A) and saccular (B) popliteal venous aneurysms. (Reprinted from Irwin C, Synn A, Kraiss L, et al. Metalloproteinase expression in venous aneurysms. *J Vasc Surg.* 2008;48:1278-1285, with permission from The Society for Vascular Surgery.)

and the remaining patients aneurysm ruptured spontaneously. The mesenteric VA, an incidental finding at laparotomy was excised. Thrombus was present in 2 popliteal, 1 upper extremity and in the mesenteric aneurysm. Histologically, VA and VV were characterized by fragmentation of the elastic lamellae, loss of smooth muscle cells (SMCs) and attenuation of the venous wall when compared to NSV. Varicose veins and VA also demonstrated increased expression of MMP-2, MMP-9 and MMP-13 in endothelial cells (ECs), SMCs and adventitial microvessels compared to NSV. Both pro-MMP-2 and pro-MMP-9 were detected by zymography in VA,VV and NSV but only MMP-2 activity was demonstrable.

Conclusions.—The structural changes in the venous wall in addition to the increased expression of MMP-2, MMP-9 and MMP-13 in VA compared to NSV and VV suggests a possible causal role for these MMPs in their pathogenesis (Figs 2a and b).

▶ Venous aneurysms are uncommon. They exist in both saccular and fusiform configurations. They appear to have no particular sex predilection and can occur at any age. They are not associated with trauma or previous arteriovenous communications. Most venous aneurysms in the upper extremity or the neck are asymptomatic, and come to treatment because of cosmetic concerns. Venous aneurysms involving thoracic or abdominal veins are usually asymptomatic and detected as incidental findings on CT or MRI examinations. Such aneurysms, along with venous aneurysms, present in the lower extremities (Figs 2A and 2B) are sometimes considered for repair because of scattered reports of thrombosis and associated pulmonary embolism.

The etiology of venous aneurysms is unknown, but it makes sense that matrix metalloproteinases (MMPs) are possibly involved because of their association with aneurysms in the arterial system. The authors documentation of these differential expressions of MMP-2, -9, and -13 in venous aneurysms, combined with the morphologic changes of the extracellular matrix that they observed, suggests a possible causal role of MMPs in the pathogenesis of venous aneurysms.

A bit of information that may be important clinically is that the morphologic changes observed in venous aneurysms may only involve part of the circumference of the venous wall. The authors point out that this asymmetry of the disease process makes lateral venorrhaphy a feasible technique for repair of venous aneurysms.

G. L. Moneta, MD

Sox18 induces development of the lymphatic vasculature in mice
François M, Caprini A, Hosking B, et al (The Univ of Queensland, Brisbane, Australia; FIRC Inst of Molecular Oncology, Milan, Italy)
Nature 456:643-647, 2008

The lymphatic system plays a key role in tissue fluid regulation and tumour metastasis, and lymphatic defects underlie many pathological states including lymphoedema, lymphangiectasia, lymphangioma and lymphatic dysplasia. However, the origins of the lymphatic system in the embryo, and the mechanisms that direct growth of the network of lymphatic vessels, remain unclear. Lymphatic vessels are thought to arise from endothelial precursor cells budding from the cardinal vein under the influence of the lymphatic hallmark gene *Prox1* (prospero homeobox 1; ref. 4). Defects in the transcription factor gene *SOX18* (SRY (sex determining region Y) box 18) cause lymphatic dysfunction in the human syndrome hypotrichosis-lymphoedema-telangiectasia, suggesting that Sox18 may also play a role in lymphatic development or function. Here we use molecular, cellular and genetic assays in mice to show that Sox18 acts as a molecular switch to induce differentiation of lymphatic endothelial cells. Sox18 is expressed in a subset of cardinal vein cells that later co-express Prox1 and migrate to form lymphatic vessels. Sox18 directly activates *Prox1* transcription by binding to its proximal promoter. Overexpression of Sox18 in blood vascular endothelial cells induces them to express Prox1 and other lymphatic endothelial markers, while *Sox18*-null embryos show a complete blockade of lymphatic endothelial cell differentiation from the cardinal vein. Our findings demonstrate a critical role for Sox18 in developmental lymphangiogenesis, and suggest new avenues to investigate for therapeutic management of human lymphangiopathies.

▶ This article provides an exquisite demonstration of in vivo molecular analysis. Using an evaluation of the gene expression in embryos that have genetic deletion of the *SOX18* gene, the authors identify downstream molecular targets, which are relevant to lymphatic differentiation. The structure of the mature lymphatic vascular network in adult mice with heterozygous *Sox18* mutations (RaOp/1 and Sox181/2 B6) were evaluated by immunofluorescence analysis of whole ear tissue using antibodies specific for the marker LYVE-1. The authors demonstrate defects in gene expression, lymphatic cell differentiation, and tissue edema, which correlate with *SOX18* expression. Using an in vitro system of *SOX18* overexpression, the authors observed a significant upregulation of the lymphatic markers Prox1, ephrinB2 and Vegfr3. The convincing biochemical and anatomic changes associated mutations and overexpression of the *SOX18* gene provides rationale for investigating the relative expression of these genes in humans with lymphatic abnormalities.

M. T. Watkins, MD

2 Coronary Disease

General and Abdominal Adiposity and Risk of Death in Europe
Pischon T, Boeing H, Hoffmann K, et al (German Inst of Human Nutrition, Potsdam-Rehbruecke, Germany; et al)
N Engl J Med 359:2105-2120, 2008

Background.—Previous studies have relied predominantly on the body-mass index (BMI, the weight in kilograms divided by the square of the height in meters) to assess the association of adiposity with the risk of death, but few have examined whether the distribution of body fat contributes to the prediction of death.

Methods.—We examined the association of BMI, waist circumference, and waist-to-hip ratio with the risk of death among 359,387 participants from nine countries in the European Prospective Investigation into Cancer and Nutrition (EPIC). We used a Cox regression analysis, with age as the time variable, and stratified the models according to study center and age at recruitment, with further adjustment for educational level, smoking status, alcohol consumption, physical activity, and height.

Results.—During a mean follow-up of 9.7 years, 14,723 participants died. The lowest risks of death related to BMI were observed at a BMI of 25.3 for men and 24.3 for women. After adjustment for BMI, waist circumference and waist-to-hip ratio were strongly associated with the risk of death. Relative risks among men and women in the highest quintile of waist circumference were 2.05 (95% confidence interval [CI], 1.80 to 2.33) and 1.78 (95% CI, 1.56 to 2.04), respectively, and in the highest quintile of waist-to-hip ratio, the relative risks were 1.68 (95% CI, 1.53 to 1.84) and 1.51 (95% CI, 1.37 to 1.66), respectively. BMI remained significantly associated with the risk of death in models that included waist circumference or waist-to-hip ratio (P<0.001).

Conclusions.—These data suggest that both general adiposity and abdominal adiposity are associated with the risk of death and support the use of waist circumference or waist-to-hip ratio in addition to BMI in assessing the risk of death.

▶ Adipose tissue, especially adipose tissue associated with visceral fat deposits, can secrete mediators that are likely important in the development of chronic diseases. These mediators are thought to potentiate inflammation that has been associated with respiratory ailments, cancer, and atherosclerosis. Indeed, a recent report suggests that the increased risk of death associated with a high body-mass index (BMI) is driven by cancer and cardiovascular causes.[1]

BMI, however, is not the whole story when it comes to the impact of adipose tissue on life span. The study results suggest that in patients with low BMI, measurements of waist circumference or waist-to-hip ratio are more important predictors of the risk of death than the BMI itself. The study also challenges the use of precise cut-off points to define the risk of death associated with abdominal obesity. The risk imposed by the presence of adipose tissue exists essentially as a continuous rather than as a categorical variable, and it now appears important to assess distribution of body fat even in persons of normal weight.

G. L. Moneta, MD

Reference

1. Jee SH, Sull JW, Park J, et al. Body-mass index and mortality in Korean men and women. N Engl J Med. 2005;355:779-787.

Prevalence and extent of dyslipidemia and recommended lipid levels in US adults with and without cardiovascular comorbidities: The National Health and Nutrition Examination Survey 2003-2004
Ghandehari H, Kamal-Bahl S, Wong ND, et al (Univ of California, Irvine, CA; Global Outcomes Res, West Point, PA)
Am Heart J 156:112-119, 2008

Background.—Despite improvements in low-density lipoprotein cholesterol (LDL-C) levels, recent national data are limited regarding the proportion of adults at recommended lipid levels according to the presence of cardiovascular disease (CVD) and related comorbidities. We evaluated the proportion of US adults with and without these conditions at (and distance to) recommended levels of LDL-C, non–high-density lipoprotein cholesterol (non–HDL-C), HDL-C, and triglycerides.

Methods.—We analyzed data from adults aged ≥20 who had fasted for 8 or more hours (n = 2,883, weighted to a US population of 128.5 million) in the National Health and Nutrition Examination Survey 2003-2004, a nationally representative cross-sectional survey. The number of adults at National Cholesterol Education Program recommended levels for LDL-C, non–HDL-C, HDL-C, triglycerides, and combined lipids, stratified by sex, age group, ethnicity, and the presence of CVD comorbidities was determined.

Results.—Although 85% to 89% of persons without CVD or related comorbidities were at recommended levels for LDL-C, non–HDL-C, HDL-C, and triglycerides, only 36% to 37% of those with CVD or related comorbidities were at recommended levels for LDL-C and non–HDL-C, and only 17% were at recommended levels for all lipids. Treated persons compared with those untreated had significantly lower LDL-C (112.3 vs 156.7 mg/dL, $P < .001$) and non–HDL-C levels (145.9 vs 188.7 mg/dL, $P < .001$), but similar HDL-C (52.0 vs 50.1 mg/dL, $P = .09$) and triglyceride (160.1 vs 148.7 mg/dL, $P = .20$) levels.

Conclusions.—Despite improved LDL-C levels, many adults, especially with CVD or related comorbidities, are not at recommended levels for all lipids. Improved treatment efforts to target the spectrum of dyslipidemia are needed.

▶ The National Cholesterol Education Program promotes guidelines for goal lipid levels. Data suggest that the extent of treatment and control of hypercholesterolemia in the United States is poor, with only 35% of adults in 1999-2000 being aware of their hypercholesterol, only 12% on treatment, and 5% controlled.[1] Only one fifth of high-risk secondary prevention patients were at goal LDL cholesterol of less than 100 mg/dL.[2] Treatment recommendations have primarily focused on management of LDL-C. This emphasis has resulted in improvements in LDL-C levels in the United States. The new data here, however, point out that those patients, perhaps in most, need control of their lipid levels, that is, those with cardiovascular disease or related comorbidities had really quite poor overall control of their lipid levels. In patients with cardiovascular disease, diabetes, or chronic kidney disease, only one third were at goal LDL-C and non-HDL-C levels. Only 20% were at recommended levels for all lipids. Lack of achieving lipid levels in this population may reflect a lack of awareness, not being treated despite awareness, or inadequate treatment. It appears that there needs to be even greater use of efficacious dosages of lipid-lowering agents and likely greater use of combination therapy to address patients with multiple lipid disorders, especially if such patients have cardiovascular disease or significant comorbidities for cardiovascular disease.

G. L. Moneta, MD

References

1. Ford ES, Mokdad AH, Giles WH, Mensah GA. Serum total cholesterol concentrations and awareness, treatment, and control of hypercholesterolemia among US adults: findings from the National Health and Nutrition Examination Survey, 1999 to 2000. *Circulation.* 2003;107:2185-2189.
2. Expert Panel on Detection, Evaluation, and Treatment of High Blood Cholesterol in Adults. Executive Summary of The Third Report of The National Cholesterol Education Program (NCEP) Expert Panel on Detection, Evaluation, And Treatment of High Blood Cholesterol In Adults (Adult Treatment Panel III). *JAMA.* 2001;285:2486-2497.

Telmisartan, Ramipril, or Both in Patients at High Risk for Vascular Events
Yusuf S, Teo KK, Pogue J, et al (McMaster Univ, Hamilton Health Sciences, Ontario, Canda; et al)
N Engl J Med 358:1547-1559, 2008

Background.—In patients who have vascular disease or high-risk diabetes without heart failure, angiotensin-converting–enzyme (ACE) inhibitors reduce mortality and morbidity from cardiovascular causes, but the role of angiotensin-receptor blockers (ARBs) in such patients is unknown. We compared the ACE inhibitor ramipril, the ARB telmisartan, and the combination of the two drugs in patients with vascular disease or high-risk diabetes.

Methods.—After a 3-week, single-blind run-in period, patients underwent double-blind randomization, with 8576 assigned to receive 10 mg of ramipril per day, 8542 assigned to receive 80 mg of telmisartan per day, and 8502 assigned to receive both drugs (combination therapy). The primary composite outcome was death from cardiovascular causes, myocardial infarction, stroke, or hospitalization for heart failure.

Results.—Mean blood pressure was lower in both the telmisartan group (a 0.9/0.6 mm Hg greater reduction) and the combination-therapy group (a 2.4/1.4 mm Hg greater reduction) than in the ramipril group. At a median follow-up of 56 months, the primary outcome had occurred in 1412 patients in the ramipril group (16.5%), as compared with 1423 patients in the telmisartan group (16.7%; relative risk, 1.01; 95% confidence interval [CI], 0.94 to 1.09). As compared with the ramipril group, the telmisartan group had lower rates of cough (1.1% vs. 4.2%, $P < 0.001$) and angioedema (0.1% vs. 0.3%, $P = 0.01$) and a higher rate of hypotensive symptoms (2.6% vs. 1.7%, $P < 0.001$); the rate of syncope was the same in the two groups (0.2%). In the combination-therapy group, the primary outcome occurred in 1386 patients (16.3%; relative risk, 0.99; 95% CI, 0.92 to 1.07); as compared with the ramipril group, there was an increased risk of hypotensive symptoms (4.8% vs. 1.7%, $P < 0.001$), syncope (0.3% vs. 0.2%, $P = 0.03$), and renal dysfunction (13.5% vs. 10.2%, $P < 0.001$).

Conclusions.—Telmisartan was equivalent to ramipril in patients with vascular disease or high risk diabetes and was associated with less angioedema. The combination of the two drugs was associated with more adverse events without an increase in benefit.

▶ Over 150 000 patients have been involved in randomized trials, establishing the benefits of angiotensin converting exzyme (ACE) inhibitors in reducing cardiovascular events. Because ACE inhibitors do not completely block production of angiotensin II, there is also interest in directly blocking the receptor for angiotensin II, so-called angiotensin receptor blockers (ARBs). The data in this article indicate that the ARB inhibitor, telmisartan, is equivalent to the ACE inhibitor, ramipril, in patients with vascular disease or high-risk diabetes, in reducing cardiovascular events. However, the combination of the 2 drugs does not provide increased benefit and, in fact, is associated with more adverse events. This is the fourth trial indicating that the ARBs are equivalent to ACE inhibitors in reducing cardiovascular events. The clinical role of ARBs, however, is still being defined. These drugs are more costly than ACE inhibitors and, in general, have more side effects. At this point, their primary value seems to be patients who cannot tolerate ACE inhibitors because of cough.

G. L. Moneta, MD

Effect of PCI on Quality of Life in Patients with Stable Coronary Disease
Weintraub WS, Spertus JA, Kolm P, et al (Christiana Care Health System, Newark, DE; Univ of Missouri–Kansas City; et al)
N Engl J Med 359:677-687, 2008

Background.—It has not been clearly established whether percutaneous coronary intervention (PCI) can provide an incremental benefit in quality of life over that provided by optimal medical therapy among patients with chronic coronary artery disease.

Methods.—We randomly assigned 2287 patients with stable coronary disease to PCI plus optimal medical therapy or to optimal medical therapy alone. We assessed angina-specific health status (with the use of the Seattle Angina Questionnaire) and overall physical and mental function (with the use of the RAND 36-item health survey [RAND-36]).

Results.—At baseline, 22% of the patients were free of angina. At 3 months, 53% of the patients in the PCI group and 42% in the medical-therapy group were angina-free (P<0.001). Baseline mean ($\pm SD$) Seattle Angina Questionnaire scores (which range from 0 to 100, with higher scores indicating better health status) were 66 ± 25 for physical limitations, 54 ± 32 for angina stability, 69 ± 26 for angina frequency, 87 ± 16 for treatment satisfaction, and 51 ± 25 for quality of life. By 3 months, these scores had increased in the PCI group, as compared with the medical-therapy group, to 76 ± 24 versus 72 ± 23 for physical limitation (P=0.004), 77 ± 28 versus 73 ± 27 for angina stability (P=0.002), 85 ± 22 versus 80 ± 23 for angina frequency (P<0.001), 92 ± 12 versus 90 ± 14 for treatment satisfaction (P<0.001), and 73 ± 22 versus 68 ± 23 for quality of life (P<0.001). In general, patients had an incremental benefit from PCI for 6 to 24 months; patients with more severe angina had a greater benefit from PCI. Similar incremental benefits from PCI were seen in some but not all RAND-36 domains. By 36 months, there was no significant difference in health status between the treatment groups.

Conclusions.—Among patients with stable angina, both those treated with PCI and those treated with optimal medical therapy alone had marked improvements in health status during follow-up. The PCI group had small, but significant, incremental benefits that disappeared by 36 months. (ClinicalTrials.gov number, NCT00007657.)

▶ Up to one-third of percutaneous coronary interventions (PCIs) have been performed in patients with stable angina. This is despite the fact that patients with chronic coronary disease do not have a reduction in major cardiovascular events when treated with PCI versus best medical management. The argument has been made that PCI reduces angina symptoms more effectively than best medical management and therefore improves the quality of life. In this study, the authors analyzed quality-of-life data to determine whether quality of life was enhanced by a strategy of PCI in patients with chronic coronary artery disease. The study was not a "head-to-head" trial of medical therapy versus

PCI. The trial, in fact, compared a strategy of initial PCI plus optimal medical therapy with optimal medical therapy alone initially. Eventually, 21% of the patients in the medical therapy alone group crossed over and received PCI. Therefore, what this trial tells us is that in patients with stable coronary disease, initial management should be optimal medical therapy and, if this is ineffective, patients should then be treated with coronary intervention.

G. L. Moneta, MD

Drug-Eluting or Bare-Metal Stents for Acute Myocardial Infarction

Mauri L, Silbaugh TS, Garg P, et al (Brigham and Women's Hosp, Boston, MA; Harvard Med School, Boston, MA; et al)
N Engl J Med 359:1330-1342, 2008

Background.—Studies comparing percutaneous coronary intervention (PCI) with drug-eluting and bare-metal coronary stents in acute myocardial infarction have been limited in size and duration.

Methods.—We identified all adults undergoing PCI with stenting for acute myocardial infarction between April 1, 2003, and September 30, 2004, at any acute care, nonfederal hospital in Massachusetts with the use of a state-mandated database of PCI procedures. We performed propensity-score matching on three groups of patients: all patients with acute myocardial infarction, all those with acute myocardial infarction with ST-segment elevation, and all those with acute myocardial infarction without ST-segment elevation. Propensity-score analyses were based on clinical, procedural, hospital, and insurance information collected at the time of the index procedure. Differences in the risk of death between patients receiving drug-eluting stents and those receiving bare-metal stents were determined from vital-statistics records.

Results.—A total of 7217 patients were treated for acute myocardial infarction (4016 with drug-eluting stents and 3201 with bare-metal stents). According to analysis of matched pairs, the 2-year, risk-adjusted mortality rates were lower for drug-eluting stents than for bare-metal stents among all patients with myocardial infarction (10.7% vs. 12.8%, P=0.02), among patients with myocardial infarction with ST-segment elevation (8.5% vs. 11.6%, P=0.008), and among patients with myocardial infarction without ST-segment elevation (12.8% vs. 15.6%, P=0.04). The 2-year, risk-adjusted rates of recurrent myocardial infarction were reduced in patients with myocardial infarction without ST-segment elevation who were treated with drug-eluting stents, and repeat revascularization rates were significantly reduced with the use of drug-eluting stents as compared with bare-metal stents in all groups.

Conclusions.—In patients presenting with acute myocardial infarction, treatment with drug-eluting stents is associated with decreased 2-year

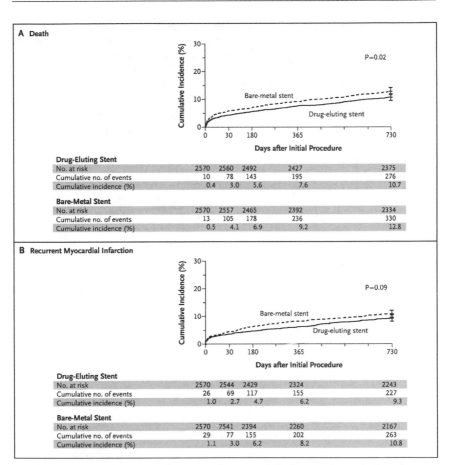

FIGURE 1.—Clinical Outcomes after Stenting for Myocardial Infarction. The graphs show the cumulative 2-year incidence of death (Panel A), myocardial infarction (Panel B), and repeat target-vessel revascularization (Panel C) in the matched sample of patients receiving bare-metal or drug-eluting stents. Error bars are 95% confidence intervals. P values were calculated by the paired t test. (Reprinted from Mauri L, Silbaugh TS, Garg P, et al. Drug-eluting or bare-metal stents for acute myocardial infarction. *N Engl J Med.* 2008;359:1330-1342, with permission from Massachusetts Medical Society.)

mortality rates and a reduction in the need for repeat revascularization procedures as compared with treatment with bare-metal stents (Fig 1).

▶ The Massachusetts Department of Public Health in 2002 established a requirement that hospitals in that state providing interventional cardiology services collect data on percutaneous coronary interventions (PCIs). Data are collected by trained data collectors and are submitted electronically to the Massachusetts Data Analysis Center. Analysis of this data forms the basis of this study. During this study, patients with myocardial infarction accounted for 40% of coronary stent procedures in Massachusetts. Drug-eluting stents appeared to reduce restenosis in the coronary circulation following stent treatment. Previous studies have reported an association between restenosis and risk of death for myocardial infarction. Therefore, the findings of the study make inherent sense. However, this data was observational, and although the authors tried to make their groups comparable, there are potential confounding variables. In particular, drug-eluting stents were not available in the same size ranges as nondrug-eluting stents. Small vessel stenting is associated with higher risks during the follow-up and during the procedure. Therefore, because the study was not randomized, treatment choices may have been influenced by stent availability.

G. L. Moneta, MD

3 Epidemiology

Angina pectoris is a stronger indicator of diffuse vascular atherosclerosis than intermittent claudication: Framingham study
Kannel WB, Evans JC, Piper S, et al (NHLBI's Framingham Heart Study, MA; Boston Univ, MA; Univ of Houston, TX)
J Clin Epidemiol 61:951-957, 2008

Objective.—To compare implications of Angina Pectoris (AP) and Intermittent Claudication (IC) as indicators of clinical atherosclerosis in other vascular territories.

Study Design and Setting.—Prospective cohort study of cardiovascular disease (CVD) in 5,209 men and women of Framingham, MA, aged 28–62 years at enrollment in 1948–1951, who received biennial examinations during the first 36 years of follow-up. Comparative 10-year incidence of subsequent atherosclerotic CVD in participants with IC and AP relative to a reference sample free of CVD was determined.

Results.—On follow-up, 95 CVD events occurred in 186 participants with IC and 206 of 413 with AP. After age, sex, and risk-factor adjustment, the proportion acquiring other CVD was 34.0% for IC and 43.4% for AP. Relative to the reference sample, those with IC had a 2.73-fold higher age and sex-adjusted 10-year hazard of CVD (95% CI 2.21, 3.38) and for AP was 3.17 (95% CI 2.73, 3.69). CVD hazard ratios remained more elevated for AP and statistically significant after standard risk factor adjustment. Risk factors accounted for more of the excess CVD risk associated with IC (34.8%) than AP (9.5%).

Conclusion.—AP is as useful as IC as a hallmark of diffuse atherosclerotic CVD and an indication for comprehensive preventive measures (Fig 1).

▶ Intermittent claudication is an accepted marker of the presence of diffuse atherosclerosis and conveys an increased risk for mortality, primarily from cardiovascular causes. Angina pectoris (AP) is another condition provoked by exertion. AP, however, is generally regarded only as a hallmark of impending myocardial infarction or a coronary fatality. As an example, the Rose angina questionnaire, a tool for epidemiological investigation of angina, has been tested chiefly as a predictor of coronary morbidity and mortality. Given that the underlying risk factors for AP and intermittent claudication are largely the same, it is surprising that the relative abilities of these conditions to predict subsequent cardiovascular events of all sorts has not been previously studied in detail. Clearly, angina and intermittent claudication are both hallmarks of

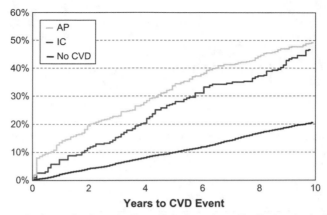

FIGURE 1.—Cardiovascular disease incidence in the Intermittent Claudication, Angina Pectoris, and Reference Group: Results of Age- and Sex-adjusted Kaplan–Meier Survival Analysis. (Reprinted from Kannel WB, Evans JC, Piper S, et al. Angina pectoris is a stronger indicator of diffuse vascular atherosclerosis than intermittent claudication: Framingham study. *J Clin Epidemiol*. 2008;61:951-957.)

diffuse atherosclerotic vascular disease. The data indicate that both impart a 2- to 3-fold increased risk of cardiovascular disease compared with a reference group (Fig 1). Patients with AP should therefore have as much attention as those with intermittent claudication with respect to instituting aggressive preventative measures against diffuse or accelerated atherosclerosis. It is interesting that the factors increasing the risk for clinical events in other vascular territories are apparently not chiefly a product of the shared risk factors of patients with intermittent claudication and those with AP. Coexistent risk factors only accounted for about 35% of the cardiovascular risk for intermittent claudication and 9.5% of the hazard associated with AP. The mechanism of this somewhat unexpected effect is uncertain. It is also important to note the limitations of the study, in that the Framingham Study has few African-Americans or other minority populations and the data presented, therefore, cannot be generalized to the entire United States population.

G. L. Moneta, MD

Patients with peripheral arterial disease in the CHARISMA trial

Cacoub PP, for the CHARISMA Investigators (La Pitié-Salpêtrière Hospital, Paris Cedex, France; VA Boston Healthcare System and Brigham and Women's Hospital, Boston, MA; Bichat Hospital, Paris, France; et al)
Eur Heart J 30:192-201, 2009

Aims.—The aim of this study was to determine whether clopidogrel plus aspirin provides greater protection against major cardiovascular events than aspirin alone in patients with peripheral arterial disease (PAD).

Methods and Results.—This is a *post hoc* analysis of the 3096 patients with symptomatic (2838) or asymptomatic (258) PAD from the

CHARISMA trial. The rate of cardiovascular death, myocardial infarction (MI), or stroke (primary endpoint) was higher in patients with PAD than in those without PAD: 8.2% vs. 6.8% [hazard ratio (HR), 1.25; 95% CI 1.08, 1.44; $P = 0.002$]. Among the patients with PAD, the primary endpoint occurred in 7.6% in the clopidogrel plus aspirin group and 8.9% in the placebo plus aspirin group (HR, 0.85; 95% CI, 0.66–1.08; $P = 0.18$). In these patients, the rate of MI was lower in the dual antiplatelet arm than the aspirin alone arm: 2.3% vs. 3.7% (HR, 0.63; 95% CI, 0.42–0.96; $P = 0.029$), as was the rate of hospitalization for ischaemic events: 16.5% vs. 20.1% (HR, 0.81; 95% CI, 0.68–0.95; $P = 0.011$). The rates of severe, fatal, or moderate bleeding did not differ between the groups, whereas minor bleeding was increased with clopidogrel: 34.4% vs. 20.8% (odds ratio, 1.99; 95% CI, 1.69–2.34; $P < 0.001$).

Conclusion.—Dual therapy provided some benefit over aspirin alone in PAD patients for the rate of MI and the rate of hospitalization for ischaemic events, at the cost of an increase in minor bleeding.

▶ The Antithrombotic Trialist Collaboration involved a meta-analysis of 42 trials that included 9717 patients. This analysis found that in peripheral arterial disease (PAD) patients there was a 22% odds reduction for adverse cardiovascular events (stroke, vascular death, or myocardial infarction) when they were treated with antiplatelet therapy versus those who were not treated with antiplatelet agents. In the Clopidogrel Versus Aspirin in Patients at Risk for Ischemic Events (CAPRIE) trial of 6452 patients, clopidogrel reduced risk of stroke, vascular death, or myocardial infarction by 23.8% more than aspirin in patients with PAD.[1] There are also certain subgroups of patients, such as those undergoing percutaneous coronary interventions, who are known to fare better with a combination of aspirin and clopidogrel versus aspirin alone. It is not know however, whether in patients with PAD the combination of aspirin and clopidogrel is more effective in reducing cardiovascular events than a single antiplatelet agent. This combination was evaluated in the Clopidogrel for High Atherothrombotic Risk and Ischemic Stabilization, Management and Avoidance (CHARISMA) trial. The trial enrolled patients with either atheroembolic disease or multiple risk factors for atheroembolic events. In CHARISMA, dual antiplatelet therapy versus aspirin alone produced only a nonsignificant 7.1% relative risk reduction in MI, cardiovascular death, or stroke over a median of 28 months.[2] Post hoc subgroup analysis of CHARISMA suggested perhaps increased benefit in those patients with PAD. This article is a post hoc analysis of the PAD patients from CHARISMA.

With respect to cardiovascular risk, patients with PAD are clearly the worst among the bad. Both symptomatic and asymptomatic PAD patients have a worse outcome with respect to the CHARISMA end points than those patients with coronary artery disease or those patients with multiple risk factors for vascular disease, but without the actual development of detectable PAD. This post hoc analysis shows some benefit of dual antiplatelet therapy in the PAD patients, but it is certainly not the results dreams are made of. Given increasing evidence that there are genetic determinants of responses to antiplatelet therapies, whether that be aspirin or clopidogrel, it would seem that further investigations should focus on identifying which patients with PAD are likely to benefit the most from dual antiplatelet therapy, and where such benefit clearly exceeds the increased risk of bleeding.

G. L. Moneta, MD

References

1. CAPRIE Steering Committee. A randomised, blinded, trial of clopidogrel versus aspirin in patients at risk of ischaemic events (CAPRIE). CAPRIE Steering Committee. *Lancet.* 1996;348:1329-1339.
2. Bhatt DL, Bhatt DL, Bhatt DL, et al. Clopidogrel and aspirin versus aspirin alone for the prevention of atherothrombotic events. *N Engl J Med.* 2006;354: 1706-1717.

Symptomatic Peripheral Arterial Disease in Women: Nontraditional Biomarkers of Elevated Risk
Pradhan AD, Shrivastava S, Cook NR, et al (Brigham and Women's Hosp, Harvard Med School, Boston, MA; et al)
Circulation 117:823-831, 2008

Background.—Most investigations of novel biomarkers for prediction of cardiovascular disease pertain to coronary artery disease. Few large-scale prospective studies have critically assessed plasma-based factors as predictors of peripheral arterial disease (PAD), and comparative data between individual biomarkers and lipid levels are sparse, especially among women.

Methods and Results.—We evaluated the relationship between baseline levels of several novel biomarkers and confirmed incident symptomatic PAD (n = 100) in a prospective cohort study (median follow-up, 12.3 years) involving 27 935 US female health professionals ≥45 years of age without diagnosed vascular disease at baseline. Biomarkers assessed were high-sensitivity C-reactive protein, fibrinogen, soluble intercellular adhesion molecule-1 (sICAM-1), homocysteine, lipoprotein(a), hemoglobin A_{1c}, creatinine, and conventional lipid levels. In univariate analyses, levels of high-sensitivity C-reactive protein, fibrinogen, sICAM-1, homocysteine, lipoprotein(a), creatinine clearance, high-density lipoprotein cholesterol (HDL-C), non–HDL-C, and the ratio of total cholesterol to HDL-C (TC:HDL-C) were significantly related to PAD (all $P<0.05$). However, after multivariable adjustment, risk associations were significant only for high-sensitivity C-reactive protein (adjusted hazard ratio [HR] extreme tertiles, 2.1; 95% confidence interval, 1.2 to 3.7), sICAM-1 (adjusted HR, 4.0; 95% confidence interval, 1.9 to 8.6), HDL-C (adjusted HR, 0.4; 95% confidence interval, 0.3 to 0.8), and TC:HDL-C (adjusted HR, 2.2; 95% confidence interval, 1.2 to 3.9). In a model simultaneously controlling for traditional risk factors plus these significant biomarkers, sICAM-1 remained independently predictive of PAD (adjusted HR in each tertile, 1.0 [reference], 2.3, and 3.5).

Conclusions.—Among a broad range of biomarkers of cardiovascular risk, only 4 factors, sICAM-1, high-sensitivity C-reactive protein, HDL-C, and TC:HDL-C, were significantly associated with incident symptomatic PAD in women. Findings pertaining to novel biomarkers provide clinical confirmation of a prominent role of endothelial activation and leukocyte recruitment in lower-extremity arterial disease.

▶ It is generally accepted that traditional cardiovascular risk factors such as smoking, diabetes, hyperlipidemia, and hypertension are clinical predictors of peripheral arterial disease (PAD). There is, however, emerging interest in the use of nontraditional markers of biologic processes such as subclinical inflammation, thrombosis, and endothelial dysfunction to further stratify clinical risk factors with respect to overall cardiovascular risk and to delineate site-specific cardiovascular risk, that is cerebrovascular versus coronary versus PAD. This was the first prospective study in women to evaluate so-called biomarkers reflective of subclinical inflammation or endothelial dysfunction against other risk factors for PAD. The biomarker with the strongest association with PAD was sICAM-1. This is a pro-inflammatory adhesion molecule reflecting leukocyte recruitment in endothelial activation. The authors astutely point out that factors leading to more gradual encroachment of luminal vessels in PAD may differ from those leading to the sudden plaque rupture that is so important in coronary artery disease-associated events.

G. L. Moneta, MD

Von Willebrand Factor, Type 2 Diabetes Mellitus, and Risk of Cardiovascular Disease: The Framingham Offspring Study

Frankel DS, Meigs JB, Massaro JM, et al (Univ of Pennsylvania, Philadelphia; Harvard Med School, Boston, MA; the Natl Heart, Lung, and Blood Inst's Framingham Heart Study, MA; et al)
Circulation 118:2533-2539, 2008

Background.—Von Willebrand factor (vWF) is inconsistently associated with cardiovascular disease (CVD). This might be explained by associations of vWF with type 2 diabetes mellitus and insulin resistance.

Methods and Results.—We tested whether vWF predicted incident CVD in 3799 Framingham Offspring Study participants, and in particular, among those with type 2 diabetes mellitus or insulin resistance. During 11 years of follow-up, 351 participants developed CVD. In proportional hazards models (with adjustment for age, sex, blood pressure, smoking, body mass index, total and high-density lipoprotein cholesterol, and treatment with aspirin, insulin, antihypertensives, and lipid-lowering medications) with the lowest quartile of the vWF distribution as the referent, the hazard ratio (HR) for CVD was 0.94 in the second quartile, 0.98 in

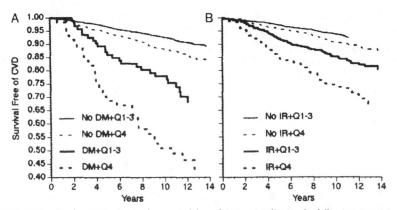

FIGURE 2.—Kaplan–Meier curves for survival free of CVD according to the following strata: A, No diabetes–low vWF; no diabetes–high vWF; diabetes–low vWF; diabetes–high vWF (Wilcoxon rank sum $P<0.0001$). B, Insulin sensitive–low vWF; insulin sensitive–high vWF; Insulin resistant–low vWF; insulin resistant–high vWF ($P<0.001$). Low vWF is defined as the lower 3 quartiles of the vWF distribution. High vWF is the top quartile. Insulin sensitive is defined as the lower 3 quartiles of HOMA-IR. Insulin resistant is the top quartile. DM indicates diabetes mellitus; Q, quartile; and IR, insulin resistance. (Reprinted from Frankel DS, Meigs JB, Massaro JM, et al. Von Willebrand factor, type 2 diabetes mellitus, and risk of cardiovascular disease: the Framingham offspring study. *Circulation.* 2008;118:2533-2539.)

the third, and 1.32 in the highest ($P = 0.04$ for trend). Additional adjustment for type 2 diabetes mellitus or insulin resistance (homeostasis model) partially attenuated the association (multivariable HRs for top quartile 1.28 and 1.21, respectively). We then stratified the models by diabetes status or the homeostasis model of insulin resistance distribution (top quartile versus lower 3 quartiles). vWF was associated with CVD among participants with diabetes mellitus (HR for top quartile relative to bottom 1.47, $P = 0.04$ for trend) but not among nondiabetic participants (HR 1.15, $P = 0.5$) and similarly among insulin-resistant (HR 1.50, $P = 0.01$) but not insulin-sensitive (HR 1.02, $P = 0.9$) participants.

Conclusions.—Higher levels of vWF were associated with risk of CVD in people with type 2 diabetes mellitus or insulin resistance, which suggests that vWF may be a risk factor unique to these populations (Fig 2).

▶ About 35% of deaths in the United States results from cardiovascular disease. Cardiovascular disease is associated with biomarkers of endothelial dysfunction, including interleukin-6, C-reactive protein, fibrinogen, fibrin D-dimer and plasminogen active inhibitor-1, as well as cellular adhesion molecules. Von Willebrand Factor (vWF) is a large glycoprotein produced by endothelial cells. It participates in the initial steps of thrombus formation by mediating platelet adhesion to injured endothelium. Because it interacts with endothelium it is thought that vWF may be a biomarker of endothelial damage. vWF is also known to be associated with insulin resistance and type 2 diabetes. Therefore vWF may be a risk factor for cardiovascular disease with increased significance in patients with insulin resistance or type 2 diabetes. The authors therefore sought to examine whether vWF serves as a particularly important risk factor for cardiovascular disease in patients with type 2 diabetes or insulin resistance.

The data suggest vWF may be a risk factor unique in patients with type 2 diabetes mellitus or insulin resistance (Fig 2). While diabetes mellitus and insulin resistance are clear risk factors for cardiovascular disease, patients with these risk factors have varying severities of clinical manifestations of atherosclerosis. This study offers the possibility of additional risk stratification among these patients. Because vWF may act through adverse modulation of endothelial dysfunction, cardiovascular risk in patients with diabetes, or insulin resistance may be lowered by therapies targeting levels of vWF, or endothelial dysfunction potentially mediated by elevated levels of vWF.

G. L. Moneta, MD

The Obesity Paradox in Patients With Peripheral Arterial Disease
Galal W, van Gestel YRBM, Hoeks SE, et al (Erasmus Med Ctr, Rotterdam, The Netherlands; et al)
Chest 134:925-930, 2008

Background.—Cardiac events are the predominant cause of late mortality in patients with peripheral arterial disease (PAD). In these patients, mortality decreases with increasing body mass index (BMI). COPD is identified as a cardiac risk factor, which preferentially affects underweight individuals. Whether or not COPD explains the obesity paradox in PAD patients is unknown.

Methods.—We studied 2,392 patients who underwent major vascular surgery at one teaching institution. Patients were classified according to COPD status and BMIs (*ie*, underweight, normal, overweight, and obese), and the relationship between these variables and all-cause mortality was determined using a Cox regression analysis. The median follow-up period was 4.37 years (interquartile range, 1.98 to 8.47 years).

Results.—The overall mortality rates among underweight, normal, overweight, and obese patients were 54%, 50%, 40%, and 31%, respectively (p < 0.001). The distribution of COPD severity classes showed an increased prevalence of moderate-to-severe COPD in underweight patients. In the entire population, BMI (continuous) was associated with increased mortality (hazard ratio [HR], 0.96; 95% confidence interval [CI], 0.94 to 0.98). In addition, patients who were classified as being underweight were at increased risk for mortality (HR, 1.42; 95% CI, 1.00 to 2.01). However, after adjusting for COPD severity the relationship was no longer significant (HR, 1.29; 95% CI, 0.91 to 1.93).

Conclusions.—The excess mortality among underweight patients was largely explained by the overrepresentation of individuals with moderate-to-severe COPD. COPD may in part explain the "obesity paradox" in the PAD population.

▶ There is a paradox in patients with peripheral arterial disease (PAD) with respect to weight. In the population with PAD, overweight or obese patients have a better survival rate than those patients of normal weight, with the highest mortality seen in the so-called underweight patient.[1] Chronic obstructive pulmonary disease (COPD) is emerging as an independent risk factor for cardiovascular mortality.[2] Given COPD is a potential independent risk factor for cardiovascular mortality, the authors sought to investigate whether the presence of COPD may in part explain the so-called obesity paradox of increased mortality in underweight patients with PAD. Other studies have also found that underweight patients, especially those with severe COPD, have an increased risk of mortality. Why there should be an inverse relationship between body mass index (BMI) and mortality is uncertain. It has been suggested that underweight patients may have higher metabolic rates, lower antioxidant capacity in skeletal muscles, and perhaps increased systemic inflammatory responses that may contribute to the combination of lower BMI and morbidity. Underweight patients may also have overt or occult malignancy. It should also be noted that heart failure patients with elevated BMIs have lower mortality than those with normal or reduced BMIs. This study suggests that part of the obesity paradox may be related to increased prevalence of more significant COPD in underweight patients. It is important to note that spirometry, which was used routinely in this study to classify COPD, is not routinely obtained in vascular disease patients. The fact that 50% of the patients in this study had COPD when examined with spirometry, and that only 10% to 15% of patients were treated for COPD, indicates a possible screening role for spirometry in patients with PAD undergoing vascular surgery.

G. L. Moneta, MD

References

1. Galal W, van Domburg RT, Feringa HH, et al. Relation of body mass index to outcome in patients with known or suspected coronary artery disease. *Am J Cardiol.* 2007;99:1485-1490.
2. Sinn DD, Anthonisen NR, Soriano JB, Agusti AG. Mortality in COPD: Role of comorbidities. *Eur Respir J.* 2006;28:1245-1257.

Progression of Peripheral Arterial Disease Predicts Cardiovascular Disease Morbidity and Mortality
Criqui MH, Ninomiya JK, Wingard DL, et al (Univ of California, San Diego; et al)
J Am Coll Cardiol 52:1736-1742, 2008

Objectives.—The purpose of this study was to examine the association of progressive versus stable peripheral arterial disease (PAD) with the risk of future cardiovascular disease (CVD) events.

Background.—An independent association between PAD, defined by low values of the ankle-brachial index (ABI), and future CVD risk has been demonstrated. However, the prognostic significance of declining versus stable ABI has not been studied.

Methods.—We recruited 508 subjects (59 women, 449 men) from 2 hospital vascular laboratories in San Diego, California. ABI and CVD risk factors were measured at Visit 2 (1990 to 1994). ABI values from each subject's earliest vascular laboratory examination (Visit 1) were abstracted from medical records. Mortality and morbidity were tracked for 6 years after Visit 2 using vital statistics and hospitalization data.

Results.—In multivariate models adjusted for CVD risk factors, very low (<0.70) and, in some cases, low (0.70 ≤ ABI <0.90) Visit 2 ABIs were associated with significantly elevated all-cause mortality, CVD mortality, and combined CVD morbidity/mortality at 3 and 6 years. Decreases in ABI of more than 0.15 between Visit 1 and Visit 2 were significantly associated with an increased risk of all-cause mortality (risk ratio [RR]: 2.4) and CVD mortality (RR: 2.8) at 3 years, and CVD morbidity/mortality (RR: 1.9) at 6 years, independent of Visit 2 ABI and other risk factors.

Conclusions.—Progressive PAD (ABI decline >0.15) was significantly and independently associated with increased CVD risk. Patients with decreasing ABI may be candidates for more intensive cardiovascular risk factor management.

▶ Peripheral arterial disease (PAD) is clearly associated with future cardiovascular disease events and cardiovascular disease total mortality. Other studies have demonstrated that the ankle-brachial index (ABI) is a risk factor for cardiovascular mortality and is independent of traditional cardiovascular disease risk factors. Studies examining the association of PAD with cardiovascular disease outcomes have used ABI obtained at baseline and have not addressed the potential additional significance of changes in ABI over time. In this study, the association between PAD, as measured by ABI with cardiovascular disease mortality and morbidity, was examined in a group of patients recruited from a vascular laboratory. These data provide the first evaluation of the relationship between PAD progression and cardiovascular disease morbidity and mortality. There was a consistent association between PAD progression and cardiovascular disease morbidity and mortality independent of the severity of PAD and traditional cardiovascular disease risk factors. There are some problems with the study. It is important to note that progression of ABI is relatively insensitive in detection of progression of PAD. PAD can clearly progress without a change in ABI; the study did not examine the association of any progression of PAD, including that it was not associated with a fall in ABI, with cardiovascular disease morbidity and mortality. The data also were not stratified for the location of atherosclerotic disease. There were not enough patients with very severe PAD to determine whether there is a plateau effect. It may be that once a patient's PAD has become sufficiently severe, the further progression adds no incremental risk to overall mortality.

G. L. Moneta, MD

The epidemiology of abdominal aortic diameter
Allison MA, Kwan K, DiTomasso D, et al (Univ of California, San Diego)
J Vasc Surg 48:121-127, 2008

Background.—The diameter of the abdominal aorta is central to the diagnosis of abdominal aortic aneurysm. This study aimed to determine the associations between the diameter of the abdominal aorta at three distinct locations and the traditional cardiovascular disease risk factors as well as calcified atherosclerosis.

Methods.—A total of 504 patients (41% women) underwent whole body scanning by electron beam computed tomography (EBCT) and a standardized assessment for cardiovascular disease risk factors. The resulting EBCT images were retrospectively interrogated for the diameter of the abdominal aorta just inferior to the superior mesenteric artery (SMA), just superior to the aortic bifurcation, and at the midpoint between the SMA and bifurcation.

Results.—Mean patient age was 57.8 years. The mean (SD) diameter was 21.3 (2.9) mm at the SMA, 19.3 (2.5) mm at the midpoint, and 18.6 (2.2) mm at the bifurcation. In a model containing the traditional cardiovascular disease risk factors, age (standardized $\beta = 0.96$), male sex ($\beta = 3.06$), and body mass index (standardized $\beta = 0.68$) were significantly associated with increasing aortic diameter at the SMA ($P < .01$ for all). The significance of the associations for these variables was the same for aortic diameter at the midpoint and bifurcation. Furthermore, a 1-unit increment in the calcium score in the abdominal aorta and iliac arteries was associated with 0.13-mm ($P < .01$) and 0.09-mm ($P = .02$) increases, respectively, in aortic diameter at the SMA. The results were similar for the midpoint ($\beta = 0.19$, $P < .01$; $\beta = 0.12$, $P = .01$, respectively) and bifurcation ($\beta = 0.09$, $P < .04$; $\beta = 0.09$, $P = .03$, respectively).

Conclusions.—Age, sex, body mass index, and the presence and extent of calcified atherosclerosis in both the abdominal aorta and iliac arteries are significantly associated with increasing aortic diameter independent of the other cardiovascular disease risk factors.

▶ The epidemiologic data presented here are interesting and, I suspect, quite accurate. However, like all epidemiologic data, one must consider the potential to apply the data to the general population. Patients in this study were derived from a university affiliated disease prevention center in San Diego, California. Participants were either self-referred or referred by their physicians. The very large majority were asymptomatic and most were free of cardiovascular risk factors. Only 6.5% were current smokers and < 3% had diabetes. The sample here, therefore, may apply more to the "worried well" than to the general population. It may very well be that additional risk factors for increased aortic diameter would be present in a population more representative of those with vascular disease.

G. L. Moneta, MD

Carotid artery stenting has increased rates of postprocedure stroke, death, and resource utilization than does carotid endarterectomy in the United States, 2005

McPhee JT, Schanzer A, Messina LM, et al (Univ of Massachusetts Med School, Worcester)
J Vasc Surg 48:1442-1450, 2008

Objective.—Carotid endarterectomy (CEA) remains the procedure of choice for treatment of patients with severe carotid artery stenosis. The role of carotid artery stenting (CAS) in this patient group is still being defined. Prior single and multicenter studies have demonstrated economic savings associated with CEA compared with CAS. The purpose of this study was to compare surgical outcomes and resource utilization associated with these two procedures at the national level in 2005, the first year in which a specific ICD-9 procedure code for CAS was available.

Methods.—All patient discharges for carotid revascularization for the year 2005 were identified in the Nationwide Inpatient Sample based on ICD9-CM procedure codes for CEA (38.12) and CAS (00.63). The primary outcome measures of interest were in-hospital mortality and postoperative stroke; secondary outcome measures included total hospital charges and length of stay (LOS). All statistical analyses were performed using SAS version 9.1 (Cary, NC), and data are weighted according to the Nationwide Inpatient Sample (NIS) design to draw national estimates. Univariate analyses of categorical variables were performed using Rao-Scott χ^2, and continuous variables were analyzed by survey weighted analysis of variance (ANOVA). Multivariate logistic regression was performed to evaluate independent predictors of postoperative stroke and mortality.

Results.—During 2005, an estimated 135,701 patients underwent either CEA or CAS nationally. Overall, 91% of patients underwent CEA. The mean age overall was 71 years. Postoperative stroke rates were increased for CAS compared with CEA (1.8% vs 1.1%, $P < .05$), odds ratio (OR) 1.7; (95% confidence interval [CI] 1.2-2.3). Overall, mortality rates were higher for CAS compared with CEA (1.1% vs 0.57%, $P < .05$) this difference was substantially increased in regard to patients with symptomatic disease (4.6% vs 1.4%, $P < .05$). By logistic regression, CAS trended toward increased mortality, OR 1.5; (95% CI .96-2.5). Overall, the median total hospital charges for patients that underwent CAS were significantly greater than those that underwent CEA ($30,396 vs $17,658 $P < .05$).

Conclusions.—Based on a large representative sample during the year 2005, CEA was performed with significantly lower in-hospital mortality, postoperative stroke rates, and lower median total hospital charges than CAS in US hospitals. As the role for CAS becomes defined for the management of patients with carotid artery stenosis, clinical as well as economic outcomes must be continually evaluated.

▶ This article is among a number of recent publications suggesting that there may be significant disadvantages to carotid artery stenting for treatment of carotid artery stenotic disease versus the use of standard carotid endarterectomy. These large database analyses have significant limitations, the primary one of which is lack of comprehensive risk stratification. In this study, carotid artery stenting was inferior to carotid endarterectomy for treatment of both symptomatic and asymptomatic carotid stenosis. In addition, it was also significantly more expensive. Cost analyses from this type of data are notoriously difficult. One cannot really infer the potential source of the increased cost of carotid artery stenting versus carotid endarterectomy. It may be that this cost is due to the increased complication rates noted with carotid artery stenting. I tend to agree with the author's conclusions but, unfortunately, I don't think it proves my biased position.

G. L. Moneta, MD

Endovenous laser ablation: Does standard above-knee great saphenous vein ablation provide optimum results in patients with both above- and below-knee reflux? A randomized controlled trial
Theivacumar NS, Dellagrammaticas D, Mavor AID, et al (General Infirmary at Leeds, UK)
J Vasc Surg 48:173-178, 2008

Background.—Following above-knee (AK) great saphenous vein (GSV) endovenous laser ablation (EVLA) 40% to 50% patients have residual varicosities. This randomized controlled trial (RCT) assesses whether more extensive GSV ablation enhances their resolution and influences symptom improvement.

Method.—Sixty-eight limbs (65 patients) with varicosities and above and below-knee GSV reflux were randomized to Group A: AK-EVLA (n = 23); Group B: EVLA mid-calf to groin (n = 23); and Group C: AK-EVLA, concomitant below-knee GSV foam sclerotherapy (n = 22). Primary outcomes were residual varicosities requiring sclerotherapy (6 weeks), improvement in Aberdeen varicose vein severity scores (AVVSS, 12 weeks), patient satisfaction, and complication rates.

Results.—EVLA ablated the treated GSV in all limbs. Sclerotherapy requirements were Group A: 14/23 (61%); Group B: 4/23 (17%); and Group C: 8/22 (36%); $\chi^2 = 9.3$ (2 df) $P = .01$ with $P_{A-B} = 0.006$; $P_{B-C} = 0.19$; $P_{A-C} = 0.14$. AVVSS scores improved in all groups as follows: A: 14.8 (9.3-22.6) to 6.4 (3.2-9.1), $(P < .001)$; B: 15.8 (10.2-24.5) to 2.5 (1.1-3.7), $(P < .001)$; and C: 15.1 (9.0-23.1) to 4.1 (2.3-6.8), $(P < .001)$

and $P_{A-B} = 0.011$, $P_{A-C} = 0.042$. Patient satisfaction was highest in Group B. BK-EVLA was not associated with saphenous nerve injury.

Conclusions.—Extended EVLA is safe, increases spontaneous resolution of varicosities, and has a greater impact on symptom reduction. Similar benefits occurred after concomitant BK-GSV foam sclerotherapy.

▶ This study represents a bit of potential fine-tuning of the endovenous laser ablation technique of the greater saphenous vein (GSV). Widespread teaching is to confine endovenous laser therapy (EVLT) to the above knee segment of the GSV to avoid thermal injury to the saphenous nerve, which is in closer proximity to the GSV below the knee. (The logic is similar to that employed where stripping of the GSV is also confined to the above knee segment.) The study grows out of the fact varicosities associated with the GSV frequently become smaller or disappear after EVLT alone. It therefore would seem logical that if reflux in the GSV extends below the knee ablation of that segment of vein in addition to the above knee segment would provide better resolution of varicosities than just ablating the above knee segment alone. The results of this article do indeed suggest that is the case and that it can be achieved without thermal injury to the saphenous nerve. The amount of laser energy delivered was the same above and below the knee (60-70 J/cm). Laser therapist should consider this technique in patients with above and below knee GSV reflux and associated GSV varicosities.

G. L. Moneta, MD

A Predictive Model for Identifying Surgical Patients at Risk of Methicillin-Resistant *Staphylococcus aureus* Carriage on Admission

Harbarth S, Sax H, Uckay I, et al (Univ of Geneva Hosps and Med Schools, Geneva, Switzerland)
J Am Coll Surg 207:683-689, 2008

Background.—Legislative mandates and current guidelines for control of nosocomial transmission of methicillin-resistant *Staphylococcus aureus* (MRSA) recommend screening of patients at risk of MRSA carriage on hospital admission. Indiscriminate application of these guidelines can result in a large number of unnecessary screening tests.

Study Design.—This study was conducted to develop and validate a prediction model to define surgical patients at risk of previously unknown MRSA carriage on admission. We used data from two prospective studies to derivate and validate predictors of previously unknown MRSA carriage on admission, using logistic regression analysis.

Results.—A total of 13,262 patients (derivation cohort, 3,069; validation cohort, 10,193) were admitted to the surgery department and screened for MRSA. Prevalence of MRSA carriage at time of admission increased from 3.2% in 2003 to 5.1% in the period 2004 to 2006, with a majority of newly identified MRSA carriers (64%). Three independent factors were correlated with previously unknown MRSA carriage: recent antibiotic treatment (adjusted odds ratio [OR]: 4.5; p < 0.001), history of hospitalization (adjusted OR: 2.7; p = 0.03), and age older than 75 years (adjusted OR: 1.9; p = 0.048). A score (range 0 to 9 points) calculated from these variables was developed. Probability of previously unknown MRSA carriage was 5% (8 of 152) in patients with a low score (< 2 points), 11% (19 of 166) in those with an intermediate score (2 to 6 points), and 34% (30 of 87) in those with a high score (≥ 7 points). Limiting screening to patients with all 3 risk factors (21% and 26% of patients in the derivation and validation cohort, respectively) would have correctly identified 53% and 37% of MRSA carriers in both cohorts.

Conclusions.—A predictive model using three easily retrievable determinants might help to better target surgical patients at risk of MRSA carriage on admission.

▶ There are guidelines for control of nosocomial transmission of methicillin-resistant *Staphylococcus aureus* (MRSA).[1] The spread of MRSA is facilitated by cross-transmission via health care workers' hands and broad-spectrum antibiotic treatment selection for MRSA. MRSA infections are associated with increased treatment cost and excess morbidity and mortality. MRSA is now present in the community and patients without previous MRSA infection are being increasingly recognized upon admission to the hospital. The authors sought to develop and validate a prediction model to confine surgical patients with previously unknown MRSA who are, in fact, carriers of MRSA on admission to the hospital. The data indicate that most MRSA carriers are unknown at the time of hospital admission. The 3 variables found to be predictive of unsuspected MRSA infection, namely previous hospitalization, recent antibiotic use, and age greater than 75 years, are extremely common in patients with vascular disease admitted to the hospital. Vascular surgeons should be aware that many of their patients without previously recognized MRSA infection are very likely to be carriers of MRSA at the time of their admission to the hospital.

G. L. Moneta, MD

Reference

1. Muto CA, Jernigan JA, Ostrowsky BE, et al. SHEA guideline for preventing nosocomial transmission of multidrug-resistant strains of *Staphylococcus aureus* and enterococcus. *Infect Control Hosp Epidemiol.* 2003;24:362-386.

4 Vascular Lab and Imaging

Reappraisal of velocity criteria for carotid bulb/internal carotid artery stenosis utilizing high-resolution B-mode ultrasound validated with computed tomography angiography
Shaalan WE, Wahlgren CM, Desai T, et al (Univ of Chicago, IL)
J Vasc Surg 48:104-113, 2008

Objective.—Reliability of the most commonly used duplex ultrasound (DUS) velocity thresholds for internal carotid artery (ICA) stenosis has been questioned since these thresholds were developed using less precise methods to grade stenosis severity based on angiography. In this study, maximum percent diameter carotid bulb ICA stenosis (European Carotid Surgery Trial [ECST] method) was objectively measured using high resolution B-mode DUS validated with computed tomography angiography (CTA) and used to determine optimum velocity thresholds for ≥50% and ≥80% bulb internal carotid artery stenosis (ICA).

Methods.—B-mode DUS and CTA images of 74 bulb ICA stenoses were compared to validate accuracy of the DUS measurements. In 337 mild, moderate, and severe bulb ICA stenoses (n = 232 patients), the minimal residual lumen and the maximum outer bulb/proximal ICA diameter were determined on longitudinal and transverse images. This in contrast to the North American Symptomatic Carotid Endarterectomy Trial (NASCET) method using normal distal ICA lumen diameter as the denominator. Severe calcified carotid segments and patients with contralateral occlusion were excluded. In each study, the highest peak systolic (PSV) and end-diastolic (EDV) velocities as well as ICA/common carotid artery (CCA) ratio were recorded. Using receiver operating characteristic (ROC) analysis, the optimum threshold for each hemodynamic parameter was determined to predict ≥50% (n = 281) and ≥80% (n = 62) bulb ICA stenosis.

Results.—Patients mean age was 74 ± 8 years; 49% females. Clinical risk factors for atherosclerosis included coronary artery disease (40%), diabetes mellitus (32%), hypertension (70%), smoking (34%), and hypercholesterolemia (49%). Thirty-three percent of carotid lesions (n = 110) presented with ischemic cerebrovascular symptoms and 67% (n = 227) were asymptomatic. There was an excellent agreement between B-mode DUS and CTA ($r = 0.9$, $P = .002$). The inter/intraobserver agreement (κ) for B-mode imaging measurements were 0.8 and 0.9, respectively, and for CTA measurements 0.8 and 0.9, respectively. When both PSV of ≥155 cm/s and ICA/CCA ratio of ≥2 were combined for the detection of ≥50% bulb ICA stenosis, a positive predictive value (PPV) of 97% and an accuracy of 82% were obtained. For a ≥80% bulb ICA stenosis, an EDV of ≥140 cm/s, a PSV of ≥370 cm/s and an ICA/CCA ratio of ≥6 had acceptable probability values.

Conclusion.—Compared with established velocity thresholds commonly applied in practice, a substantially higher PSV (155 vs 125 cm/s) was more accurate for detecting ≥50% bulb/ICA stenosis. In combination, a PSV of ≥155 cm/s and an ICA/CCA ratio of ≥2 have excellent predictive value for this stenosis category. For ≥80% bulb ICA stenosis (NASCET 60% stenosis), an EDV of 140 cm/s, a PSV of ≥370 cm/s, and an ICA/CCA ratio of ≥6 are equally reliable and do not indicate any major change from the established criteria. Current DUS ≥50% bulb ICA stenosis criteria appear to overestimate carotid bifurcation disease and may predispose patients with asymptomatic carotid disease to untoward costly diagnostic imaging and intervention.

▶ The debate of how to measure carotid stenosis continues and is becoming a bit tiresome. Should the diameter of the internal carotid artery (ICA) bulb or the diameter of the distal ICA be used as the reference vessel (ie, denominator) in calculations of ICA stenosis? I think both are valuable. Bulb-based measurements will tell you about the presence of atherosclerosis in the carotid bulb. Calculations of stenosis using the distal ICA as the reference vessel reflect the methodology used in the North American trials of carotid endarterectomy for both symptomatic and asymptomatic patients. Such measurements are more useful for selection of patients for intervention without additional imaging studies. What are the implications of accepting Dr Bassiouny's criteria of 155 cm/s as indicative of a > 50% ICA stenosis using the bulb as the reference vessel? If one looks at Table 3 in the original article, the cutoff of 125 cm/s would provide 96% sensitivity for detection of a > 50% bulb-based calculation of ICA stenosis. Sensitivity drops to 82% if one uses a cutoff of 155 cm/s. Overall accuracy is greatest with the 155 cm/s value, but this occurs at a price of decreased sensitivity. In this range of carotid stenosis what is really important is not whether or not there is 50% stenosis but whether there is plaque in the ICA bulb. No one should treat a 50% ICA stenosis in an asymptomatic patient. In symptomatic patients, ICA velocities in the range under discussion (125-155 cm/s) are very uncommon. Dr Bassiouny may be correct that 125 cm/s is too low a cutoff value for 50% bulb-based calculations of ICA stenosis. However, I would urge interpreters of vascular laboratory studies to supplement their reading of a < 50% ICA stenosis with whether or not there is plaque present in the carotid bulb. For many primary care physicians caring for patients at risk for atherosclerotic disease, the presence of carotid plaque, even in the absence of a > 50% stenosis, may influence the decision to recommend aspirin or statin therapy.

G. L. Moneta, MD

Color Doppler Ultrasonography in Occlusive Diseases of the Brachiocephalic and Proximal Subclavian Arteries

Yurdakul M, Tola M, Uslu OS (Türkiye Yüksek Ihtisas Hospital, Ankara, Turkey)
J Ultrasound Med 27:1065-1070, 2008

Objective.—The purpose of this study was to investigate the capability of color Doppler ultrasonography (CDU) in showing the brachiocephalic and proximal subclavian arteries and to determine the accuracy of CDU for diagnosis of occlusive diseases of those arteries.

Methods.—Two groups of patients were examined. The first group was examined with CDU to determine whether the brachiocephalic and subclavian artery origins could be seen. The second group, including patients with occlusive arterial disease, was examined with CDU before digital subtraction angiography (DSA). Results of CDU and DSA were compared.

Results.—In the first group, the origins of 42 (84%) of 50 brachiocephalic arteries, 48 (96%) of 50 right subclavian arteries, and 25 (50%) of 50 left subclavian arteries could be displayed by CDU. In the second group, 8 (89%) of 9 lesions on the right and 23 (96%) of 24 lesions on the left were diagnosed correctly. Color Doppler ultrasonography had sensitivity, specificity, positive predictive value, negative predictive value, and accuracy values of 88%, 94%, 78%, 97%, and 94%, respectively, for detecting major stenosis and 100%, 98%, 94%, 100%, and 99% for detecting occlusion. Agreement between the CDU and DSA findings was substantial for stenosis ($\kappa = 0.78$) and almost perfect for occlusion ($\kappa = 0.96$).

Conclusions.—The percentage of proximal left subclavian arteries shown on CDU was considerably lower compared with the right subclavian and brachiocephalic arteries. However, there was no significant difference between the two sides in diagnosing occlusive arterial diseases. With CDU, occlusion can be diagnosed more accurately than stenosis.

▶ The authors describe excellent results in identifying occlusive lesions of the origin of the subclavian and brachiocephalic arteries. This was despite the fact that the equipment they used in this study was a bit dated. A newer machine with smaller footprint probes using the sterna notch as a window likely would be even more accurate in assessing the great vessels of the aortic arch. It is not surprising that the left subclavian artery was the most difficult to visualize as it originates more posteriorly than the other vessels and can be obscured by the apex of the left lung. It should also be noted that criteria for stenosis of these vessels is slightly different than that used elsewhere, whereas the authors used a peak systolic velocity ratio of > 2 to indicate stenosis; stenosis was also determined by the presence of monophasic flow in the brachiocephalic or subclavian artery without actual visualization of a high velocity jet. The presence of reverse flow in a vertebral artery was also used as an indicator of stenosis or occlusion (Figs 2A and 2B in the original article). These additional criteria must be used to assess the brachiocephalic vessels. If only peak systolic velocity ratios are used, there will be higher numbers of both false positive and false negative results.

G. L. Moneta, MD

Duplex ultrasound velocity criteria for the stented carotid artery
Lal BK, Hobson RW II, Tofighi B, et al (Division of Vascular Surgery, Univ of Medicine, Dentistry–New Jersey Medical School, Newark, NJ, et al)
J Vasc Surg 47:63-73, 2008

Objectives.—Ultrasound velocity criteria for the diagnosis of in-stent restenosis in patients undergoing carotid artery stenting (CAS) are not well established. In the present study, we test whether ultrasound velocity measurements correlate with increasing degrees of in-stent restenosis in patients undergoing CAS and develop customized velocity criteria to identify residual stenosis ≥20%, in-stent restenosis ≥50%, and high-grade in-stent restenosis ≥80%.

Methods.—Carotid angiograms performed at the completion of CAS were compared with duplex ultrasound (DUS) imaging performed immediately after the procedure. Patients were followed up with annual DUS imaging and underwent both ultrasound scans and computed tomography angiography (CTA) at their most recent follow-up visit. Patients with suspected high-grade in-stent restenosis on DUS imaging underwent diagnostic carotid angiograms. DUS findings were therefore available for comparison with luminal stenosis measured by carotid angiograms or CTA in all these patients. The DUS protocol included peak-systolic (PSV) and end-diastolic velocity (EDV) measurements in the native common carotid artery (CCA), proximal stent, mid stent, distal stent, and distal internal carotid artery (ICA).

Results.—Of 255 CAS procedures that were reviewed, 39 had contralateral ICA stenosis and were excluded from the study. During a mean follow-up of 4.6 years (range, 1 to 10 years), 23 patients died and 64 were lost. Available for analysis were 189 pairs of ultrasound and procedural carotid angiogram measurements; 99 pairs of ultrasound and CTA measurements during routine follow-up; and 29 pairs of ultrasound and carotid angiograms measurements during follow-up for suspected high-grade in-stent restenosis ≥80% (n = 310 pairs of observations, ultrasound vs carotid angiograms/CTA). The accuracy of CTA vs carotid angiograms was confirmed ($r^2 = 0.88$) in a subset of 19 patients. Post-CAS PSV ($r^2 = .85$) and ICA/CCA ratios ($r^2 = 0.76$) correlated most with the degree of stenosis. Receiver operating characteristic analysis demonstrated the following optimal threshold criteria: residual stenosis ≥20% (PSV ≥150 cm/s and ICA/CCA ratio ≥2.15), in-stent restenosis ≥50% (PSV ≥220 cm/s and ICA/CCA ratio ≥2.7), and in-stent restenosis ≥80% (PSV 340 cm/s and ICA/CCA ratio ≥4.15).

Conclusions.—Progressively increasing PSV and ICA/CCA ratios correlate with evolving restenosis within the stented carotid artery. Ultrasound velocity criteria developed for native arteries overestimate the degree of in-stent restenosis encountered. These changes persist during long-term follow-up and across all grades of in-stent restenosis after CAS. The proposed new velocity criteria accurately define residual stenosis ≥20%, in-stent restenosis ≥50%, and high-grade in-stent restenosis ≥80% in the stented carotid artery.

▶ The need to establish new criteria for detecting restenosis in stented carotid arteries is now clearly apparent, but also of unclear importance. This study is relatively small but confirms my, and many others', impression that stented carotid arteries have higher velocities than native vessels of comparable levels of angiographic stenosis. Different series have slightly different numbers, but the over estimation of stenosis in stented carotid arteries by traditional duplex criteria appears to apply, primarily, to more moderate lesions and stented arteries with minimal or detectable angiographic stenosis. Very high velocities indicate a significant lesion in both native and stented arteries. Unless it turns out that we can identify which mild or moderate lesions progress to high-grade lesions, and more importantly, symptomatic lesions, much of the current debate may not turn out to be all that important in the long run.

G. L. Moneta, MD

Grading Carotid Intrastent Restenosis: A 6-Year Follow-Up Study
Setacci C, Chisci E, Setacci F, et al (Univ of Siena, Italy)
Stroke 39:1189-1196, 2008

Background and Purpose.—The accuracy of carotid ultrasound has not been well established in predicting intrastent restenosis (ISR) after carotid artery stenting (CAS). The aim of this study is to determine different degrees of ISR using ultrasound velocity criteria compared to percentage of stenosis at angiography.

Methods.—This is a 6-year prospective study. After CAS procedure, each patient underwent angiography for measuring ISR (NASCET method) which was compared to peak systolic velocity (PSV), end diastolic velocity (EDV), and the ratio between PSV of internal carotid artery and common carotid artery (ICA/CCA). This was done within 48 hours, thus, creating a baseline value. Ultrasound (US) examination was performed at day 30, at 3, 6, 9, and 12 months, and then yearly. Patients with an increase in PSV greater than 3 times the baseline value or in presence of PSV ≥200 cm/s underwent angiography.

Results.—814 CAS procedures, 6427 US examinations, and 1123 angiographies were performed. ISR ≥70% and ISR ≥50% was detected, respectively, in 22 patients and in 73 patients. We defined velocity criteria for grading carotid ISR: PSV ≤104 cm/s, if <30% stenosis; PSV:105 to 174 cm/s if 30% to 50% stenosis; PSV:175 to 299 cm/s if a 50% to 70% stenosis; PSV ≥300 cm/s, EDV ≥140 cm/s, and ICA/CCA ≥3.8 if a ≥70% stenosis. Receiver operator characteristic (ROC) curves for ISR ≥70% were, respectively, for PSV, EDV, and ICA/CCA: 0.99, 0.98, and 0.99.

Conclusions.—US grading of carotid ISR can guarantee a correct follow-up after CAS if new customized velocity criteria are validated by skilled operators, using a specific protocol of follow-up in a certified laboratory.

▶ This is arguably the most comprehensive article to date assessing ultrasound evaluation of intrastent restenosis after carotid artery stenting (CAS). The strength of the article is the large number of CAS patients followed (814), the large number of duplex scans performed (6427), and the large number of angiograms performed (1123) in follow-up for suspected restenosis of the stented carotid artery. Like smaller, previous articles on this subject, the authors concluded that velocities in stented arteries are higher than in native vessels with similar degrees of angiographic stenosis. However, it appears that this applies primarily to more moderate lesions as suggested criteria for high grade (>70%) restenotic stented arteries, essentially mirroring those reported for high-grade native artery stenosis. Nevertheless, the criteria suggested here deserves serious consideration for use in vascular laboratories that perform follow-up duplex examinations of stented carotid arteries.

G. L. Moneta, MD

Validation of a method for determination of the ankle-brachial index in the seated position
Gornik HL, Garcia B, Wolski K, et al (Cleveland Clinic Foundation, Cleveland, Ohio)
J Vasc Surg 48:1204-1210, 2008

Objective.—To validate a method for determination of the ankle-brachial index (ABI) in the seated position.

Background.—Peripheral arterial disease (PAD) is a prevalent disorder that is associated with quality of life impairment and increased risk of a major cardiovascular event. The ABI is the initial test for screening and diagnosis of PAD. To prevent error due hydrostatic pressure, accurate measurement of the ABI requires supine patient positioning. Access to ABI measurement is limited for patients who are immobilized or unable to lie flat.

Methods.—Patients presenting to a vascular laboratory for suspected arterial disease were enrolled. Arm and ankle blood pressures were measured in the supine and seated positions. Seated ankle pressures were corrected by the following physiology-based formula: Corrected ankle pressure = Measured ankle pressure − D*(.078), where D = the vertical distance between the arm and ankle cuffs (mm). This formula equates to a correction factor of 78 mm Hg per meter distance between

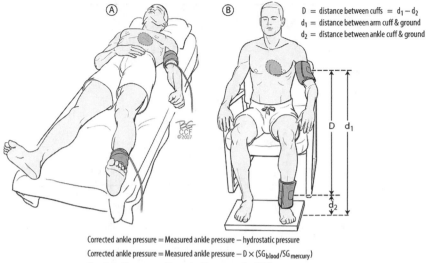

D = distance between cuffs = $d_1 - d_2$
d_1 = distance between arm cuff & ground
d_2 = distance between ankle cuff & ground

Corrected ankle pressure = Measured ankle pressure − hydrostatic pressure
Corrected ankle pressure = Measured ankle pressure − D × ($SG_{blood}/SG_{mercury}$)
Corrected ankle pressure = Measured ankle pressure − D × (.078)

FIGURE 1.—Method of determining an accurate ankle pressure in the supine (**A**) and seated (**B**) positions. Blood pressure is measured at the ankles using a hand-held Doppler scan device. The measured pressure is corrected for the effects of hydrostatic pressure using the physiology-based formula, as shown (see Methods). A two ruler technique is used to accurately determine the vertical distance (height) between the cuffs. The distance from the center of the ankle cuff to the floor (d_2) is subtracted from the distance between from the center of the arm cuff to the floor (d_1) to determine the distance between the two cuffs (D). For each meter distance between the ankle and the brachial cuffs, 78 mm Hg is subtracted from the seated ankle pressure to correct for hydrostatic pressure. The corrected seated ankle pressures are used for calculation of the seated ankle-brachial index (ABI), using standard methods. Reprinted with the permission of The Cleveland Clinic Center for Medical Art & Photography © 2008. All Rights Reserved. (Reprinted from Gornik HL, Garcia B, Wolski K, et al. Validation of a method for determination of the ankle-brachial index in the seated position. *J Vasc Surg.* 2008; 48:1204-1210, with permission from The Society for Vascular Surgery.)

the arm and ankle cuffs. Corrected ankle pressure measurements were used for seated ABI calculation.

Results.—Complete data were available for 100 patients. Mean ABI was 0.97, and 31% of patients had an ABI ≤0.9. There was excellent correlation between supine and corrected seated ankle pressure measurements (r = 0.884-0.936, P < .001). The difference between measurements was negligible (<5 mm Hg). Similarly, there was excellent correlation between supine and seated ABI measures (r = 0.936, P < .001). There was no significant difference between the supine and seated ABI measures.

Conclusion.—We have developed and validated a method for determination of the ABI in the seated position which can be used to broaden availability of PAD testing. This method could also be incorporated into new technologies for ABI determination in the seated position (Figs 1 and 4).

▶ There are patients with suspected peripheral arterial disease (PAD) or with established PAD who are unable to lie supine on the examining table because

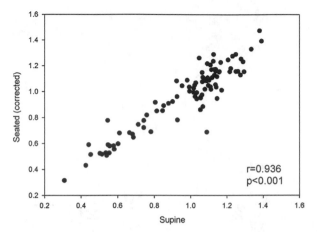

FIGURE 4.—Association of ankle-brachial index (ABI) measurement in the supine and seated positions. Scatter plots for supine vs seated ABI measurements. The ABI in the seated position was calculated using corrected ankle pressures. The degree of association between the two measures was excellent (Pearson correlation coefficient 0.936, $P < .001$). (Reprinted from Gornik HL, Garcia B, Wolski K, et al. Validation of a method for determination of the ankle-brachial index in the seated position. *J Vasc Surg.* 2008; 48:1204-1210, with permission from The Society for Vascular Surgery.)

of degenerative diseases of the spine, advanced cardiopulmonary disease, or perhaps inability to transfer from a wheelchair. The authors' technique for determining ankle-brachial indices (ABIs) under such circumstances is therefore quite useful and will be applauded by vascular laboratory technicians everywhere who struggle to obtain accurate measurements on patients who cannot tolerate the supine position (Figs 1 and 4). The authors' formula requires only determining the vertical distance between the arm cuff and the ankle cuff. The formula should theoretically be applicable to patients in both the full upright and partially upright positions. The simple formula presented in this article should be widely distributed to vascular surgeons, vascular residents, and vascular technologists.

G. L. Moneta, MD

Duplex ultrasound of the superficial femoral artery is a better screening tool than ankle-brachial index to identify at risk patients with lower extremity atherosclerosis

Flanigan DP, Ballard JL, Robinson D, et al (St Joseph Hosp Vascular Inst, Orange; et al)
J Vasc Surg 47:789-793, 2008

Objectives.—The purpose of vascular disease screening is early identification of atherosclerotic disease and the aim of an ankle-brachial index (ABI) is to identify lower extremity (LE) atherosclerosis as a marker for coronary artery disease (CAD). However, early evidence of atherosclerosis may be present in the superficial femoral artery (SFA) with a normal resting ABI. This study was performed to determine if SFA duplex ultrasound (DUS) could detect more patients with LE atherosclerosis than an ABI; be performed in the same or less time as the ABI measurement; and be associated with similar vascular disease markers as the ABI.

Methods.—From January through November 2006, 585 patients were screened for peripheral arterial disease. SFA DUS was included in this Institutional Review Board approved program and demographic/ultrasound data were collected prospectively. SFA DUS findings were divided into six categories. Plaque w/o color change or worse and ABI <0.90 or >1.20 were considered to be abnormal. Data were evaluated using decision matrix and logistical regression analysis.

Results.—Sensitivity and specificity of SFA DUS using the ABI as the benchmark was 100% and 88%, respectively. Sensitivity and specificity of ABI was 17% and 100%, respectively, using DUS as the standard. DUS detected atherosclerotic disease in 143 SFAs (93 patients) in which the ipsilateral ABI was normal, and there were no false negative SFA DUS studies. Multivariate logistic regression analysis demonstrated the following variables to be significantly and independently associated with an abnormal SFA DUS as well as an abnormal ABI: history of claudication, history of myocardial infarction, and an abnormal carotid DUS. Additional variables (current or past smoker and age >55) were also independently associated with an abnormal SFA DUS but not with an abnormal ABI. Mean time to complete bilateral testing was essentially the same for both tests.

Conclusions.—SFA DUS is an accurate screening tool and can be utilized in screening protocols in place of the time-honored ABI without prolonging the examination. Traditional vascular disease markers that are found in patients with an abnormal ABI are also associated with an abnormal SFA DUS. SFA DUS identifies more patients with early LE atherosclerosis than does ABI without missing significant popliteal/tibial artery occlusive disease. Finally, an abnormal SFA DUS can be used as an indirect marker to identify more potentially at risk patients with CAD.

▶ The authors conclude that duplex ultrasound of the superficial femoral artery is more sensitive than the calculation of the ankle-brachial index in detecting arterial changes consistent with the presence of peripheral arterial disease (PAD). The ankle-brachial index (ABI) has long been the standard for PAD screening. Because it can be used in the office setting and because it requires minimal time and equipment, it is unlikely to be displaced any time soon as the primary screening modality for PAD. The authors' conclusion, in this study, that duplex ultrasound is a more sensitive test than ABI in detecting PAD should not be surprising. After all, the closer you look, the more you see. ABI is an indirect test assessing distal hemodynamic effects of arterial disease and is really a marker of arterial disease of sufficient magnitude to produce a pressure drop at the ankle. In essence, the authors' data suggest the screening of the superficial femoral artery, in a manner analogous to obtaining intimal medial thickness of the carotid artery to predict the presence of PAD, potentially predicts late cardiovascular risk. I think the observations here are interesting but I doubt they will go anywhere. After all, carotid intimal medial thickness has been around for years and is still not widely practiced or reimbursed for risk stratification in cardiovascular disease.

G. L. Moneta, MD

Assessment of the medial head of the gastrocnemius muscle in functional compression of the popliteal artery

Pillai J, Levien LJ, Haagensen M, et al (Univ of the Witwatersrand, Johannesburg, South Africa)
J Vasc Surg 48:1189-1196, 2008

Objective.—Nonfunctional popliteal entrapment is due to embryologic maldevelopment within the popliteal fossa. Functional entrapment occurs in the apparent absence of an anatomic abnormality. Gastrocnemius hypertrophy has been associated with the latter. Both forms of entrapment may cause arterial injury and lower limb ischemia. This study assessed the attachment of the medial head of the gastrocnemius muscle in healthy occluders and healthy nonoccluders.

Methods.—Provocative tests were used to identify 58 nonoccluders and 16 occluders. Ten subjects from each group underwent magnetic resonance imaging evaluation of the popliteal fossa. The medial head of the gastrocnemius muscle attachment was assessed in the supracondylar, pericondylar, and intercondylar areas.

Results.—In the occluder group, significantly more muscle was attached towards the femoral midline (supracondylar), around the lateral border of the medial condyle (pericondylar), and within the intercondylar fossa.

Conclusion.—The more extensive midline position of the medial head of the gastrocnemius in occluders is likely to be a normal embryological variation. Forceful contraction results in compression and occlusion of the adjacent popliteal artery. The clinical significance of these anatomic variations remains unclear. However, these new observations may provide insight for future analysis of the causes and natural history of functional compression and the potential progression to clinical entrapment (Fig 1).

▶ This is a complicated article and one must study the figures closely to have an appreciation for what the authors are saying. Nevertheless, what it boils down to is that adult patients who can functionally occlude their popliteal artery during forceful plantar flexion of the foot tend to have attachment sites of the medial head of the gastrocnemius muscle that extend toward the midline above the medial condyle within the intercondylar notch (Area C in Fig 1).

I like articles like this. They provide an explanation for a common observation, which in this case is that many healthy people without signs of clinical popliteal entrapment syndrome apparently can, when studied in the vascular laboratory, occlude their popliteal artery with forced plantar flexion of the foot. Common

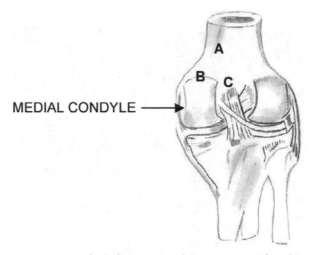

MEDIAL CONDYLE ⟶

FIGURE 1.—Posterior aspect of right femur. *A, B,* and *C* represent areas of attachment of the medial head of the gastrocnemius muscle that were examined by magnetic resonance imaging. (Reprinted from Pillai J, Levien LJ, Haagensen M, et al. Assessment of the medial head of the gastrocnemius muscle in functional compression of the popliteal artery. *J Vasc Surg.* 2008;48:1189-1196, with permission from The Society for Vascular Surgery.)

practice in vascular laboratories is to evaluate the pedal pulses with forced plantar flexion in patients with possible popliteal artery entrapment. Based on the data here this would lack specificity for detecting clinically important popliteal entrapment and is a worthless test.

Patients with suspected popliteal artery entrapment syndrome should have an MRI of the knee to evaluate the attachment sites of the medial head of gastrocnemius muscle. If the clinical symptoms are appropriate, exercise testing on the treadmill reveals a decreased ankle pressure with exercise, and there is medial deviation of the attachment of the medial head of the gastrocnemius muscle, then the diagnosis of popliteal artery entrapment syndrome can be made.

G. L. Moneta, MD

Duplex criteria for determination of in-stent stenosis after angioplasty and stenting of the superficial femoral artery
Baril DT, Rhee RY, Kim J, et al (Univ of Pittsburgh Med Ctr, PA)
J Vasc Surg 49:133-139, 2009

Objective.—Endovascular intervention is considered first-line therapy for most superficial femoral artery (SFA) occlusive disease. Duplex ultrasound (DU) criteria for SFA in-stent stenosis and correlation with angiographic data remain poorly defined. This study evaluated SFA-specific DU criteria for the assessment of SFA in-stent stenosis.

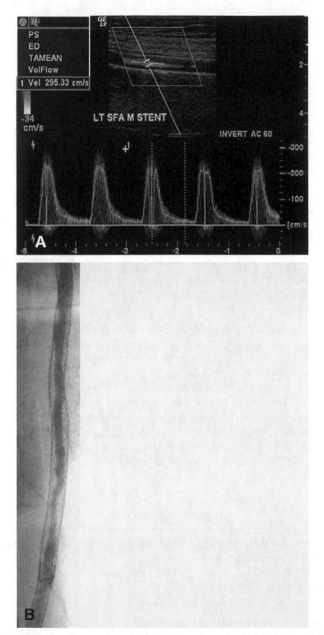

FIGURE 1.—A, Duplex ultrasound results demonstrate elevated velocity of 295 cm/s in the middle portion of a superficial femoral artery stent. B, Arteriogram demonstrates a superficial femoral artery mid-stent 70% stenosis. (Reprinted from Baril DT, Rhee RY, Kim J, et al. Duplex criteria for determination of in-stent stenosis after angioplasty and stenting of the superficial femoral artery. *J Vasc Surg.* 2009;49:133-139, with permission from The Society for Vascular Surgery.)

Methods.—From May 2003 to May 2008, 330 limbs underwent SFA angioplasty and stenting and were monitored by serial DU imaging. Suspected stenotic lesions underwent angiography and intervention when appropriate. Data pairs of DU and angiographically estimated stenosis ≤30 days of each other were analyzed. Seventy-eight limbs met these criteria, and 59 underwent reintervention. In-stent peak systolic velocity (PSV), the ratio of the stented SFA velocity/proximal SFA velocity, changes in ankle-brachial indices (ABIs), and the percentage of angiographic stenosis were examined. Linear regression and receiver operator characteristic (ROC) curve analyses were used to compare angiographic stenosis with PSV and velocity ratios (Vrs) to establish optimal criteria for determining significant in-stent stenosis.

Results.—Mean follow-up was 16.9 ± 8.3 months. Of the 59 limbs that underwent reintervention, 37 (63%) were symptomatic, and 22 (37%) underwent reintervention based on DU findings alone. Linear regression models of PSV and Vr vs degree of angiographic stenosis showed strong adjusted correlation coefficients ($R^2 = 0.60$, $P < .001$ and $R^2 = 0.55$, $P < 0.001$, respectively). ROC curve analysis showed that to detect a ≥50% in-stent stenosis, a PSV ≥190 had 88% sensitivity, 95% specificity, a 98% positive predictive value (PPV), and a 72% negative predictive value (NPV); for Vr, a ratio of >1.50 had 93% sensitivity, 89% specificity, a 96% PPV, and a 81% NPV. To detect ≥80% in-stent stenosis, a PSV ≥275 had 97% sensitivity, 68% specificity, a 67% PPV, and a 97% NPV; a Vr ratio ≥3.50 had 74% sensitivity, 94% specificity, a 77% PPV, and a 88% NPV. Combining a PSV ≥275 and a Vr ≥3.50 to determine ≥80% in-stent stenosis had 74% sensitivity, 94% specificity, a 88% PPV, and a 85% NPV; odds ratio was 42.17 (95% confidence interval, 10.20-174.36, $P < .001$) to predict ≥80% in-stent stenosis. A significant drop in ABI (>0.15) correlated with a >62% in-stent stenosis, although the adjusted correlation coefficients was low ($R^2 = 0.31$, $P = .02$).

Conclusion.—PSV and Vr appear to have a significant role in predicting in-stent stenosis. To determine ≥80% stenosis, combining PSV ≥275 cm/s and Vr ≥3.50 is highly specific and predictive (Fig 1).

▶ The data here are not a lot different than one would expect from previous articles looking at vein grafts or stenoses associated with native atherosclerotic lesion in the superficial femoral artery (SFA). The authors found that a decrease in ankle brachial indices (ABI) did not always accompany a significant in-stent restenosis. This is similar to stenoses in vein grafts. A peak systolic velocity of about 200 cm/s predicted a 50% in-stent SFA stenosis, and a peak systolic velocity of > 275 cm/s (Fig 1a and b) or a velocity ratio of > 3.5 predicted pretty well a > 80% in-stent SFA stenosis. Values are again similar to those used in native arteries or vein grafts. One might therefore ask, so what?

Despite the expected findings, the article has value in that detecting stenoses in stented arteries is a bit problematic using traditional native artery criteria. I believe the problem with stented arteries is primarily false positives for more minor degrees of stenosis that actually have little clinical relevance. Traditional criteria for native arteries work pretty well for detecting high-grade stenoses in stented carotid and renal arteries but probably not so well for stented superior mesenteric arteries. We therefore need to examine stents in all locations for assessment of stenoses of stented arteries. Hence the value of this article.

G. L. Moneta, MD

Efficacy of duplex ultrasound surveillance after infrainguinal vein bypass may be enhanced by identification of characteristics predictive of graft stenosis development

Tinder CN, Chavanpun JP, Bandyk DF, et al (Univ of South Florida College of Med, Tampa, FL)
J Vasc Surg 48:613-618, 2008

Objective.—Controversy regarding the efficacy of duplex ultrasound surveillance after infrainguinal vein bypass led to an analysis of patient and bypass graft characteristics predictive for development of graft stenosis and a decision of secondary intervention.

Methods.—Retrospective analysis of a contemporary, consecutive series of 353 clinically successful infrainguinal vein bypasses performed in 329 patients for critical (n = 284; 80%) or noncritical (n = 69; 20%) limb ischemia enrolled in a surveillance program to identify and repair duplex-detected graft stenosis. Variables correlated with graft stenosis and bypass repair included: procedure indication, conduit type (saphenous vs nonsaphenous vein; reversed vs nonreversed orientation), prior bypass graft failure, postoperative ankle-brachial index (ABI) < 0.85, and interpretation of the first duplex surveillance study as "normal" or "abnormal" based on peak systolic velocity (PSV) and velocity ratio (Vr) criteria.

Results.—Overall, 126 (36%) of the 353 infrainguinal bypasses had 174 secondary interventions (endovascular, 100; surgery, 74) based on duplex surveillance; resulting in 3-year Kaplan-Meier primary (46%), assisted-primary (80%), and secondary (81%) patency rates. Characteristics predictive of duplex-detected stenosis leading to intervention (PSV: 443 ± 94 cm/s; Vr: 8.6 ± 9) were: "abnormal" initial duplex testing indicating moderate (PSV: 180-300 cm/s, Vr: 2-3.5) stenosis ($P < .0001$), non-single segment saphenous vein conduit ($P < .01$), warfarin drug therapy ($P < .01$), and redo bypass grafting ($P < .001$). Procedure indication, postoperative ABI level, statin drug therapy, and vein conduit orientation were not predictive of graft revision. The natural history of 141 (40%) bypasses with an abnormal first duplex scan differed from "normal" grafts by more frequent (51% vs 24%, $P < .001$) and earlier (7 months vs 11 months) graft revision for severe stenosis and a lower 3-year assisted primary patency (68% vs 87%; $P < .001$). In 52 (15%) limbs, the bypass graft failed and 20 (6%) limbs required amputation.

Conclusions.—The efficacy of duplex surveillance after infrainguinal vein bypass may be enhanced by modifying testing protocols, eg, rigorous surveillance for "higher risk" bypasses, based on the initial duplex scan results and other characteristics (warfarin therapy, non- single segment saphenous vein conduit, redo bypass) predictive for stenosis development.

▶ These authors from the University of South Florida are among the most vociferous in advocating postoperative duplex surveillance of infrainguinal bypass grafts. Their findings that an abnormal initial duplex scan, non-single segment saphenous vein conduits, or a redo bypass graft are associated with higher rates of graft stenosis are really no surprise. These things have been reported before. They also report use of warfarin is a marker of increased risk of graft stenosis. We have also noticed in our practice that warfarin is a marker for increased risk of vein graft failure. I am quite sure warfarin itself does not have a detrimental effect on graft patency. Warfarin likely serves as a marker for a high risk graft and indicates that surgeons are fairly astute in identifying patients whose grafts are at risk of failure. Perhaps more interesting were factors not predictive of increased risk of graft stenosis. These included a lower than expected postoperative ankle-brachial index (ABI), nonuse of statin medications, and the indication for the procedure. What it all boils down to is what matters the most in infrainguinal arterial reconstruction is the vein used as the conduit. A good vein will do well and a suboptimal vein will not do well. Infrainguinal arterial reconstructions are all about the vein with the arteries being of secondary importance.

G. L. Moneta, MD

Bleeding into the intraluminal thrombus in abdominal aortic aneurysms is associated with rupture
Roy J, Labruto F, Beckman MO, et al (Capio St. Görans Hosp, Stockholm, Sweden; Karolinska Univ Hosp and Karolinska Institutet, Stockholm, Sweden)
J Vasc Surg 48:1108-1113, 2008

Objective.—The aim of this study was to determine signs of bleeding in the intraluminal thrombus and the site of rupture using multislice computed tomography (CT) imaging in patients with abdominal aortic aneurysms (AAA).

Methods.—We analyzed CT images of 42 patients with ruptured infrarenal AAA in two hospitals in Stockholm, Sweden during a 3-year period. A "crescent sign" or localized areas with higher attenuation in the thrombus were interpreted as signs of bleeding in the thrombus. A localized area of hyperattenuation did not have the typical crescent shape and was distinguished from calcifications in the thrombus. We measured the attenuation in Hounsfield units in the intraluminal thrombus using CT software to quantify the presence of blood in the thrombus. As controls, we analyzed 36 patients with intact AAA and a comparable aneurysm diameter and age.

Results.—The crescent sign was more frequent in the ruptured group (38% vs 14%, *P* =.02), but there was no significant difference in the

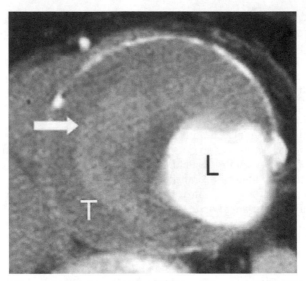

FIGURE 1.—CT scans showing the crescent sign (*white arrow*) in a ruptured AAA (**A**) and a localized area of high attenuation (*white arrow*) in an intact AAA. (Reprinted from Roy J, Labruto F, Beckman MO, et al. Bleeding into the intraluminal thrombus in abdominal aortic aneurysms is associated with rupture. *J Vasc Surg.* 2008;48:1108-1113, with permission from the Society for Vascular Surgery.)

presence of localized areas of hyperattenuation in the two groups. The attenuation in the thrombus was significantly higher in patients with rupture than in those with intact aneurysms ($P = .02$). The site of rupture could be localized in 29/42 patients. Ruptures occurred both through the thrombus-covered and the thrombus free wall. In 45% of the patients, the rupture site was localized in the left lateral wall, in 24% in the anterior wall, in 24% in the right lateral wall, but only in 7% in the posterior wall.

Conclusion.—The site of rupture could be identified in a majority of cases of AAA with routine multislice CT. This study demonstrates an association between the presence of blood in the thrombus as suggested by higher attenuation levels and a crescent sign and AAA rupture. If these findings also predict AAA rupture, remains to be established (Fig 1A).

▶ The only widely acknowledged and accepted predictor of abdominal aortic aneurysm (AAA) rupture is aneurysm diameter. Most AAAs of any significant size contain intraluminal thrombus and the growth of intraluminal thrombus may be associated with rupture risk.[1,2] This may relate to a thinner aneurysm wall underlying areas with thrombus and/or increased levels of inflammatory cells in the aortic wall underlying the intraluminal thrombus. If in fact the aortic wall underlying the thrombus is weaker, for rupture to occur through this site bleeding must occur into the thrombus. This study demonstrates an association between bleeding in the thrombus and rupture of AAAs. The study does not prove a definite relationship between bleeding into the thrombus and rupture. The authors point out 2 possible explanations for the crescent sign (Fig 1A) and its possible association with rupture. One is that it represents blood eventually reaching the underlying weakened aortic wall segment. Conversely, it may occur when the aneurysm wall expands faster than the thrombus with the resulting fissures within the intraluminal thrombus.

The data suggest that the presence of bleeding within an intraluminal thrombus may portend rupture of an AAA. The timing of repair of AAAs with a crescent sign is controversial. However, it would seem that expedient, although not necessarily emergent, repair should be considered.

G. L. Moneta, MD

References

1. Satta J, Läärä E, Juvonen T. Intraluminal thrombus predicts rupture of an abdominal aortic aneurysm. *J Vasc Surg.* 1996;23:737-739.
2. Stenbaek J, Kalin B, Swedenborg J. Growth of thrombus may be a better predictor of rupture than diameter in patients with abdominal aortic aneurysms. *Eur J Vasc Endovasc Surg.* 2000;20:466-469.

Assessment of renal artery stenosis: side-by-side comparison of angiography and duplex ultrasound with pressure gradient measurements
Drieghe B, Madaric J, Sarno G, et al (Cardiovascular Ctr, Moorselbaan, Belgium; et al)
Eur Heart J 29:517-524, 2008

Aims.—A ratio of distal renal pressure to aortic pressure (P_d/P_a) <0.90 can be considered a threshold for defining a significant renal artery stenosis (RAS). The aim of this study was to compare renal angiography (QRA) and colour duplex ultrasound (CDUS) to pressure measurements in assessing RAS.

Methods and Results.—In 56 RAS, percent diameter stenosis (DS_{angio}), minimal luminal diameter (MLD), Doppler-derived peak systolic velocity (PSV), end-diastolic velocity (EDV), and renal-to-aortic ratio (RAR) were obtained and compared with the P_d/P_a measured with a 0.014" pressure wire. P_d/P_a correlated with angiography- and CDUS-derived parameters. The best correlation was observed with EDV $(R = -0.61)$. To identify stenosis associated with a $P_d/P_a < 0.90$, the diagnostic accuracy of $DS_{angio} > 50\%$, MLD < 2 mm, PSV > 180 cm/s, EDV > 90 cm/s and RAR > 3.5 were, respectively, 60%, 77%, 45%, 77% and 79%, yet, with a high proportion of false positives (38%, 15%, 55%, 11% and 15%, respectively), indicating an overestimation of the severity of the RAS by both QRA and CDUS. New cut-off values for QRA- and CDUS-derived indices were proposed.

Conclusion.—Generally accepted QRA and CDUS-derived indices of RAS severity overestimate the actual severity of RAS. This 'overdiagnosis'

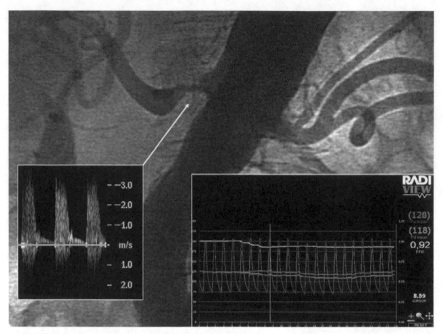

FIGURE 2.—Representative example of angiography, ultrasound measurements and trans-stenotic pressure gradient in a right-sided renal artery stenosis (RAS). Angiography clearly demonstrates a >50% stenosis. The left insert shows Doppler signals at the level of the stenosis (300 cm/s). Both suggest a 'significant' RAS, while an invasive pressure gradient measurement only documents a very mild gradient (P_d/P_a ratio 0.92—hence haemodynamically not significant). (Reprinted from Drieghe B, Madaric J, Sarno G, et al. Assessment of renal artery stenosis: side-by-side comparison of angiography and duplex ultrasound with pressure gradient measurements. *Eur Heart J.* 2008;29:517-524, with permission from Author 2008.)

TABLE 4.—Receiver-operating characteristic curves of different parameters compared with P_d/P_a ratio

	Optimal cut-off value	Sensitivity (%)	Specificity (%)	PPV (%)	NPV (%)	Accuracy (%)	AUC
DS$_{angio}$	>65%	63 (49–75)	90 (78–96)	77	86	83	0.82 ± 0.072 (0.67–0.91)
MLD	<1.74 mm	63 (49–75)	94 (83-98)	91	83	85	0.81 ± 0.062 (0.67–0.91)
PSV	>318 cm/s	88 (76–95)	77 (63–87)	57	88	74	0.88 ± 0.060 (0.75–0.96)
EDV	>70 cm/s	88 (76–95)	77 (63–87)	62	92	79	0.85 ± 0.066 (0.71–0.94)
RAR	>3.74	75 (61–85)	97 (88–99)	92	89	89	0.94 ± 0.043 (0.83–0.99)

PPV, positive predictive value; NPV, negative predictive value; AUV, area under the curve; DS$_{angio}$, percentage stenosis dervied from quantitative renal angiography; MLD, minimal luminal diameter; PSV, peak systolic Velocity; EDV, end-diastolic velocity; RAR, renal-to-aortic ratio; values in brackets represent 95% confidence intervals.

(Reprinted from Drieghe B, Madaric J, Sarno G, et al. Assessment of renal artery stenosis: side-by-side comparison of angiography and duplex ultrasound with pressure gradient measurements. *Eur Heart J.* 2008;29:517-524, with permission from Author 2008.)

is, likely, the main cause of the disappointing results of renal angioplasty for renovascular hypertension (Fig 2), (Table 4).

▶ Basically, this study says angiographic and duplex criteria for renal artery stenosis (RAS) correlate with invasively measured pressure gradients across a renal artery stenosis. However, there are many false positives, in that a 50% stenosis by angiography alone does not have a significant pressure gradient 38% of the time. A stenosis, producing a renal to aortic peak systolic velocity ratio of > 3.5, will not have a significant pressure gradient 15% of the time (Fig 2). The authors proposed revised duplex criteria for hemodynamically significant lesions, based on pressure gradients (Table 4), deserve careful consideration. The old ultrasound criteria are not bad. They do what they say they do; identify high-grade angiographic diameter reductions. These diameter reductions may not correlate with pressure gradients and are an entirely different matter that may or may not have clinical relevance. I am, however, not yet fully convinced, as the authors are, that use of their criteria will improve the ability to select patients who will benefit from renal artery stenting. However, I am in favor of anything that will make people more selective in their decision to perform a procedure with very little proven benefit.

G. L. Moneta, MD

Magnetic resonance angiography of collateral blood supply to spinal cord in thoracic and thoracoabdominal aortic aneurysm patients
Backes WH, Nijenhuis RJ, Mess WH, et al (Maastricht Univ Hosp, The Netherlands; et al)
J Vasc Surg 48:261-271, 2008

Objective.—Preservation of spinal cord blood supply during descending thoracic (TAA) and thoracoabdominal aortic aneurysm (TAAA) surgery is mandatory to prevent neurologic complications. Although collateral arteries have been identified occasionally and are considered crucial for maintaining spinal cord function in the individual patient, their critical functionality is poorly understood and very little experience exists with visualization. This study investigated whether the preoperative and post-operative presence or absence of collateral arteries detected by magnetic resonance angiography (MRA) is related to spinal cord function during the intraoperative exclusion of the segmental supply to the Adamkiewicz artery.

Methods.—Spinal cord MRA was used to localize the Adamkiewicz artery and its segmental supplier in 85 patients scheduled for open elective surgery for TAA or TAAA. The segmental artery to the Adamkiewicz artery was inside the cross-clamped aortic area in 55 patients, and spinal cord supply was consequently dependent on collateral supply. In these 55 patients the presence of collaterals originating from arteries outside the cross-clamped aortic segment was related to changes in the intraoperative

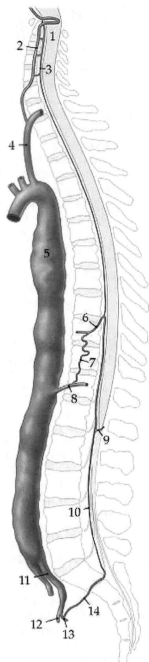

motor-evoked potentials (MEPs) that occurred before corrective measures. Twenty-one patients returned for postoperative MRA.

Results.—A highly significant ($P < .0015$) relation was found between the presence of collaterals and intraoperative spinal cord function. In 30 of 31 patients (97%) in whom collaterals were identified, MEPs remained stable. The collaterals in most patients originated caudally to the distal clamp (eg, from the pelvic arteries), which were perfused by means of extracorporeal circulation during cross-clamping. The MEPs declined in 9 of 24 patients (38%) in whom no collaterals were preoperatively visualized. Postoperatively, the 21 patients who had MRA, including 10 in whom preoperatively no collaterals were found, displayed a well-developed collateral network.

Conclusion.—Collateral arteries supplying the spinal cord can be systematically visualized using MRA. Spinal cord blood supply during open aortic surgery may crucially depend on collateral arteries. Preoperatively identified collateral supply was 97% predictive for stable intraoperative spinal cord function. Patients in whom no collaterals can be depicted preoperatively are at increased risk for spinal cord dysfunction (Fig 1).

▶ This beautifully illustrated study shows that it is possible, using magnetic resonance angiography (MRA), to visualize the artery of Adamkiewicz and collateral blood supply to the spinal cord in patients undergoing repair of thoracoabdominal and thoracic aneurysms. Fig 1 identifications of such collaterals appears highly predictive of stable intraoperative spinal cord function. Preoperative MRA may aid the surgeon in counseling the patient as to their risk of spinal cord dysfunction in conjunction with thoracic or thoracoabdominal aneurysm surgery. It is very unlikely that the beautiful MR angiograms depicted in this article can be obtained at all institutions. Nevertheless, it would seem reasonable to try and develop appropriate expertise in this technique of MRA in institutions choosing to perform open repairs of thoracic and thoracoabdominal aneurysms.

G. L. Moneta, MD

FIGURE 1.—Anatomic drawing shows the different blood-supplying trajectories to the thoracolumbar spinal cord in thoracoabdominal aortic aneurysm patients. The segmental artery directly connecting to the Adamkiewicz artery is partially occluded. The Adamkiewicz artery is supplied by a proximal intersegmental collateral, which originates from a segmental artery two vertebral levels below. This trajectory does not represent the only route for the blood to reach the spinal cord. Alternative original trajectories include the anterior radiculomedullary arteries deriving from the vertebral arteries and the filum terminale artery originating from the iliolumbar artery. *1,* Spinal cord; *2,* vertebral artery; *3,* anterior spinal cord; *4,* left subclavian artery; *5,* aneurysmatic aorta; *6,* Adamkiewicz artery; *7,* intersegmental collateral; *8,* segmental artery indirectly supplying the Adamkiewicz artery; *9,* anastomotic loop to the posterior spinal artery; *10,* filum terminale artery; *11,* common iliac artery; *12,* external iliac artery; *13,* internal iliac artery (hypogastric artery); *14,* iliolumbar artery. (Reprinted from Backes WH, Nijenhuis RJ, Mess WH, et al. Magnetic resonance angiography of collateral blood supply to spinal cord in thoracic and thoracoabdominal aortic aneurysm patients. *J Vasc Surg.* 2008;48:261-271, with permission from the Society for Vascular Surgery.)

5 Perioperative Considerations

Effects of extended-release metoprolol succinate in patients undergoing non-cardiac surgery (POISE trial): a randomised controlled trial
POISE Study Group (McMaster Univ, Faculty of Health Sciences, Clinical Epidemiology and Biostatistics, Hamilton, ON, Canada)
Lancet 371:1839-1847, 2008

Background.—Trials of β blockers in patients undergoing non-cardiac surgery have reported conflicting results. This randomised controlled trial, done in 190 hospitals in 23 countries, was designed to investigate the effects of perioperative β blockers.

Methods.—We randomly assigned 8351 patients with, or at risk of, atherosclerotic disease who were undergoing non-cardiac surgery to receive extended-release metoprolol succinate (n=4174) or placebo (n=4177), by a computerised randomisation phone service. Study treatment was started 2–4 h before surgery and continued for 30 days. Patients, health-care providers, data collectors, and outcome adjudicators were masked to treatment allocation. The primary endpoint was a composite of cardiovascular death, non-fatal myocardial infarction, and non-fatal cardiac arrest. Analyses were by intention to treat. This trial is registered with ClinicalTrials.gov, number NCT00182039.

Findings.—All 8351 patients were included in analyses; 8331 (99·8%) patients completed the 30-day follow-up. Fewer patients in the metoprolol group than in the placebo group reached the primary endpoint (244 [5·8%] patients in the metoprolol group *vs* 290 [6·9%] in the placebo group; hazard ratio 0·84, 95% CI 0·70–0·99; p=0·0399). Fewer patients in the metoprolol group than in the placebo group had a myocardial infarction (176 [4·2%] vs 239 [5·7%] patients; 0·73, 0·60–0·89; p=0·0017). However, there were more deaths in the metoprolol group than in the placebo group (129 [3·1%] *vs* 97 [2·3%] patients; 1·33, 1·03–1·74; p=0·0317). More patients in the metoprolol group than in the placebo group had a stroke (41 [1·0%] *vs* 19 [0·5%] patients; 2·17, 1·26–3·74; p=0·0053).

Interpretation.—Our results highlight the risk in assuming a perioperative β-blocker regimen has benefit without substantial harm, and the importance and need for large randomised trials in the perioperative setting. Patients are unlikely to accept the risks associated with perioperative extended-release metoprolol (Fig 2).

▶ The study has potentially huge implications but needs to be interpreted with caution. Although it is routine to treat patients with atherosclerotic risk factors undergoing high-risk surgery with perioperative β-blockers, β blockade was begun only 2 to 4 hours before surgery in this study. The results may not apply to patients with more extended periods of treatment with preoperative β-blockers. The data indicate that under the conditions of the trial, extended release metoprolol can reduce the risk of myocardial infarction. This, however, is at a cost of an increased risk of death, stroke, and clinically significant hypotension. The authors also performed a number of meta-analyses of trials of β-blockers. Analysis of 9 trials, including PeriOperative ISchemic Evaluation

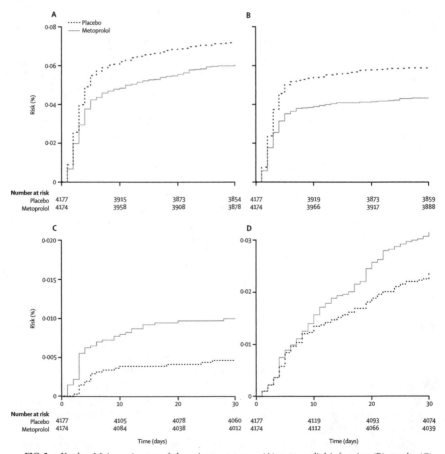

FIG 2.—Kaplan-Meier estimates of the primary outcome (A), myocardial infarction (B), stroke (C), and death (D). (Reprinted from POISE Study Group, Effects of extended-release metoprolol succinate in patients undergoing non-cardiac surgery (POISE trial): a randomised controlled trial. *Lancet.* 2008;371:1839-1847.)

(POISE), in which at least 1 patient had a fatal myocardial infarction, also indicated that β-blockers reduced the risk of myocardial infarction and increased the risk of nonfatal stroke (hazard ratio 2.19, 1.26-3.78, $P = 0.005$). The authors point out that for every 1000 patients undergoing noncardiac surgery, and with similar risk profiles to those in POISE, extended release metoprolol can be expected to prevent 15 myocardial infarctions and prevent 7 patients from undergoing new clinically significant atrial fibrillation. However, extended release metoprolol will also result in an excess of 8 deaths and 5 additional patients having a stroke, with 53 experiencing clinically significant hypotension and 42 experiencing clinically significant bradycardia.

Once again an accepted axiom of perioperative care is questioned by the results of a large randomized trial. Vascular surgeons may need to reconsider the use of routine perioperative β blockade in their patients. There are very few single-edged swords in medicine.

G. L. Moneta, MD

Predictors and outcomes of a perioperative myocardial infarction following elective vascular surgery in patients with documented coronary artery disease: Results of the CARP trial
McFalls EO, Ward HB, Moritz TE, et al (VA Med Ctr, Minneapolis, MN)
Eur Heart J 29:394-401, 2008

Aims.—The predictors and outcomes of patients with a peri-operative elevation in cardiac troponin I above the 99th percentile of normal following an elective vascular operation have not been studied in a homogeneous cohort with documented coronary artery disease.

Methods and Results.—The Coronary Artery Revascularization Prophylaxis (CARP) trial was a randomized trial that tested the benefit of coronary artery revascularization prior to vascular surgery. Among 377 randomized patients, core lab samples for peak cardiac troponin I concentrations were monitored following the vascular operation and the blinded results were correlated with outcomes. A peri-operative myocardial infarction (MI), defined by an increase in cardiac troponin I greater than the 99th percentile reference (≥ 0.1 μg/L), occurred in 100 patients (26.5%) and the incidence was not dissimilar in patients with and without pre-operative coronary revascularization (24.2 vs. 28.6%; $P = 0.32$). By logistic regression analysis, predictors of MI (odds risk; 95%CI; P-value) were age >70 (1.84; 1.14–2.98; $P = 0.01$), abdominal aortic surgery (1.82; 1.09–3.03; $P = 0.02$), diabetes (1.86; 1.11–3.11; $P = 0.02$), angina (1.67; 1.03–2.64; $P = 0.04$), and baseline STT abnormalities (1.62; 1.00–2.6; $P = 0.05$). At 2.5 years post-surgery, the probability of survival in patients with and without the MI was 0.73 and 0.84, respectively ($P = 0.03$, log-rank test). Using a Cox proportional hazards regression analysis, a peri-operative MI in diabetic patients was a strong predictor of long-term mortality (hazards ratio: 2.43; 95% CI: 1.31–4.48; $P < 0.01$).

Conclusion.—Among patients with coronary artery disease who undergo vascular surgery, a peri-operative elevation in cardiac troponin levels is common and in combination with diabetes, is a strong predictor of long-term mortality. These data support the utility of cardiac troponins as a means of stratifying high-risk patients following vascular operations.

▶ Data indicate perioperative myocardial infarction, at least as defined by this study, occurs in 27% of patients undergoing a peripheral vascular operation, and the incidence is not influenced by preoperative coronary revascularization. Mortality at 1 year following vascular surgery in patients with peak cardiac troponin 1 concentrations (> 0.1 mg/L) was a surprising 20%. This was compared with 4.7% in those patients with a peak concentration (< 0.1 mg/ L, P < 0.001). These are certainly dramatic numbers.

It is always difficult to know what to do with data collected after the fact. Postoperative troponin levels may turn out to be a valuable prognostic factor. They, of course, obviously cannot influence the decision to perform the initial index operation. However, such information may influence a decision to perform subsequent elective vascular surgery in patients with myocardial infarction (MI) following a previous vascular operation.

G. L. Moneta, MD

Intensive Blood Glucose Control and Vascular Outcomes in Patients with Type 2 Diabetes

Patel A, The ADVANCE Collaborative Group (Univ of Sydney, Australia)
N Engl J Med 358:2560-2572, 2008

Background.—In patients with type 2 diabetes, the effects of intensive glucose control on vascular outcomes remain uncertain.

Methods.—We randomly assigned 11,140 patients with type 2 diabetes to undergo either standard glucose control or intensive glucose control, defined as the use of gliclazide (modified release) plus other drugs, as required, to achieve a glycated hemoglobin value of 6.5% or less. Primary end points were composites of major macrovascular events (death from cardiovascular causes, nonfatal myocardial infarction, or nonfatal stroke) and major microvascular events (new or worsening nephropathy or retinopathy), assessed both jointly and separately.

Results.—After a median of 5 years of follow-up, the mean glycated hemoglobin level was lower in the intensive-control group (6.5%) than in the standard-control group (7.3%). Intensive control reduced the incidence of combined major macrovascular and microvascular events (18.1%, vs. 20.0% with standard control; hazard ratio, 0.90; 95% confidence interval [CI], 0.82 to 0.98; P = 0.01), as well as that of major microvascular events (9.4% vs. 10.9%; hazard ratio, 0.86; 95% CI, 0.77 to 0.97; P = 0.01), primarily because of a reduction in the incidence of nephropathy (4.1% vs. 5.2%; hazard ratio, 0.79; 95% CI, 0.66 to 0.93;

P = 0.006), with no significant effect on retinopathy (P = 0.50). There were no significant effects of the type of glucose control on major macrovascular events (hazard ratio with intensive control, 0.94; 95% CI, 0.84 to 1.06; P = 0.32), death from cardiovascular causes (hazard ratio with intensive control, 0.88; 95% CI, 0.74 to 1.04; P = 0.12), or death from any cause (hazard ratio with intensive control, 0.93; 95% CI, 0.83 to 1.06; P = 0.28). Severe hypoglycemia, although uncommon, was more common in the intensive-control group (2.7%, vs. 1.5% in the standard-control group; hazard ratio, 1.86; 95% CI, 1.42 to 2.40; P < 0.001).

Conclusions.—A strategy of intensive glucose control, involving gliclazide (modified release) and other drugs, as required, that lowered the glycated hemoglobin value to 6.5%, yielded a 10% relative reduction in the combined outcome of major macrovascular and microvascular events, primarily as a consequence of a 21% relative reduction in nephropathy.

▶ This is one of the 2 companion articles on the effects of intensive glucose control in patients with type 2 diabetes that appeared in the same issue of the *New England Journal of Medicine*. In this article, we are disappointed to learn that intensive glucose control did not result in a reduction in macrocardiovascular events in patients with type 2 diabetes. It may be, however, that longer follow-up is needed to detect such an effect. The clear improvement in nephropathy, with longer follow-up, perhaps, could be expected to have benefit over time in reducing macrovascular events. This is, however, only speculation, and the idea that intensive glucose control is beneficial in patients with type 2 diabetes must be seriously questioned, especially given the companion article.[1] In that study, over 10,000 patients with type 2 diabetes were randomized to standard or intensive diabetic control. The study was stopped after 3.5 years because of an increased mortality rate in the intensively treated patients. Once again, when subjected to the rigors of a randomized trial, a commonly held belief appears to have been incorrect. These studies will be intensely debated, but the bottom line is there was no clear benefit from intensive glucose control in reducing macrovascular events in patients with type 2 diabetes.

G. L. Moneta, MD

Reference

1. The Action to Control Cardiovascular Risk in Diabetes Study Group. Effects of intensive glucose lowering in type 2 diabetes. *N Engl J Med.* 2008;358: 2545-2559.

Effect of Statin Therapy on Mortality in Patients With Peripheral Arterial Disease and Comparison of Those With Versus Without Associated Chronic Obstructive Pulmonary Disease

van Gestel YRBM, Hoeks SE, Sin DD, et al (Dept of Anesthesiology, Thoraxcenter, Erasmus MC, Rotterdam; Univ of British Columbia, Canada;)
Am J Cardiol 102:192-196, 2008

Chronic obstructive pulmonary disease (COPD) and peripheral arterial disease (PAD) are both inflammatory conditions. Statins are commonly used in patients with PAD and have anti-inflammatory properties, which may have beneficial effects in patients with COPD. The relation between statin use and mortality was investigated in patients with PAD with and without COPD. From 1990 to 2006, we studied 3,371 vascular surgery patients. Statin use was noted at baseline and, if prescribed, converted to <25% (low dose) and ≥25% (intensified dose) of the maximum recommended therapeutic dose. The diagnosis of COPD was based on the Global Initiative for Chronic Obstructive Lung Disease guidelines using pulmonary function test. End points were short- (30-day) and long-term (10-year) mortality. A total of 330 patients with COPD (25%) used statins, and 480 patients (23%) without COPD. Statin use was independently associated with improved short- and long-term survival in patients with COPD (odds ratio 0.48, 95% confidence interval [CI] 0.23 to 1.00; hazard ratio 0.67, 95% CI 0.52 to 0.86, respectively). In patients without COPD, statins were also associated with improved short- and long-term survival (odds ratio 0.42, 95% CI 0.20 to 0.87; hazard ratio 0.76, 95% CI 0.60 to 0.95, respectively). In patients with COPD, only an intensified dose of statins was associated with improved short-term survival. However, for the long term, both low-dose and intensive statin therapy were beneficial. In conclusion, statin use was associated with improved short- and long-term survival in patients with PAD with and without COPD. Patients with COPD should be treated with an intensified dose of statins to achieve an optimal effect on both the short and long term (Figs 1 and 2).

▶ This is another of the rapidly expanding pile of publications confirming the benefits of statin therapy in vascular surgical patients. (Vascular surgeons may not be aware that statins also benefit patients with chronic obstructive pulmonary disease [COPD] as well.) Like virtually all articles investigating the pleiotropic effects of statins, this one is retrospective and, therefore, has significant limitations. Nevertheless, a couple of things are especially worth noting here. The first, not unique to this study, is that there is increasing focus on the anti-inflammatory effects of statin therapy, as the mechanism of pleiotropy has favorable effect on survival in patients with vascular disease and/or COPD. The second is that we are now beginning to get some idea as to what specific dose of a statin medication is required to achieve benefit. It has been our practice for several years to start all our vascular surgical patients on perioperative low-dose statin therapy if they were not already on the medication preoperatively. The data here suggest that approach will work for most

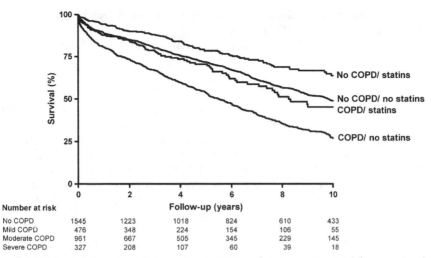

Number at risk

No COPD	1545	1223	1018	824	610	433
Mild COPD	476	348	224	154	106	55
Moderate COPD	961	667	505	345	229	145
Severe COPD	327	208	107	60	39	18

FIGURE 1.—Long-term mortality according to COPD and statin use. (Reprinted from van Gestel YRBM, Hoeks SE, Sin DD, et al. Effect of statin therapy on mortality in patients with peripheral arterial disease and comparison of those with versus without associated chronic obstructive pulmonary disease. *Am J Cardiol.* 2008;102:192-196, with permission from Elsevier.)

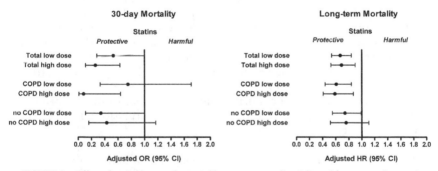

FIGURE 2.—Effect of statin dose on short- and long-term mortality. Adjusted for age, gender, previous myocardial infarction, previous coronary revascularization (coronary artery bypass graft or percutaneous coronary intervention), previous heart failure, previous angina pectoris, previous cerebrovascular accident or transient ischemic attack, hypertension, hypercholesterolemia, diabetes mellitus, impaired renal function, smoking status, body mass index, type of surgery (AAA, CEA, or LLR), year of surgery, and use of β blockers, aspirin, bronchodilators, and corticosteroids. (Reprinted from van Gestel YRBM, Hoeks SE, Sin DD, et al. Effect of statin therapy on mortality in patients with peripheral arterial disease and comparison of those with versus without associated chronic obstructive pulmonary disease. *Am J Cardiol.* 2008;102:192-196, with permission from Elsevier.)

patients but that perhaps higher doses are needed to optimize short-term perioperative survival in the vascular surgical patient with COPD (Figs 1 and 2).

G. L. Moneta, MD

Clinical outcome in patients with peripheral artery disease. Results from a prospective registry (FRENA)

Monreal M, Alvarez L, Vilaseca B, et al (Hospital Universitari Germans Trias i Pujol, Badalona, Spain; et al)
Eur J Intern Med 19:192-197, 2008

Background.—The risk of future cardiovascular events in patients with peripheral artery disease (PAD) is often underestimated.

Patients and Methods.—FRENA is an ongoing, observational registry of consecutive outpatients with symptomatic PAD, coronary artery disease (CAD) or cerebrovascular disease (CVD). We compared the incidence of major cardiovascular events (i.e., myocardial infarction, ischemic stroke, critical limb ischemia, or cardiovascular death) during a 12-month follow-up period in a series of consecutive outpatients with PAD, CAD or CVD.

Results.—As of December 2006, 1265 patients had been enrolled in FRENA who completed the 12-month follow-up. Of these, 417 patients (33%) had PAD, 474 (37%) had CAD, 374 (30%) had CVD. Patients with PAD had an increased incidence of major cardiovascular events per 100 patient-years: 17 (95% CI: 13–22) vs. 7.9 (5.5–11) in those with CAD, or 8.9 (6.1–13) in those with CVD. Compared to patients with CAD or CVD those with PAD had a similar incidence of myocardial infarction or stroke, but a higher incidence of critical limb ischemia, limb amputation and death. This incidence increased with the severity of the symptoms: 8.7 (95% CI: 5.3–13) in patients in Fontaine stage IIa; 25 (95% CI: 16–38) in stage IIb; 26 (95% CI: 13–47) in stage III; 42 (95% CI: 24–67) in stage IV.

Conclusions.—Our data confirm a higher incidence of major cardiovascular events for patients with PAD, as well as a correlation of these events with the severity of PAD.

▶ This is an observational study and, therefore, has a number of limitations. They include that it cannot answer questions on the efficacy of different treatment modalities, and it may underestimate incidence of events in those patients lost to follow-up, and there is no information on patients that were considered for the study but were excluded. We, therefore, do not truly know how representative the patients included in the study are to those in the community with various manifestations of vascular disease. Nevertheless, what is quite interesting is the type of morbid events that the patients with peripheral arterial disease (PAD) suffer in comparison with those patients with coronary artery disease (CAD) and cerebral vascular disease (CVD). The patients with PAD had the same incidence of myocardial infarction, or stroke, as the patients with CAD and CVD, but had a higher rate of death and limb specific complications that correlates with the severity of their PAD. I suppose this makes sense, but the study will change how I talk to my patients, in that I will now emphasize a bit more the adverse natural history of PAD, with respect to limb specific complications. This is, of course, in addition to reminding my PAD patients that their leg artery disease is a marker of their risk of stroke and myocardial infarction.

G. L. Moneta, MD

Are patients with thrombophilia and previous venous thromboembolism at higher risk to arterial thrombosis?
Linnemann B, Schindewolf M, Zgouras D, et al (Johann Wolfgang Goethe Univ Hosp, Germany)
Thromb Res 121:743-750, 2008

Introduction.—Whether thrombophilic disorders, which are established risk factors for venous thromboembolism (VTE), also increase the risk of arterial thrombosis is still unknown.

Materials and Methods.—We analyzed data from 1081 consecutive patients (649 F/432 M, 16–93 years of age) with previous VTE registered in the MAISTHRO (MAin-ISar-THROmbosis) database with regard to arterial thrombotic events and contributing risk factors. Screening for thrombophilia included testing for factor V Leiden and prothrombin G20210A mutation, antiphospholipid antibodies and activities of factor VIII, protein C, protein S and antithrombin.

Results.—Of the entire study cohort, 40 patients (3.7%) had a prior myocardial infarction (MI), and 41 (3.8%) suffered a stroke. Other arterial thrombotic events were rare. Elevated factor VIII levels were more prevalent in MI patients than in controls (44.4 vs. 25.9%, $p = 0.044$), but after adjusting for the traditional cardiovascular risk factors, this relationship was no longer significant. We observed a higher rate of lupus anticoagulant in MI patients with an adjusted odds ratio of 3.3 (95%CI 0.84–12.8, $p = 0.090$). No difference in any other tested thrombophilia was observed in patients with MI or stroke relative to those without.

Conclusion.—The cumulative incidence of arterial thrombotic events in VTE patients is low, and the inherited thrombophilias do not seem to substantially increase the risk of arterial thrombosis.

▶ Vascular surgeons sometimes see that patients feel they are "hypercoagulable." I am sure that very few of them are, but most are just victims of a technically imperfect open or endovascular surgical procedure, rather than the victim of a genetic thrombophilia. Nevertheless, testing for hypercoagulable states is common in vascular surgical patients. This article tells us that native artery events, induced by recognized thrombophilias, is rare. It does not tell us if thrombophilias contribute to failed arterial reconstructions. My belief is, genetically based thrombophilias are a very infrequent cause of a failed arterial reconstruction. Just as abnormal anatomy is often the indicator of a confused surgeon, so is the likelihood that postoperative "hypercoagulable states" are the result of surgical imperfections than genetic abnormalities of the coagulation system.

G. L. Moneta, MD

A comparison of recombinant thrombin to bovine thrombin as a hemostatic ancillary in patients undergoing peripheral arterial bypass and arteriovenous graft procedures
Weaver FA, Lew W, Granke K, et al (USC CardioVascular Thoracic Inst, Los Angeles, CA; Detroit VA Med Ctr, MI; et al)
J Vasc Surg 47:1266-1273, 2008

Objectives.—Recombinant thrombin (rThrombin) is a potential hemostatic alternative to bovine and human plasma-derived thrombin. This report examines the clinical results for the vascular surgery subgroup of patients enrolled in a larger double-blind, randomized, multicenter trial, which evaluated the comparative safety and efficacy of rThrombin and bovine plasma-derived thrombin (bThrombin) when used as adjuncts to surgical hemostasis.

Methods.—Data from the 164 vascular patients, who underwent either a peripheral arterial bypass (PAB) or arteriovenous graft (AV) procedure, are included in this analysis. Time to hemostasis at proximal and distal anastomotic sites at 1.5-, 3-, 6-, and 10-minute intervals was determined by procedure (PAB or AV) and overall (PAB + AV). Baseline and day 29 immunologic sera were analyzed. The incidences of postoperative adverse events were compared between treatment groups. Categorical adverse events were evaluated in relation to thrombin product antibody formation.

Results.—Patients were randomized to either bThrombin (n = 82) or rThrombin (n = 82). Procedures included PAB (n = 88) and AV (n = 76). The bThrombin and rThrombin groups were well matched for demographics and baseline characteristics. A comparable incidence of anastomotic hemostasis was observed in both treatment groups at 10 minutes (94% bThrombin, 91% rThrombin). The incidence of hemostasis was lower at all time points for PAB procedures compared with AV procedures. In the PAB group, a significantly greater proportion of patients receiving rThrombin (55%) achieved hemostasis at 3 minutes compared with bThrombin (39%; $P < .05$). Adverse event profiles and laboratory findings were similar between groups. No patients in the rThrombin group developed anti-rThrombin product antibodies at day 29, whereas 27% of patients in the bThrombin group developed antibodies to bThrombin product ($P < .0001$).

Conclusions.—rThrombin or bThrombin used as a hemostatic ancillary for anastomotic bleeding was equally effective at 10 minutes; however, rThrombin compared with bThrombin may provide a more rapid onset of hemostasis at 3 minutes in PAB procedures. Adverse events were similar between the two thrombins. In patients undergoing vascular surgery, both treatments were similarly well tolerated, although rThrombin demonstrated a superior immunogenicity profile.

▶ Bovine thrombin has been used for years and has gained widespread acceptance as an adjunct to achieving hemostasis in many vascular and nonvascular surgical procedures. There may be as much as 250 million dollars spent annually in the United States alone for the use of topical thrombin. There are a number of complications associated with bovine thrombin, including anaphylaxis and coagulopathy but they are vanishingly infrequent. There is, however, an available recombinant thrombin product that appears to work with bovine thrombin in achieving local hemostasis but is not associated with development of antibodies. This trial, sponsored by the recombinant thrombin people and first authored by a consultant to the recombinant thrombin people, was a well designed, randomized study that proves all of this—clinically irrelevant differences in local hemostasis, more antibodies to bovine thrombin, no differences in hard serious clinical adverse events. However, no trial of the 2 thrombins is likely to differ in hard, adverse end points, as they are too infrequent. The recombinant thrombin people will, therefore, point to the high incidence of antibodies with bovine thrombin. The bovine thrombin people will point out clinical adverse events associated with bovine thrombin and are too few to matter, and they will use long-established relationships and marketing experience to promote their product. Let the thrombin wars begin! Try not to be influenced by the free lunches, and let the safest and most cost-effective product win.

G. L. Moneta, MD

Femoral vs Jugular Venous Catheterization and Risk of Nosocomial Events in Adults Requiring Acute Renal Replacement Therapy: A Randomized Controlled Trial

Parienti J-J, for Members of the Cathedia Study Group (Côte de Nacre Univ Hosp Ctr, Caen CEDEX, France; et al)
JAMA 299:2413-2422, 2008

Context.—Based on concerns about the risk of infection, the jugular site is often preferred over the femoral site for short-term dialysis vascular access.

Objective.—To determine whether jugular catheterization decreases the risk of nosocomial complications compared with femoral catheterization.

Design, Setting, and Patients.—A concealed, randomized, multicenter, evaluator-blinded, parallel-group trial (the Cathedia Study) of 750 patients from a network of 9 tertiary care university medical centers and 3 general hospitals in France conducted between May 2004 and May 2007. The severely ill, bed-bound adults had a body mass index (BMI) of less than 45 and required a first catheter insertion for renal replacement therapy.

Intervention.—Patients were randomized to receive jugular or femoral vein catheterization by operators experienced in placement at both sites.

Main Outcome Measures.—Rates of infectious complications, defined as catheter colonization on removal (primary end point), and catheter-related bloodstream infection.

Results.—Patient and catheter characteristics, including duration of catheterization, were similar in both groups. More hematomas occurred in the jugular group than in the femoral group (13/366 patients [3.6%] vs 4/370 patients [1.1%], respectively; $P = .03$). The risk of catheter colonization at removal did not differ significantly between the femoral and jugular groups (incidence of 40.8 vs 35.7 per 1000 catheter-days; hazard ratio [HR], 0.85; 95% confidence interval [CI], 0.62-1.16; $P = .31$). A pre-specified subgroup analysis demonstrated significant qualitative heterogeneity by BMI (P for the interaction term $< .001$). Jugular catheterization significantly increased incidence of catheter colonization vs femoral catheterization (45.4 vs 23.7 per 1000 catheter-days; HR, 2.10; 95% CI, 1.13-3.91; $P = .017$) in the lowest tercile (BMI <24.2), whereas jugular catheterization significantly decreased this incidence (24.5 vs 50.9 per 1000 catheter-days; HR, 0.40; 95% CI, 0.23-0.69; $P < .001$) in the highest tercile (BMI >28.4). The rate of catheter-related bloodstream infection was similar in both groups (2.3 vs 1.5 per 1000 catheter-days, respectively; $P = .42$).

Conclusion.—Jugular venous catheterization access does not appear to reduce the risk of infection compared with femoral access, except among adults with a high BMI, and may have a higher risk of hematoma.

Trial Registration.—clinicaltrials.gov Identifier: NCT00277888.

▶ It is widely believed that infectious complications associated with acute renal replacement therapy are reduced with jugular access versus femoral access for short-term dialysis. In this study, the authors sought to determine whether jugular catheterization actually decreases the risk of nosocomial complications compared with femoral catheterization. The authors' data is inconsistent with the widely accepted belief of avoiding femoral catheterization to prevent risk of catheter-related infection in patients undergoing acute renal replacement therapy. The 1 exception appears to be those individuals with a significantly increased body mass index (BMI). This was, however, a large, multi-center randomized trial and the data therefore must be taken seriously. Except for patients with elevated BMI, there appears to be no particular advantage, and perhaps a disadvantage in terms of hematoma formation, of using the jugular site versus the femoral site for acute renal replacement therapy.

G. L. Moneta, MD

Oral Vitamin K Versus Placebo to Correct Excessive Anticoagulation in Patients Receiving Warfarin: A Randomized Trial
Crowther MA, Ageno W, Garcia D, et al (McMaster Univ, Hamilton, Ontario, Canada; Univ of Insubria, Varese, Italy; Univ of New Mexico, Albuquerque; et al)
Ann Intern Med 150:293-300, 2009

Background.—Low-dose oral vitamin K decreases the international normalized ratio (INR) in overanticoagulated patients who receive warfarin therapy. Its effects on bleeding events are uncertain.

Objective.—To see whether low-dose oral vitamin K reduces bleeding events over 90 days in patients with warfarin-associated coagulopathy.

Design.—Multicenter, randomized, placebo-controlled trial. Randomization was computer-generated, and participants were allocated to trial groups by using sequentially numbered study drug containers. Patients, caregivers, and those who assessed outcomes were blinded to treatment assignment.

Setting.—14 anticoagulant therapy clinics in Canada, the United States, and Italy.

Patients.—Nonbleeding patients with INR values of 4.5 to 10.0.

Intervention.—Oral vitamin K, 1.25 mg (355 patients randomly assigned; 347 analyzed), or matching placebo (369 patients randomly assigned; 365 analyzed).

Measurements.—Bleeding events (primary outcome), thromboembolism, and death (secondary outcomes).

Results.—56 patients (15.8%) in the vitamin K group and 60 patients (16.3%) in the placebo group had at least 1 bleeding complication (absolute difference, −0.5 percentage point [95% CI, −6.1 to 5.1 percentage points]); major bleeding events occurred in 9 patients (2.5%) in the vitamin K group and 4 patients (1.1%) in the placebo group (absolute difference, 1.5 percentage points [CI, −0.8 to 3.7 percentage points]). Thromboembolism occurred in 4 patients (1.1%) in the vitamin K group and 3 patients (0.8%) in the placebo group (absolute difference, 0.3 percentage point [CI, −1.4 to 2.0 percentage points]). Other adverse effects were not assessed. The day after treatment, the INR had decreased by a mean of 1.4 in the placebo group and 2.8 in the vitamin K group ($P < 0.001$).

Limitation.—Patients who were actively bleeding were not included, and warfarin dosing after enrollment was not mandated or followed.

Conclusion.—Low-dose oral vitamin K did not reduce bleeding in warfarin recipients with INRs of 4.5 to 10.0.

Funding.—Canadian Institutes of Health Research and Italian Ministry of Universities and Research.

▶ Warfarin, although very effective for primary and secondary prevention of arterial and venous thromboembolism, has highly unpredictable dose-response characteristics. Response to warfarin therapy may vary both within and among individuals over time. Bleeding risk increases when international normalized ratio (INR) exceeds 4.5.[1] In addition, INRs outside the therapeutic range can occur up to one third to one half of the time.[2] When patients present with an INR greater than 4.5, clinicians may either elect to treat with vitamin K therapy administered intravenously or orally, or just withhold warfarin treatment and allow the INR to drift down over time.

The data indicate that active reduction of the INR by administration of vitamin K does not reduce bleeding episodes in patients with supratherapeutic INR levels. Conversely, the data also indicate that administration of vitamin K did not result in increased episodes of thromboembolism. The results have significant implications for clinical practice. Patients with INRs between 4.5 to 10 should simply have warfarin therapy withheld with reinstitution of warfarin therapy once the INR has returned to the desired range. It is important to note which patients were also not studied in this trial. The data cannot be extrapolated to those patients who are bleeding or who present with INRs greater than 10. Overall, the results of the trial should help simplify the management of most patients treated with warfarin who present with supratherapeutic INR levels.

G. L. Moneta, MD

References

1. Ansell J, Hirsh J, Hylek E, et al. Pharmacology and management of the vitamin K antagonists: American College of Chest Physicians Evidence-Based Clinical Practice Guidelines (8th Edition). *Chest.* 2008;133:160S-198S.
2. Witt DM, Sadler MA, Shanahan RL, Mazzoli G, Tillman DJ. Effect of a centralized clinical pharmacy anticoagulation service on the outcomes of anticoagulation therapy. *Chest.* 2005;127:1515-1522.

Preoperative Shower Revisited: Can High Topical Antiseptic Levels Be Achieved on the Skin Surface Before Surgical Admission?
Edmiston CE Jr, Krepel CJ, Seabrook GR, et al (Med College of Wisconsin, Milwaukee, WI)
J Am Coll Surg 207:233-239, 2008

Background.—Skin asepsis is a sentinel strategy for reducing risk of surgical site infections. In this study, chlorhexidine gluconate (CHG) skin concentrations were determined after preoperative showering/skin cleansing using 4% CHG soap or 2% CHG-impregnated polyester cloth.

Study Design.—Subjects were randomized to one of three shower (4% soap)/skin cleansing (2% cloth) groups (n = 20 per group): (group 1 A/B) evening, (group 2 A/B) morning, or (group 3 A/B) evening and morning. After showering or skin cleansing, volunteers returned to the investigator's laboratory where CHG skin surface concentrations were determined at five separate skin sites. CHG concentrations were compared with CHG minimal inhibitory concentration that inhibits 90% (MIC$_{90}$) of staphylococcal skin isolates.

Results.—CHG MIC_{90} for 61 skin isolates was 4.8 parts per million (ppm). In group 1A, 4% CHG skin concentrations ranged from 17.2 to 31.6 ppm, and CHG concentrations were 361.5 to 589.5 ppm ($p < 0.0001$) in group 1B (2%). In group 2A (4%), CHG levels ranged from 51.6 to 119.6 ppm and 848.1 to 1,049.6 ppm in group 2B (2%), respectively ($p < 0.0001$). CHG levels ranged from 101.4 to 149.4 ppm in the 4% CHG group (group 3A) compared with 1,484.6 to 2,031.3 ppm in 2% CHG cloth (group 3B) group ($p < 0.0001$). Effective CHG levels were not detected in the 4% CHG group in selected sites in seven (35%) subjects in group 1A, three (15%) in group 2A, and five (25%) in group 3A.

Conclusions.—Effective CHG levels were achieved on most skin sites after using 4% CHG; gaps in antiseptic coverage were noted at selective sites even after repeated application. Use of the 2% CHG polyester cloth resulted in considerably higher skin concentrations with no gaps in antiseptic coverage. Effective decolonization of the skin before hospital admission can play an important role in reducing risk of surgical site infections.

▶ The Cochrane Collaborative has appropriately pointed out the gap between preoperative skin antisepsis and evidence-based outcomes to reduce surgical site infection. We still do not know the impact of a carefully administered preoperative program of skin decolonization on actual reduction in surgical site infection. As in this study, the surrogate end point of chlorhexidine gluconate (CHG) concentrations does not reflect the clinical end point of surgical site infection. In addition, none of the volunteers in this study had a body mass index greater than 40. Comorbidities such as diabetes, renal failure, and nutritional status that may affect surgical site infection were not assessed. Nevertheless, it does appear possible to achieve CHG concentrations in the skin that considerably exceed the minimal inhibitory concentration that inhibits 90% (MIC_{90}) of staphylococcal isolates. Therefore, although the data is not perfect, there seems little downside in the use of preoperative antiseptic shower or skin cleansing and it appears that a 2% CHG-impregnated polyester cloth is superior to 4% CHG soap in achieving effective MIC's on the skin.

G. L. Moneta, MD

Five Day Antibiotic Prophylaxis for Major Lower Limb Amputation Reduces Wound Infection Rates and the Length of In-hospital Stay
Sadat U, Chaudhuri A, Hayes PD, et al (Addenbrooke's Hosp, Cambridge, UK)
Eur J Vasc Endovasc Surg 35:75-78, 2008

Objective.—To compare wound infection, revision rates and hospital stay after major lower limb amputation between patients receiving 24 hours versus 5 days of prophylactic antibiotics.

Methods.—The outcomes of a consecutive series of 40 major lower limb amputations in patients receiving a short 24-hour course of combined prophylactic antibiotics (flucloxacillin/vancomycin + gentamicin/ciproxin + metronidazole) were retrospectively analysed. Following this a further consecutive group of 40 major lower limb amputations were studied prospectively following the institution of a 5-day combined regime using the same antibiotics.

Results.—The 2 groups of patients were similar in terms of demographics, vascular risk factors and level of amputation. The 5-day antibiotic regime led to a significant reduction in wound infection rates (5% vs. 22.5%, $P = 0.023$) and a reduced length of hospital stay (22 vs. 34 days, $P = 0.001$). Revision rates were lower (2.5% vs. 10%) but did not reach statistical significance ($P = 0.36$). More patients in the prospective 5-day antibiotic series were operated on by the vascular trainee. (77.5% vs. 55% $P = 0.033$).

Conclusions.—This data supports the use of a prolonged 5-day course of combined antibiotics after major lower limb amputation. This appears to reduce stump infection rates leading to shorter in-hospital stay.

▶ This is a small report with controversial conclusions. It will likely offend the "perioperative antiobiotic police"! There are, of course, legitimate concerns about the development of antimicrobial resistance and *Clostridium difficile* infections with prolonged antibiotic prophylaxis. Clearly, there must be a balance in patients with major lower limb amputations between the need to minimize often high rates of stump infection with the detrimental effects of prolonged antibiotic usage. However, the significant reduction in wound infection rates in this study, with 5 days of routine antibiotic prophylaxis, cannot be dismissed lightly. We should keep an open mind and consider that there may well be a place for more intense antibiotic regimes in patients undergoing major limb amputation. Getting this by your hospital infection control committee is an entirely different matter.

G. L. Moneta, MD

Use of vacuum-assisted closure (VAC) therapy in treating lymphatic complications after vascular procedures: New approach for lymphoceles
Hamed O, Muck PE, Smith JM, et al (Good Samaritan Hosp, Cincinnati, OH; et al)
J Vasc Surg 48:1520-1523, 2008

Objective.—Lymphatic complications, such as lymphocutaneous fistula (LF) and lymphocele, are relatively uncommon after vascular procedures, but their treatment represents a serious challenge. Vacuum assisted closure (VAC) therapy has been reported to be an effective therapeutic option for LF, but the effectiveness of VAC therapy for lymphoceles is unclear.

Methods.—For LF, we apply the VAC directly to the skin defect after extending it to achieve a clean wound of at least one inch in length. To treat lymphocele, we convert the lymphocele to a LF in a sterile fashion by making a one inch incision in the overlying skin and applying the VAC. The setting was a community teaching hospital. We used 10 patients that we treated with VAC therapy for LF (n = 4) and lymphoceles (n = 6).

Results.—Duration of in-patient stay, duration of in-patient VAC treatment, duration of out-patient VAC treatment, total duration of VAC treatment. The median duration of in-patient stay was 4 (range, 0-18) days, the median duration of in-patient VAC treatment was 1 (range, 0-5) days, the median duration of out-patient VAC treatment was 16 (range, 7-28) days), and the median total duration of VAC therapy was 18 (range, 13-29) days. Successful wound healing was achieved in all patients with no recurrence after VAC removal. VAC therapy for treatment of both LFs and lymphoceles resulted in early control of drainage, rapid wound closure, and short hospital stays.

Conclusion.—Our results suggest that VAC therapy is a convenient and effective therapeutic option for both LFs and lymphoceles.

▶ Lymphoceles and lymphatic leaks following a vascular procedure, especially when a prosthetic graft is involved, are a real pain. Patients with lymphatic leaks are at increased risk of prosthetic graft infection and have increased hospital lengths of stay. There are many treatments for lymphocutaneous fistulas and lymphoceles. These include dressing changes, pressure dressings, drains, leg elevation, surgical re-exploration and reclosure of the wound with ligation of potential lymphatic channels, and muscle flap coverage after graft removal. The number of treatments attests to the lack of uniformity as to the best treatment for groin lymphatic complications following a vascular procedure. In our practice, we have anecdotally found that a sartorius muscle flap is a relatively simple and highly effective procedure to address groin lymphatic complications. The results here suggest that vacuum-assisted closure (VAC) therapy is also an effective treatment for lymphoceles or lymphatic fistulas that have failed outpatient conservative management. Indeed, most of us are now familiar with negative pressure therapy in many different clinical settings. The data really cannot be used to justify a uniform approach of using VAC therapy for treatment for groin lymphatic complications. There were, after all, only 10 patients in this small series. Nevertheless, a small series with uniformly good results is worth keeping in mind. VAC therapy should be added to the surgeon's armamentarium for treatment of lymphatic complications in vascular surgical patients.

G. L. Moneta, MD

Rehospitalizations among Patients in the Medicare Fee-for-Service Program

Jencks SF, Williams MV, Coleman EA (Independent consulting practice, Baltimore; Northwestern Univ Feinberg School of Medicine, Chicago; Univ of Colorado at Denver)
N Engl J Med 360:1418-1428, 2009

Background.—Reducing rates of rehospitalization has attracted attention from policymakers as a way to improve quality of care and reduce costs. However, we have limited information on the frequency and patterns of rehospitalization in the United States to aid in planning the necessary changes.

Methods.—We analyzed Medicare claims data from 2003–2004 to describe the patterns of rehospitalization and the relation of rehospitalization to demographic characteristics of the patients and to characteristics of the hospitals.

Results.—Almost one fifth (19.6%) of the 11,855,702 Medicare beneficiaries who had been discharged from a hospital were rehospitalized within 30 days, and 34.0% were rehospitalized within 90 days; 67.1% of patients who had been discharged with medical conditions and 51.5% of those who had been discharged after surgical procedures were rehospitalized or died within the first year after discharge. In the case of 50.2% of the patients who were rehospitalized within 30 days after a medical discharge to the community, there was no bill for a visit to a physician's office between the time of discharge and rehospitalization. Among patients who were rehospitalized within 30 days after a surgical discharge, 70.5% were rehospitalized for a medical condition. We estimate that about 10% of rehospitalizations were likely to have been planned. The average stay of rehospitalized patients was 0.6 day longer than that of patients in the same diagnosis-related group whose most recent hospitalization had been at least 6 months previously. We estimate that the cost to Medicare of unplanned rehospitalizations in 2004 was $17.4 billion.

Conclusions.—Rehospitalizations among Medicare beneficiaries are prevalent and costly.

▶ Rehospitalizations are paid for by Medicare. Under current rules, payment is available for rehospitalizations, except for patients rehospitalized for the same condition within 24 hours after discharge from the initial hospitalization. Policy changes are being considered that would create payment incentives to reduce rates of rehospitalization. (Reducing rehospitalization is an important component of President Obama's February 2009 proposal for financing health care reform [Washington Post, February 26, 2009]). It has been suggested by the Medicare Payment Advisory Commission (MedPAC) that hospitals receive a confidential report of risk-adjusted rehospitalization rates, which must be re-published after 2 years, from the Centers for Medicare and Medicaid Services (CMS). It has also been suggested that hospitals with high risk-adjusted rates of rehospitalization should receive lower average per-case payments. While reducing rehospitalizations is clearly a potential means of reducing costs, there is actually little information on the frequency and patterns of rehospitalization.

Vascular surgical patients had a 23.9% rate of rehospitalization within 30 days. This comprised 1.4% of all rehospitalizations of Medicare patients. The reason for rehospitalization was additional vascular surgery in 14.8% of patients, and amputation in 5.8% of patients. In comparison, 13.5% of patients undergoing cardiac stents were rehospitalized within 30 days, 15.6% of patients undergoing major bowel surgery were rehospitalized within 30 days, and 17.9% of those undergoing hip or femur surgeries were rehospitalized within 30 days. Overall rates of rehospitalization were region dependent, with the lowest rates of rehospitalization being in the Pacific Northwest and the Intermountain West, and the highest rates of rehospitalization were east of the Rocky Mountains (Fig 1 in the original article).

Rehospitalization is a huge problem. The data indicated that the risk of rehospitalization persists over time. Additional studies will be required to understand the relative contributions of inadequate discharge planning, insufficient outpatient and community care, and progression of illness as to their contribution to rates of rehospitalization. Vascular surgeons should note that, among the surgical groups analyzed, vascular surgery had the highest rates of rehospitalization. This has significant implications for the relationship between vascular surgeons and their hospital administrators, should there eventually be a financial penalty instituted for rehospitalization of surgical patients.

G. L. Moneta, MD

6 Grafts and Graft Complications

Aortic reconstruction with femoral-popliteal vein: Graft stenosis incidence, risk and reintervention

Beck AW, Murphy EH, Hocking JA, et al (Division of Vascular and Endovascular Surgery and the Univ of Texas-Southern Med Ctr, Dallas, TX)
J Vasc Surg 47:36-44, 2008

Background.—Management using femoral-popliteal vein (FPV) of aortic graft infections, failing aortofemoral bypass, and aortoiliac occlusive disease in young patients with a small aorta is now an accepted therapeutic method and is performed frequently at our institution. A high reintervention rate for FPV graft stenosis has recently been reported. The purpose of this study was to determine the incidence of FPV graft failure due to stenosis after neoaortoiliac system (NAIS) reconstruction, and to identify risk factors for this complication.

Methods.—A review was performed of 240 patients who underwent NAIS reconstruction at our institution between January 1991 and December 2005. All patients were entered into a prospective database and were evaluated for the incidence of vein graft stenosis requiring reintervention, risk factors for stenosis, and the rate and type of reintervention required to assist patency. Patients with occlusion were evaluated and reported, but excluded from detailed analysis. Risk factors assessed included gender, operative features, FPV size (diameter), smoking history, and medical comorbidities.

Results.—Of the 240 NAIS procedures performed during this time period, 11 (4.6%) patients have required 12 graft revisions (one patient required a second intervention) for stenosis using open and endovascular techniques. Over the same time period, graft occlusion occurred in nine patients (3.8%). This provided a primary patency at 2 and 5 years of 87% and 82%, and an assisted primary patency rate of 96% and 94%. Mean time to revision was 23.5 months (range 5.5 to 83.5 months). Median FPV graft size in the nonrevised patients was 7.8 mm (range 4.0 to 11.4 mm), and 6.4 mm (range 4.7 to 8.7 mm) in the revised group (P =.006). Survival analysis revealed small vein graft size (<7.2 mm), coronary artery disease (CAD), and extensive smoking history as independent predictors of time to stenosis (P =.002, .02, .01, respectively), with multivariable analysis confirming these results (P =.002, .06, .012). Patients

93

with CAD, combined with small graft size, were found to be at especially high risk for stenosis, with 8/36 (22.2%) requiring revision vs 3/184 (1.6%) of patients without both factors ($P < .0001$).

Conclusions.—FPV graft stenosis, requiring revision after NAIS reconstruction, is uncommon. Risk factors for stenosis include small graft size, history of CAD, and smoking. All patients merit aggressive counseling for smoking cessation, and patients exhibiting multiple risk factors should undergo close postoperative surveillance for graft stenosis.

▶ This is a very important article for all of us who, on occasion, use femoral-popliteal veins for aortic reconstructions. The series at Southwestern is now quite mature, and the incidence of problems encountered with these types of reconstructions are probably accurately represented by the current data. This is a valuable technique, but the incidence of late graft-related problems are somewhat higher than what has been previously suggested. The authors suggest that patients with multiple risk factors merit close postoperative surveillance for development of graft stenosis. However, I believe that virtually no vascular reconstruction is immortal, and if possible, all neoaortoiliac system procedures should be followed with periodic physical examination and duplex scanning.

G. L. Moneta, MD

Predictors for Outcome after Vacuum Assisted Closure Therapy of Peri-vascular Surgical Site Infections in the Groin

Svensson S, Monsen C, Kölbel T, et al (Malmö Univ Hosp, Sweden)
Eur J Vascular Endovasc Surg 36:84-89, 2008

Objectives.—To assess outcomes (wound healing, amputation and mortality) after vacuum assisted closure (VAC®) therapy of peri-vascular surgical site infections in the groin after arterial surgery.

Design.—Retrospective study.

Materials.—Thirty-three groins received VAC® therapy between August 2004 and December 2006 at Vascular Centre, Malmö University Hospital.

Methods.—Following surgical revision, VAC® therapy was applied in the groin at a continuous topical negative pressure of 125 mm Hg. The median follow up time was 16 months.

Results.—Median age was 75 years. Twenty-three (70%) cases underwent surgery for lower limb ischaemia. Intestinal flora was present in 88% of the wound cultures. Median duration of VAC® therapy was 20 days and 27 (82%) wounds healed within 55 days. One serious VAC® associated bleeding and three late false femoral artery aneurysms were reported. The median cost of VAC® treatment was 2.7% of the in-hospital costs. Synthetic vascular graft infection ($n = 21$) was associated with adverse infection-related events ($n = 9$; $p = 0.012$). Non-healing wounds were associated with amputation ($p = 0.005$) and death ($p < 0.001$).

Conclusions.—VAC® treated synthetic vascular graft infections in the groin were at a greater risk of developing infection-related complications. Non-healing surgical site infections after VAC® therapy were associated with amputation and death.

▶ With expanded use of vacuum assisted closure (VAC®) systems for perivascular surgical site wounds, overall healing rates as noted in this study were reasonable for these complex wounds. While all of these wounds were associated with an underlying perivascular structure after arterial exposure, not all wounds had underlying synthetic graft material. As expected, those wounds associated with synthetic graft material had higher nonhealing, complication, and limb loss rates. While perivascular wound healing and graft preservation is desirable, VAC® therapy alone in this complex subgroup may not be adequate as an isolated therapy and should not replace basic tenants of graft excision if underlying infected synthetic graft is present.

M. A. Passman, MD

7 Aortic Aneurysm

Abdominal Aortic Aneurysm Development in Men Following a "normal" Aortic Ultrasound Scan
Hafez H, Druce PS, Ashton HA (St Richard's Hosp, Chichester, West Sussex, UK)
Eur J Vasc Endovasc Surg 36:553-558, 2008

Objectives.—To determine predictors related to abdominal aortic aneurysm (AAA) development following a "normal" aortic ultrasound scan.

Design, materials & methods.—Over a 23-year period, 22 961 men participated in an AAA screening programme. Maximum aortic diameter of less than 30 mm was deemed "normal". 4308 of these "normal" individuals were later re-scanned at intervals for research purposes.

Results.—AAA prevalence was 4.4% at initial scanning. In those with a normal scan, 46 patients subsequently presented with AAAs incidentally detected and 120 (2.8%) had AAAs identified as part of the ongoing surveillance. The median initial aortic size of these 166 men was 25 mm (range 15–29 mm). Over the follow-up period, there have been 24 (14%) AAA-related deaths, 24 patients underwent successful AAA surgery and 36 died of unrelated causes. In those with an initial aortic diameter of <25 mm who later developed an AAA, the odds ratio for AAA-related mortality was 2 (95% CI 1–4.1, $p = 0.03$, x^2).

Conclusion.—AAAs can develop following an initial "normal" scan and men with an aortic diameters of 25–29 mm appear to be at greater risk. Surveillance for this sub-group may further reduce the incidence of undiagnosed AAA and AAA-related mortality.

▶ Clearly, normal now does not mean normal forever. Screening aortic studies generally use 30 mm as the upper limits of normal for the diameter of the infrarenal aorta. About 3% of men with an initial normal abdominal aortic ultrasound screening study, will eventually develop an abdominal aortic aneurysm (AAA) after about a median of 5 years. The authors noted that the mean aortic diameter of those later developing an AAA following an initial normal scan was about 25 mm. Overall, men with an initial "normal" aortic diameter of 25 to 29 mm appeared to be at increased risk of developing an AAA later in life compared with those whose aorta measured < 25 mm in diameter. (Sixty-five percent of the men who went on to develop an AAA after a normal scan had had an aortic diameter between 25-29 mm on their initial screening examination.) It seems reasonable to offer repeat screening of the abdominal aorta after 5 years if the initial screening examination demonstrated the abdominal aorta to have a diameter of 25 to 29 mm. We will have to ask the United States Preventative Services Task Force if this is medically cost-effective.

G. L. Moneta, MD

Growth predictors and prognosis of small abdominal aortic aneurysms
Schlösser FJV, Tangelder MJD, Verhagen HJM, et al (Univ Med Ctr Utrecht; Erasmus Univ Med Ctr, Rotterdam; et al)
J Vasc Surg 47:1127-1133, 2008

Objective.—Evidence regarding the influence of cardiovascular risk factors, comorbidities, and patient characteristics on the growth of small abdominal aortic aneurysms (AAA) is limited. We assessed, in an observational cohort study, rupture rates, risks of mortality, and the effects of cardiovascular risk factors and patient demographics on growth rates of small AAAs.

Methods.—Between September 1996 and January 2005, 5057 patients with manifest arterial vascular disease or cardiovascular risk factors were included in the Second Manifestation of ARTerial disease (SMART) study. Measurements of the abdominal aortic diameter were performed in all patients. All patients with an initial AAA diameter between 30 and 55 mm were selected for this study. All AAA measurements during follow-up until August 2007 were collected. Multivariate regression analysis was performed to calculate the effects of demographic patient characteristics, initial AAA diameter, and cardiovascular risk factors on AAA growth.

Results.—Included were 230 patients, with a mean age of 66 years and 90% were male. Seven AAA ruptures (six fatal) occurred in 755 patient years of follow-up (rupture rate 0.9% per patient-year). In 147 patients, AAA measurements were performed for a period of more than 6 months. The median follow-up time was 3.3 years (mean 4.0, range 0.5 to 11.1 years, standard deviation (SD) 2.5). Mean AAA diameter was 38.8 mm (SD 6.8) and mean expansion rate 2.5 mm/y. Patients using lipid-lowering drugs had a 1.2 mm/y (95% confidence interval [CI] −2.34 to −0.060 mm/y) lower AAA growth rate compared to nonusers of these drugs. Initial AAA diameter was associated with a 0.09 mm/y (95% CI 0.01 to 0.18 mm/y) higher growth rate per millimetre increase of the diameter. No other factors, including blood lipid values, were independently associated with AAA growth.

Conclusions.—Lipid-lowering drug treatment and initial AAA diameter appear to be independently associated with lower AAA growth rates. The risk of rupture of these small abdominal aortic aneurysms was low, which pleads for watchful waiting.

▶ What have we learned from this article? Higher initial abdominal aortic aneurysms (AAA) diameter appears to be associated with higher AAA expansion rates. I think we already knew that. The rupture rate of the small abdominal aortic aneurysms is low: 0.9% per patient year. We knew that as well. We also can note that an aneurysm less than 5 cm in diameter can rupture, but it is pretty rare and it is very unlikely anyone's operative results, no matter how good they think they are, can beat the natural history of AAAs < 5 cm in diameter. The most intriguing thing here is the apparent beneficial effects of statin medications in lowering expansion rates of AAAs. This is at least the third study with this finding. (Two others are by Sukhija et al[1] and Schouten et al.[2]) How statins do this is unclear, but they have clear anti-inflammatory effects and decreased levels of particular matrix metalloproteinases (MMPs) are implicated in AAA expansion and rupture. The purist will call for a randomized trial, but the evidence is so strong that people with vascular disease benefit from statins, that a randomized trial is unlikely. Bottom line: patients with AAA should be on a statin medication if possible.

G. L. Moneta, MD

References

1. Sukhija R, Aronow WS, Sandhu R, Kakar P, Babu S. Mortality and size of abdominal aortic aneurysm at long-term follow-up of patients not treated surgically and treated with and without statins. *Am J Cardiol.* 2006;97:279-280.
2. Schouten O, van Laanen JH, Boersma E, et al. Statins are associated with a reduced infrarenal abdominal aortic aneurysm growth. *Eur J Vasc Endovasc Surg.* 2006; 32:21-26.

Analysis of Expansion Patterns in 4-4.9 cm Abdominal Aortic Aneurysms
Vega de Céniga M, Gómez R, Estallo L, et al (Hosp de Galdakao-Usansolo, Barrio Labeaga S/N, spain)
Ann Vasc Surg 22:37-44, 2008

Our objective was to analyze the growth pattern of 4-4.9 cm infrarenal abdominal aortic aneurysms (AAAs). We used an observational, longitudinal, prospective study design. We followed 4-4.9 cm AAAs with 6-monthly abdominal computed tomographic (CT) scans (January 1988-August 2004). AAA growth was defined as an increase in aortic diameter ≥2 mm in each surveillance period. We established the aortic expansion pattern in AAA with three or more CT scans as continuous or discontinuous. The latter includes at least one period of nongrowth (<2 mm/6 months). We studied the influence of cardiovascular risk factors (CVRFs), comorbidity, and AAA anatomical characteristics using the chi-squared test, t-test, life tables, and Kaplan-Meier for statistical analysis. We included 195 patients: 183 (93.8%) men, age 71 ± 8.3 years (50-90). The follow-up period was 50 ± 36.4 months (6.5-193.7). The growth pattern ($n = 131$) was continuous in 15 (11.5%) and discontinuous in 116 (88.5%) AAA. The mean expansion rate was higher in AAAs with continuous expansion (7.92 ± 3.74 vs. 2.74 ± 2.94 mm/year, $p < 0.0001$). No CVRFs or comorbidity influenced the expansion pattern ($p > 0.05$). The eccentric thrombus was associated with a greater incidence of

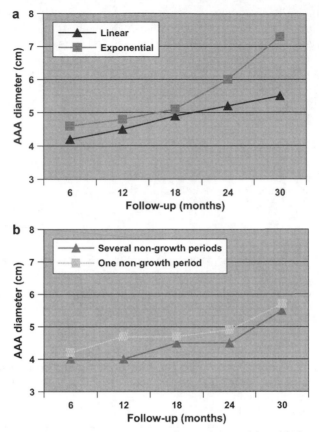

FIGURE 1.—AAA expansion patterns: (a) continuous—linear and exponential—and (b) discontinuous —one or several nongrowth periods. (Reprinted from Vega de Céniga M, Gómez R, Estallo L, et al. Analysis of expansion patterns in 4-4.9 cm abdominal aortic aneurysms. *Ann Vasc Surg.* 2008;22:37-44).

continuous growth ($p = 0.05$), with no influence of aortic calcification ($p > 0.1$). The expansion of 4-4.9 cm AAA is mostly irregular and unpredictable. We have not found any modifiable risk factors which influence their growth pattern. The eccentric distribution of the thrombus is associated with continuous expansion (Fig 1).

▶ This study confirms what most of us have observed: aneurysms expand unpredictably, thereby making continuous and regular follow-up required (Fig 1). These were relatively small aneurysms, and in my experience small aneurysms are the ones most likely to exhibit an irregular growth pattern, with larger aneurysms expanding more steadily and rapidly. It was, however, a bit surprising that the percentage of small aneurysms exhibiting an irregular growth pattern was so high (85%). With that exception, the data do not tell us anything terribly surprising or new. The data do, however, provide justification for regular follow-up of abdominal aortic aneurysms (AAAs), no matter what their previous growth pattern has been.

G. L. Moneta, MD

Abdominal aortic aneurysm events in the women's health initiative: cohort study
Lederle FA, Larson JC, Margolis KL, et al (VA Med Ctr, MN; Fred Hutchinson Cancer Research Ctr, Seattle, WA; Health Partners Research Foundation, MN; et al)
BMJ 337:a1724, 2008

Objective.—To assess the association between potential risk factors and subsequent clinically important abdominal aortic aneurysm events (repairs and ruptures) in women.

Design.—Large prospective observational cohort study with mean follow-up of 7.8 years.

Setting.—40 clinical centres across the United States.

Participants.—161 808 postmenopausal women aged 50-79 enrolled in the women's health initiative.

Main Outcome Measures.—Association of self reported or measured baseline variables with confirmed abdominal aortic aneurysm events assessed with multiple logistic regression.

Results.—Events occurred in 184 women and were strongly associated with age and smoking. Ever smoking, current smoking, and amount smoked all contributed independent risk. Diabetes showed a negative association (odds ratio 0.29, 95% confidence interval 0.13, 0.68), as did postmenopausal hormone therapy. Positive associations were also seen for height, hypertension, cholesterol lowering treatment, and coronary and peripheral artery disease.

Conclusions.—Our findings confirm the strong positive associations of clinically important abdominal aortic aneurysm with age and smoking in women and the negative association with diabetes previously reported in men.

▶ Aortic aneurysms are more common in men but may be more deadly in women. The Women's Health Initiative (WHI) involved clinical investigation of strategies of prevention of common diseases in 161 808 women. The authors used this data to assess for associations between potential risk factors for abdominal aortic aneurysm (AAA) and subsequently clinically important AAA events, rupture, and repair in postmenopausal women.

Although the incidence of AAA is significantly lower in women than in men, most risk factors for AAA and negative associations appear to be the same for men and women. The fact the authors also found a negative association between AAA in women and postmenopausal hormone therapy suggests that estrogen may have a favorable effect in reducing the development of aortic aneurysm in women. However, other studies found increased aneurysmal disease in patients treated with hormonal therapy. It therefore remains unclear why prevalence of AAA differs so much by sex. One may postulate a thus-far unknown gender-associated biologic explanation. There may also be unknown confounders of lifestyle in the WHI data. It does appear, however, that the negative association between AAA and diabetes is solid for both males and females.

G. L. Moneta, MD

Fit patients with small abdominal aortic aneurysms (AAAs) do not benefit from early intervention

Brown LC, Thompson SG, Greenhalgh RM, et al (Imperial College, London, UK; Med Res Council Biostatistics Unit, Cambridge, UK)
J Vasc Surg 48:1375-1381, 2008

Objectives.—The UK Small Aneurysm Trial (UKSAT) and the American Aneurysm Detection and Management (ADAM) trial both concluded that early elective open surgery does not confer any late survival advantage in patients with small abdominal aortic aneurysm (AAA) with diameter 4.0 to 5.5 cm. However, two trials of endovascular aneurysm repair in small AAA have started based upon speculation that a sub-group of particularly fit patients, with low operative mortality, may benefit from early intervention. Here we investigate whether the fittest patients from the UKSAT might have benefited from early intervention.

Methods.—A total of 1090 patients randomized into the UKSAT between 1991 and 1995 were followed for an average of 12 years for mortality. Baseline data were used to calculate the Customized Probability Index (CPI), a validated prognostic risk score for operative mortality after elective open aneurysm repair that assigns risk points for history of cardiac, pulmonary, and renal disease and subtracts risk points for use of statins and beta-blockers. Cox regression was used to assess any differences in all-cause or aneurysm-related mortality between policies of early surgery or surveillance across the fitness spectrum. Tests for interaction used CPI scores as a continuous variable but patients also were stratified into tertile groups for descriptive purposes. Hazard ratios were adjusted for age, gender, and aneurysm diameter.

Results.—A total of 714 deaths (95 aneurysm-related) occurred in 8485 person-years (number of patients multiplied by average years of conditional follow-up). The mean (standard deviation [SD]) CPI score was 8.1 (9.9) with similar scores between randomized groups. The tertile groups had mean (SD) scores of -1.8 (3.7) for the 389 fittest patients, 8.8 (3.3) for the 438 moderately fit, 21.4 (6.6) for the 261 least fit with missing scores in 2 patients. The tests for interaction were non-significant for both all-cause $(P=.176)$ and aneurysm-related mortality (.178). However, for the least fit patients a survival advantage was seen in the early surgery group; adjusted hazard ratios 0.73 (95% confidence interval

[CI] 0.56-0.96) and 0.46 (95% CI 0.22-0.98) for all-cause and aneurysm-related mortality respectively.

Conclusion.—Early elective surgery did not confer any survival benefit in the fittest patients. On the contrary, the possibility of a survival benefit from early intervention in patients of poor fitness merits further investigation through meta-analysis or validation in other prospective studies.

▶ It was not surprising to me that the authors found that early elective surgery does not confer survival benefit in patients with small abdominal aortic aneurysms (AAAs) when treated with open operation. The rupture rates of small AAAs are simply too low, as demonstrated by the UK Small Aneurysm Trial and the American Aneurysm Detection and Management Trial, for there to be any potential benefit for open treatment of small AAAs in fit patients. It is unclear, however, whether similar logic would apply to endovascular repair of small AAAs. We know, however, patients with small AAAs who are eligible for endovascular repair, and who are observed until the aneurysm reaches conventional size for repair, do not lose anatomic eligibility for endovascular treatment.

There are currently 2 ongoing trials, which I suspect are largely influenced by industry to expand the market, and to test the hypothesis that treatment of small AAAs in fit patients may be beneficial. I don't know what the results of these trials will be, but my suspicion is that it will be very difficult to prove benefit for endovascular treatment of small AAAs, even in fit patients. We will need to wait and see the data.

A somewhat surprising result of this article was that the least fit patients, perhaps, may benefit from early treatment of AAA. We should be very careful about potentially accepting this data as justification for treatment of small AAAs in poorly fit patients. The UK Small Aneurysm Trial was not designed to specifically address this question, and it may be that their customized probability index that forms the basis of this trial is providing erroneous results that would not be compatible with other methods of assessing prognosis and risk. I am not ready to adopt a policy that fitness, rather than aneurysm diameter, should be the primary variable of deciding when to repair an AAA, whether it be open or with an endovascular technique.

G. L. Moneta, MD

Peak wall stress measurement in elective and acute abdominal aortic aneurysms

Heng MS, Fagan MJ, Collier JW, et al (Hull Royal Infirmary; Univ of Hull)
J Vasc Surg 47:17-22, 2008

Background.—Abdominal aortic aneurysm (AAA) rupture occurs when wall stress exceeds wall strength. Engineering principles suggest that aneurysm diameter is only one aspect of its geometry that influences wall stress. Finite element analysis considers the complete geometry and determines

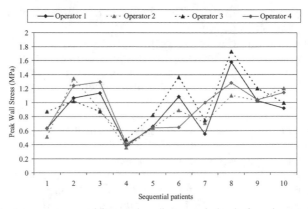

FIGURE 1.—Interoperator variability: peak wall stress calculated after edge extraction by four different operators on 10 separate aneurysms. (Reprinted from Heng MS, Fagan MJ, Collier JW, et al. Peak wall stress measurement in elective and acute abdominal aortic aneurysms. *J Vasc Surg.* 2008;47:17-22, with permission from the Society for Vascular Surgery.)

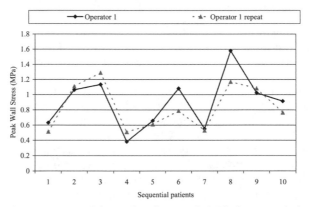

FIGURE 2.—Intraoperator variability: peak wall stress calculated after repeated edge extraction by one operator on 10 separate aneurysms. (Reprinted from Heng MS, Fagan MJ, Collier JW, et al. Peak wall stress measurement in elective and acute abdominal aortic aneurysms. *J Vasc Surg.* 2008;47:17-22, with permission from the Society for Vascular Surgery.)

wall stresses throughout the structure. This article investigates the interoperator and intraoperator reliability of finite element analysis in the calculation of peak wall stress (PWS) in AAA and examines the variation in PWS in elective and acute AAAs.

Method.—Full ethics and institutional approval was obtained. The study recruited 70 patients (30 acute, 40 elective) with an infrarenal AAA. Computed tomography (CT) images were obtained of the AAA from the renal vessels to the aortic bifurcation. Manual edge extraction, three-dimensional reconstruction, and blinded finite element analysis were performed to ascertain location and value of PWS. Ten CT data sets were analyzed by four different operators to ascertain interoperator reliability and by one operator twice to ascertain intraoperator reliability. An intraclass correlation coefficient was obtained. The Mann-Whitney U test and independent samples t test compared groups for statistical significance.

Results.—The intraclass correlation coefficient was 0.71 for interoperator reliability and 0.84 for intraoperator reliability. There was no statistically significant difference in the mean (SD) maximal AAA diameter between elective (6.47 [1.30] cm) and acute (7.08 [1.39] cm) patients ($P = .073$). The difference in PWS between elective (0.67 [0.30] MPa) and acute (1.11 [0.51] MPa) patients ($P = .008$) was statistically significant, however.

Conclusion.—Interoperator and intraoperator reliability in the derivation of PWS is acceptable. PWS, but not maximal diameter, was significantly higher in acute AAAs than in elective AAAs (Figs 1 and 2).

▶ This landmark article demonstrates that measured peak wall stress in infrarenal aortic aneurysms of acutely symptomatic patients is significantly different from the peak wall stress measured in elective asymptomatic patients. These differences were present, even though there were no significant differences in the diameter of aneurysms between these groups. While this data is quite provocative and of clinical significance, the mean size of the aneurysm in both the acutely symptomatic (7.04 cm) and the asymptomatic (6.47 cm) patients were substantially larger than the size where many clinicians would consider elective repair in good risk patients. The authors are to be congratulated because they considered very important variables such as inter- and intraoperator variability (Figs 1 and 2) in the assessment of how peak wall stress is measured. The variability is well within acceptable clinical tolerances. It is clear that this is an important issue because manual input of the external wall dimension is required. Determination of the external wall of the aneurysm may be quite difficult for the most experienced clinicians. The authors indicate that wall stress calculations are done manually, which is obviously time consuming, but do not provide any indication on how long this might be.

M. T. Watkins, MD

The Rupture Rate of Large Abdominal Aortic Aneurysms: Is This Modified by Anatomical Suitability for Endovascular Repair?
Powell JT, Brown LC, Greenhalgh RM, et al (Imperial College at Charing Cross, London, UK)
Ann Surg 247:173-179, 2008

Background.—There are no precise estimates of the rate of rupture of large abdominal aortic aneurysms (AAA). There is recent suspicion that anatomic suitability for endovascular repair may be associated with a decreased risk of AAA rupture.

Methods.—Systematic literature review of rupture rates of AAA with initial diameter ≥ 5 cm in patients not considered for open repair, with stratification by size (<6.0 cm and 6.0+ cm), and gender, combined using random-effects meta-analysis. Proportional hazards regression to analyze factors (including gender, diabetes, initial AAA diameter, aneurysm neck, and sac lengths) associated with rupture in patients anatomically suitable for endovascular repair (EVAR 2 trial).

Results.—Previous studies (2 prospective, 2 retrospective, and 1 mixed) were identified for meta-analysis and patients with elective repair excluded. The pooled rupture rates was 18.2 [95% confidence interval (CI) 13.7–24.1] per 100 person-years. There was a 2.5-fold increase in rupture rates for patients with AAA of 6.0+ cm versus <6.0 cm, rupture rates = 2.54 (95% CI 1.69–3.85). The pooled rupture rates were nonsignificantly higher in women than men, rupture rates = 1.21 (95% CI 0.77–1.90). For EVAR 2 patients with 6+ cm aneurysms, the rupture rates were 17.4 [95% CI 12.9–23.4] per 100 person-years significantly lower than the pooled rate from the meta-analysis, rupture rates = 27.0 [95% CI 21.1–34.7] per 100 person-years, $P = 0.026$. Patients with shorter neck lengths appeared to have higher rupture rates than those with longer necks, but this was of borderline significance $P = 0.10$.

Conclusions.—Rupture rates of large AAAs reported in different studies are highly variable. There is emerging evidence that patients anatomically suitable for endovascular repair have lower rupture rates.

▶ This is probably as good of an estimate as any for rupture rates of large abdominal aortic aneurysms. The data, indicating reasonably high rupture rates for abdominal aortic aneurysms (AAAs) > 6 cm, makes sense and is not unexpected. There are, however, some interesting points here. Rupture rates for men and women were not significantly different. This is a bit of a surprising find, given the current perception that aneurysms of equal diameters have a greater tendency to rupture in women compared with men. Perhaps the effects of sex differences are overwhelmed by aneurysm diameter, as the AAA grows larger in diameter. Short-necked aneurysms appear to rupture a bit more often than longer-necked aneurysms, suggesting that part of the improved natural history for aneurysm rupture in endovascular aneurysm repair (EVAR) patients may be because of the physical characteristics of AAAs that are suitable for EVAR. This article and other articles similar to it suggest a relative protective effect of diabetes on AAA rupture. The underlying biochemistry for this is unclear. Finally, a post hoc analysis, not mentioned in the abstract, suggests that statins may also greatly decrease the risk of AAA rupture. This last point, in particular, deserves greater investigation.

G. L. Moneta, MD

Anatomic Suitability of Ruptured Abdominal Aortic Aneurysms for Endovascular Repair

Slater BJ, Harris EJ, Lee JT (Stanford Univ Med Center, CA)
Ann Vasc Surg 22:716-722, 2008

Mortality from ruptured abdominal aortic aneurysms (rAAAs) remains high despite improvements in anesthesia, postoperative intensive care, and surgical techniques. Recent small series and single-center experiences suggest that endovascular aneurysm repair (EVAR) for rAAAs is feasible and may improve short-term survival. However, the applicability of EVAR to all cases of rAAA is unknown. The purpose of this study was to investigate the anatomical suitability of ruptured aneurysms for EVAR as determined by preoperative cross-sectional imaging. A contemporary consecutive series of rAAAs presenting to a tertiary academic center was retrospectively reviewed. Preoperative radiographic imaging was reviewed and assessed for endovascular compatibility based on currently available EVAR devices. Patients with aneurysm morphology demonstrating neck diameter >32 mm, neck length <10 mm, neck angulation >60 degrees, severe iliac tortuosity, or external iliac diameter <6 mm were deemed noncandidates for EVAR. Forty-seven rAAAs were treated over a 10-year period, with 47% of patients presenting with free rupture and 60% of patients transferred from outside hospitals. Five (11%) patients were treated with EVAR, all over the past 2 years, while the remaining 42 patients underwent open repair. Preoperative imaging was available for review in 43 (91%) patients, and morphological measurements indicated that 49% would have been candidates for EVAR with currently available devices. Criteria precluding EVAR in this cohort were inadequate neck length in 73%, unsuitable iliac access in 23%, large neck diameter in 18%, and severe neck angulation in 14%. Overall 30-day mortality was 34%, and 1-year mortality was 42%. Candidates for EVAR were more likely than non-EVAR candidates to be male (95% vs. 68%, $p = 0.046$) and to have smaller sac diameters (7.0 vs. 8.5 cm, $p = 0.02$) and longer neck lengths (24.1 vs. 8.6 mm, $p < 0.0001$); less likely to have a >60 degree angulated neck (10% vs. 45%, $p = 0.0002$), larger external iliac diameter (8.9 vs. 7.3 mm, $p = 0.015$), and less blood loss during surgical repair (2.4 vs. 6.0 L, $p = 0.02$); and more likely to be discharged home (71% vs. 25%, $p = 0.05$). There were no differences in 30-day, 1-year, or overall mortality between candidates for EVAR and noncandidates. Only 49% of patients with rAAAs in this consecutive series were found to be candidates for EVAR with conventional stent-graft devices. Differences in demographics, aneurysm morphology, and outcomes between candidates and noncandidates undergoing open repair suggest that differential risks apply to ruptured aneurysm patients. Protocols and future reports of EVAR for rAAAs should be tailored to these results. Device and technique modifications are necessary to increase the applicability of EVAR for rAAAs.

▶ Open surgical repair is the traditional strategy to treat patients with ruptured abdominal aortic aneurysms (rAAAs). Mortality rate is approximately 50%. There is now considerable enthusiasm for endovascular repair of rAAAs. A small case series suggests that endovascular aneurysm repair (EVAR) is feasible for rAAAs and may be associated with improved short-term morbidity and mortality compared with open repair. There has, however, been only 1 randomized controlled study comparing open versus endovascular repair of rAAAs. This study showed no difference in outcome. A previous report has also noted anatomic eligibility of EVAR in patients presenting with ruptured/symptomatic AAAs, which is less frequent than for patients with asymptomatic AAAs. This is primarily because of proximal neck anatomy. This study corroborates this previous report. It must be remembered that this is a retrospective report and based on current criteria for endovascular techniques. It is likely that some patients treated earlier in this series would not have been eligible for EVAR at the time of their presentation. Nevertheless, it is unlikely that the anatomy of ruptured aneurysms is changing much over time. The results here, using a retrospective analysis of cases up to 10 years ago, would still seem to be relatively applicable to the anatomy of patients currently with rAAAs. There are also many additional requirements that must be in place for EVAR to be a viable alternative to open repair for patients with rAAAs. Such factors include available surgical expertise, available nursing expertise, and of course, available devices at all times in the operating room. It seems unlikely, unless an institution has large exposure to patients with rAAAs, that all of these things would come together with sufficient frequency that EVAR repair of rAAAs will exceed open repair of rAAAs in the near future.

G. L. Moneta, MD

National trends in the repair of ruptured abdominal aortic aneurysms
Mureebe L, Egorova N, Giacovelli JK, et al (Weill Med College of Cornell Univ, NY; Columbia Univ College of Physicians and Surgeons, NY)
J Vasc Surg 48:1101-1107, 2008

Objective.—This study evaluated trends in hospitalizations, treatment, and mortality of ruptured abdominal aortic aneurysms (rAAAs) in the United States Medicare population.

Methods.—The Medicare inpatient database (1995 through 2006) was reviewed for patients with rAAA and AAA by using International Classification of Disease (9th Clinical Modification) codes for rAAA and AAA. Proportions and trends were analyzed by χ^2 analysis, continuous variables by t test, and trends by the Cochran-Armitage test.

Results.—During the study period, hospitalizations with the diagnoses of rAAA declined from 23.2 to 12.8 per 100,000 Medicare beneficiaries

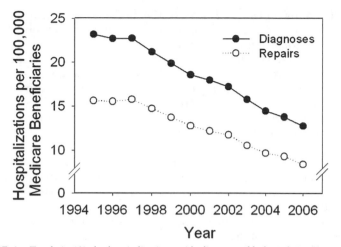

FIGURE 1.—Trends in (A) the hospitalizations with diagnoses *(black circles)* and repairs *(white circles)* of ruptured abdominal aortic aneurysms *(rAAA)*. (Reprinted from Mureebe L, Egorova N, Giacovelli JK, et al. National trends in the repair of ruptured abdominal aortic aneurysms. *J Vasc Surg.* 2008;48:1101-1107, with permission from The Society for Vascular Surgery.)

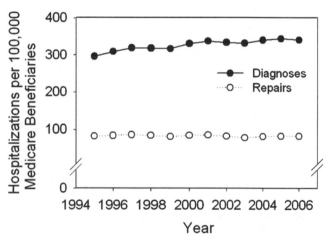

FIGURE 2.—Trend in (A) the hospitalizations with diagnoses *(black circles)* and repairs *(white circles)* of intact abdominal aortic aneurysms *(iAAA)*. (Reprinted from Mureebe L, Egorova N, Giacovelli JK, et al. National trends in the repair of ruptured abdominal aortic aneurysms. *J Vasc Surg.* 2008;48:1101-1107, with permission from The Society for Vascular Surgery.)

($P < .0001$), as did repairs of rAAA (15.6 to 8.4 per 100,000; $P < .0001$). No change was observed in AAA elective repairs. The 30-day mortality rate after open repair of rAAA decreased by 4.9% (from 39.6% to 34.7%; $P = .0007$ for trend) for the age group 65 to 74 and by 2.4% (from 52.9% to 50.5%, $P = .0008$) for the age group ≥75. Perioperative mortality after endovascular repair diminished by 13.6% (from 43.5% in 2001 to 29.9% in 2006; $P = .0020$). Mortality among women was higher than among men (51.1% vs 40.0% in 2006). The demographics of patients treated for rAAA changed to include a greater proportion of women and patients aged ≥75 years.

Conclusion.—A significant decrease has occurred in the number of patients who have a diagnosis of rAAA and undergo treatment, but there has been no change in repairs of AAA. The perioperative mortality rate has improved due to the introduction of endovascular repair and a small but progressive improvement in survival after open repair for patients aged 65 to 74 years (Figs 1A and 2A).

▶ The article indicates that there has been a decrease in the number of patients with the diagnosis of ruptured abdominal aortic aneurysms who undergo treatment, but no significant change in the rate of abdominal aortic aneurysm repair overall (Figs 1A and 2A). The lack of change in overall aneurysm repair is likely related to 2 conflicting factors. First of all, while increasing numbers of aneurysms are discovered through the widespread use of imaging studies, the threshold for aneurysm repair has risen to 5.5 cm based on the results of the VA ADAM study and the British Small Aneurysm Trial.[1,2] Ruptured aneurysm is a very frequently fatal disease, with overall mortality probably 90%, with only 50% of hospitalized patients surviving. Why repairs for ruptured aneurysm are decreasing is unknown. It may be that families and patients are declining repair given the poor prognosis. More likely, however, it is the increase in repair of larger aneurysms facilitated by imaging studies that serves as the explanation. Although the total number of AAA repairs has remained the same, those AAAs that are, in fact, repaired were the ones more likely to rupture, and therefore the incidence of ruptured AAA has decreased. This, overall, is a good thing, and indicates how well-conducted trials and the dissemination of technology can combine to provide better patient outcomes.

G. L. Moneta, MD

References

1. Lederle FA, Wilson SE, Johnson GR, et al. Immediate repair compare with surveillance of small abdominal aortic aneurysms. N Engl J Med. 2002;346:1437-1444.
2. Mortality results for randomised controlled trial of early elective surgery or ultrasonographic surveillance for small abdominal aortic aneurysms. The UK Small Aneurysm Trial Participants. *Lancet.* 1998;352:1649-1655.

Common iliac artery aneurysm: Expansion rate and results of open surgical and endovascular repair
Huang Y, Gloviczki P, Duncan AA, et al (Gonda Vascular Ctr, Mayo Clinic, Rochester, MN)
J Vasc Surg 47:1203-1211, 2008

Objectives.—To assess expansion rate of common iliac artery aneurysms (CIAAs) and define outcomes after open repair (OR) and endovascular repair (EVAR).

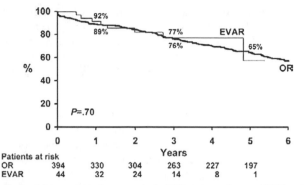

FIGURE 2.—Kaplan-Meier analysis shows survival of 438 patients after open (OR) and endovascular (EVAR) repair of common iliac artery aneurysms. The *dotted line* indicates standard error > 10%. (Reprinted from Huang Y, Gloviczki P, Duncan AA, et al. Common iliac artery aneurysm: expansion rate and results of open surgical and endovascular repair. *J Vasc Surg.* 2008;47:1203-1211. Copyright 2008, with permission from The Society for Vascular Surgery.)

Methods.—Clinical data of 438 patients with 715 CIAAs treated between 1986 and 2005 were retrospectively reviewed. Size, presentations, treatments, and outcomes were recorded. Kaplan-Meier method with log-rank tests and χ^2 test were used for analysis.

Results.—Interventions for 715 CIAAs (median, 4 cm; range, 2-13 cm) were done in 512 men (94%) and 26 women (6%); 152 (35%) had unilateral and 286 (65%) had bilateral CIAAs. Group 1 comprised 377 patients (633 CIAAs) with current or previously repaired abdominal aortic aneurysm (AAA). Group 2 comprised 15 patients (24 CIAAs) with associated internal iliac artery aneurysm (IIAA). Group 3 comprised 46 patients (58 isolated CIAAs). Median expansion rate of 104 CIAAs with at least two imaging studies was 0.29 cm/y; hypertension predicted faster expansion (0.32 vs 0.14 cm/y, $P =.01$). A total of 175 patients (29%) were symptomatic. The CIAA ruptured in 22 patients (5%, median, 6 cm; range, 3.8-8.5 cm), and the associated AAA ruptured in 20 (4%). Six (27%) ilioiliac or iliocaval fistulas developed. Repairs were elective in 396 patients (90%) and emergencies in 42 (10%). OR was performed in 394 patients (90%) and EVAR in 44 (10%). The groups had similar 30-day mortality: 1% for elective, 27% for emergency repairs ($P < .001$); 4% after OR (elective, 1%; emergency, 26%), and 0% after EVAR. No deaths occurred after OR of arteriovenous fistula. Complications were more frequent and hospitalization was longer after OR than EVAR ($P < .05$). Mean follow-up was 3.7 years (range, 1 month-17.5 years). The groups had similar 5-year primary (95%) and secondary patency rates (99.6%). At 3 years, secondary patency was 99.6% for OR and 100% for EVAR ($P =.66$); freedom from reintervention was similar after OR and EVAR (83% vs 69%, $P =.17$), as were survival rates (76% vs 77%, $P =.70$).

Conclusions.—The expansion rate of CIAAs is 0.29 cm/y, and hypertension predicts faster expansion. Because no rupture of a CIAA <3.8 cm was observed, elective repair of asymptomatic patients with CIAA ≥3.5 cm seems justified. Although buttock claudication after EVAR remains a concern, results at 3 years support EVAR as a first-line treatment for most anatomically suitable patients who require CIAA repair. Patients with compressive symptoms, or those with AVF, should preferentially be treated with OR (Fig 2).

▶ The most useful bit of information in this study is the expansion rate of iliac artery aneurysms—0.29 cm/year. That, along with the fact no iliac aneurysm under 3.8 cm in diameter ruptured, provides some guidance for when to intervene. The results, generally, fit my biases for common iliac aneurysms, in that I generally wait until they are about 4 cm in diameter before recommending repair. Endovascular repair (EVAR) appears very effective in properly selected patients, but open repair (OR) is also very effective with only a 1% mortality rate for elective open repair. So, it appears common iliac aneurysms can be observed until they are about 3.5 to 4 cm in diameter and then repaired with either open or endovascular techniques. There is no need to "push the indications" for EVAR, as OR has very low perioperative mortality and similar patency and long-term survival (Fig 2) as EVAR.

G. L. Moneta, MD

Natural history of common iliac arteries after aorto-aortic graft insertion during elective open abdominal aortic aneurysm repair: A prospective study
Ballotta E, Da Giau G, Gruppo M, et al (Univ of Padua, Padova, Italy)
Surgery 144:822-826, 2008

Background.—This study aimed to determine the natural history of common iliac arteries (CIAs) after elective open infrarenal abdominal aortic aneurysm (AAA) repair with an aorto-aortic prosthetic graft.

Methods.—All patients who had a straight tube graft inserted during elective AAA repair at our institution between 1995 and 2005 were prospectively followed up with preoperative and postoperative computed tomography (CT) scans to monitor changes in CIA diameter; their latest CT scan was performed in 2007. Based on preoperative CIA diameter, patients were divided into groups A (both CIAs normal, up to 12 mm in diameter), B (at least 1 ectatic CIA, 13–18 mm), and C (at least 1 aneurysmal CIA, 19–25 mm). The mean follow-up was 7.1 years (range, 2.1–12.3 years).

Results.—Among 201 patients eligible for the study, 92 patients (45.8%) were in group A, 63 patients (31.3%) were in group B, and 46 patients (22.9%) were in group C. Overall, the diameter increased in 119 CIAs (29.6%) by a mean of 1.1, 1.8, and 2.4 mm in groups A, B, and C, respectively. In all, 14 CIAs (5.4%) progressed from "normal" to "ectatic," and 9 CIAs (10.2%) progressed from "ectatic" to "aneurysmal."

Three aneurysmal CIAs slightly exceeded the 25-mm threshold, but none of these were repaired. No patients showed a progression or development of occlusive iliac artery disease or required repeat operation because of excessive CIA enlargement.

Conclusions.—This analysis showed that most CIAs do not expand after tube graft insertion during AAA repair, and when they do, the degree of dilation is minimal. Tube graft insertion during AAA repair is justified even for ectatic or moderately aneurysmal CIAs, and the procedure is safe and durable. The skepticism surrounding its selective use instead of a systematic bifurcated graft placement seems to be unwarranted.

▶ During an open abdominal aortic aneurysm (AAA) repair, when the common iliac arteries seem ectatic or mildly aneurismal, the surgeon must decide whether bifurcated prosthetic graft should be used. The concern arises over the possibility of progression of the iliac aneurysmal disease and late development of iliac aneurysms below the aortic tube graft. Tube graft repair has significant advantages over bi-iliac repair except, of course, when the aortic bifurcation is highly calcified. It seems tube graft repair should have a higher likelihood of preserving antegrade flow in the iliac vessels. It may be associated with lower risk of venous and ureter injury and perhaps decreased risk of postoperative erectile dysfunction. There are no criteria as to whether to place an aortic tube graft or a bifurcated graft during open AAA repair.

This is an old issue that is reasonable to revisit in the endovascular era. Obviously, the study is irrelevant to patients undergoing endovascular AAA repair, as bifurcated grafts are routinely placed with this technique. However, patients requiring open operation currently generally do so because of difficulty with the proximal neck. Such operations often require suprarenal clamping and more extensive dissection than a routine infrarenal open aneurysm operation. Because a bifurcated aortic graft adds additional time to the procedure, it would be nice to know which patients who require an open AAA repair can truly be treated with an aortic tube graft. This will help to lower the complexity of what is likely to be a more complicated open operation in the endovascular era. It appears that with reasonably long follow-up, no patient with a common iliac artery less than 25 mm in diameter will require repeat procedure for subsequent aneurysm dilatation of the iliac artery below an aortic tube graft. Indeed, most common iliac arteries do not expand after tube graft insertion during AAA repair and when they do, dilatation appears to be minimal. Overall, when used appropriately, an open AAA repair using aortic tube graft is a good operation.

G. L. Moneta, MD

Endovascular treatment of thoracoabdominal aortic aneurysms

Chuter TAM, Rapp JH, Hiramoto JS, et al (Univ of California, San Francisco)
J Vasc Surg 47:6-16, 2008

Objective.—This study assessed the role of multibranched stent grafts for thoracoabdominal aortic aneurysm (TAAA) repair.

Methods.—Self-expanding covered stents were used to connect the caudally directed cuffs of an aortic stent graft with the visceral branches of a TAAA in 22 patients (16 men, 6 women) with a mean age of 76 ± 7 years. All patients were unfit for open repair, and nine had undergone prior aortic surgery. Customized aortic stent grafts were inserted through surgically exposed femoral (n = 16) or iliac (n = 6) arteries. Covered stents were inserted through surgically exposed brachial arteries. Spinal catheters were used for cerebrospinal fluid pressure drainage in 22 patients and for and spinal anesthesia in 11.

Results.—All 22 stent grafts and all 81 branches were deployed successfully. Aortic coverage as a percentage of subclavian-to-bifurcation distance was 69% ± 20%. Mean contrast volume was 203 mL, mean blood loss was 714 mL, and mean hospital stay was 10.9 days. Two patients (9.1%) died perioperatively: one from guidewire injury to a renal arterial branch and the other from a medication error. Serious or potentially serious complications occurred in 9 of 22 patients (41%). There was no paraplegia, renal failure, stroke, or myocardial infarction among the 20 surviving patients. Two patients (9.1%) underwent successful reintervention: one for localized intimal disruption and the other for aortic dissection, type I endoleak, and stenosis of the superior mesenteric artery. One patient has a type II endoleak. Follow-up is >1 month in 19 patients, >6 months in 12, and >12 months in 8. One branch (renal artery) occluded for a 98.75% branch patency rate at 1 month. The other 80 branches remain patent. There are no signs of stent graft migration, component separation, or fracture.

Conclusions.—Multibranched stent graft implantation eliminates aneurysm flow, preserves visceral perfusion, and avoids many of the physiologic stresses associated with other forms of repair. The results support an expanded role for this technique in the treatment of TAAA.

▶ This is a landmark, Phase 1, single center prospective series evaluating the use of multi-branched stent grafts for the repair of thoracoabdominal aneurysms. This study by a group well known for innovation in this field of interest should be read by every vascular surgeon who treats this disease, as the results are impressive to say the least.

Twenty-two patients underwent repair with custom made multi-branched stent grafts with caudally oriented cuffs and bridging stents during the study interval. Eighty-one visceral branches were stented. The operative details were impressive with a mean contrast load of 203 cc and estimated blood loss of 714 cc. Two patients died within 30 days with 1 mortality directly resulting from the attempted repair. Three patients (13.6%) had transient paraparesis which all resolved with conservative measures. Most notably, there was no paraplegia, renal failure, stroke or MI in the 20 surviving patients.

The authors appropriately acknowledge that further work needs to be done to refine these techniques and to identify those patients who would benefit most from this approach. Regardless, this series serves as a bookmark in the history of vascular surgery that is truly transformative of the way in which this disease process will be managed for decades to come.

B. W. Starnes, MD

8 Abdominal Aortic Endografting

Endovascular vs. Open Repair of Abdominal Aortic Aneurysms in the Medicare Population
Schermerhorn ML, O'Malley AJ, Jhaveri A, et al (Beth Israel Deaconess Med Ctr, Boston, MA; Harvard Med School, Boston, MA; et al)
N Engl J Med 358:464-474, 2008

Background.—Randomized trials have shown reductions in perioperative mortality and morbidity with endovascular repair of abdominal aortic aneurysm, as compared with open surgical repair. Longer-term survival rates, however, were similar for the two procedures. There are currently no long-term, population-based data from the comparison of these strategies.

Methods.—We studied perioperative rates of death and complications, long-term survival, rupture, and reinterventions after open as compared with endovascular repair of abdominal aortic aneurysm in propensity-score–matched cohorts of Medicare beneficiaries undergoing repair during the 2001–2004 period, with follow-up until 2005.

Results.—There were 22,830 matched patients undergoing open repair of abdominal aortic aneurysm in each cohort. The average age of the patients was 76 years, and approximately 20% were women. Perioperative mortality was lower after endovascular repair than after open repair (1.2% vs. 4.8%, P<0.001), and the reduction in mortality increased with age (2.1% difference for those 67 to 69 years old vs. 8.5% for those 85 years or older, P<0.001). Late survival was similar in the two cohorts, although the survival curves did not converge until after 3 years. By 4 years, rupture was more likely in the endovascular-repair cohort than in the open-repair cohort (1.8% vs. 0.5%, P<0.001), as was reintervention related to abdominal aortic aneurysm (9.0% vs. 1.7%, P<0.001), although most reinterventions were minor. In contrast, by 4 years, surgery for laparotomy-related complications was more likely among patients who had undergone open repair (9.7%, vs. 4.1% among those who had undergone endovascular repair; P<0.001), as was hospitalization without surgery for bowel obstruction or abdominal-wall hernia (14.2% vs. 8.1%, P<0.001).

Conclusions.—As compared with open repair, endovascular repair of abdominal aortic aneurysm is associated with lower short-term rates of death and complications. The survival advantage is more durable among older patients. Late reinterventions, related to abdominal aortic aneurysm, are more common after endovascular repair, but are balanced by an increase in laparotomy-related reinterventions and hospitalizations after open surgery.

▶ The unique feature of this study is the population analyzed and the huge dataset evaluated. Analysis of mega datasets is difficult, and there is the possibility of real error. The authors, however, given the type of data available, have analyzed it as well as possible. Because this article appeared in the *New England Journal of Medicine*, it will be widely cited and quoted. However, with the exception of increased survival benefit for older patients with endovascular aneurysm repair (EVAR), the author's findings are neither unique nor unexpected. Perhaps, the greatest contribution of the study is that it confirms complex medical technologies that can be rapidly adapted and widely instituted with good periprocedural results. It is now time to begin taking a serious look at the cost effectiveness of EVAR versus open repair of abdominal aortic aneurysms.

G. L. Moneta, MD

Lifeline registry of endovascular aneurysm repair: Open repair surgical controls in clinical trials
Zwolak RM, Sidawy AN, Greenberg RK, et al (Dartmouth-Hitchcock Med Ctr, Lebanon, NH; Washington VA Med Ctr, Washington, DC; The Cleveland Clinic Foundation, OH; et al)
J Vasc Surg 48:511-518, 2008

Purpose.—The improvement of available endovascular aortic aneurysm repair (EVAR) devices is critical for the advancement of patient care in vascular surgery. The goal of this article is to report a highly detailed, closely monitored, audited, pooled multicenter cohort of open surgical abdominal aortic aneurysm (AAA) repairs that has potential for use in future EVAR studies as a control data set.

Methods.—Open surgical AAA repair data from four investigational device exemption clinical aortic endograft trials were tested for poolability, merged, and analyzed for the intervals of 0 to 30 days and 31 to 365 days.

Results.—The data set includes 323 open patients (83% men; mean age, 70 years). Operative mortality at 30 days was 2.8%. The mean age of women was 3 years older than men, and mortality at 30 days for women was 5.7% compared with 2.2% for men ($P = .18$). Operative mortality for patients with large AAAs (≥ 5.5 cm, 3.6%) was not different than for patients with small aneurysms (<5.5 cm, 2.4%, $P = .54$). All-cause mortality at 1 year was 6.7%, with significant predictors including age, sex, and renal failure. Women had 2.6-fold greater 1-year all-cause mortality rate (13.2%) than men (5.4%, $P = .04$), but statistical significance was lost after correction for age. Two additional AAA-related deaths occurred between days 31 and 365, resulting in a 1-year AAA-related mortality of 3.5%.

Conclusion.—This data set provides a tightly controlled, thoroughly detailed, and audited experience that has the potential to serve as an open control group for future EVAR trials.

▶ These data were compiled by the Society of Vascular Surgery Outcomes Committee. Although the 4 trials from which the data were derived had somewhat different exclusion and inclusion criteria as well as end points, statistically the data appear to be poolable to provide a contemporary group of patients of standard risk treated with open aneurysm repair. The 30-day operative mentality of 2.8% confirms that open surgical repair of an abdominal aortic aneurysm is safe. With only 2 additional aneurysm-related deaths over the first year, the trial also confirms that open repair of abdominal aortic aneurysm is effective. It may be argued, however, that institutions participating in the investigational trials of endovascular aortic aneurysm likely have a higher volume of overall aneurysm patients and because volume is related to outcomes in aortic aneurysm surgery the results here may be better than what would be expected in community practice. It should also be noted that the data set contained only 54 women. Any conclusions regarding aneurysm-related death and often mortality, with respect to female gender, are really not appropriate from this data set.

G. L. Moneta, MD

Comparison of the effects of open and endovascular aortic aneurysm repair on long-term renal function using chronic kidney disease staging based on glomerular filtration rate
Mills JL Sr, Duong ST, Leon LR Jr, et al (The Univ of Arizona Health Sciences Ctr, Tucson; Southern Arizona Veterans Affairs Health Care System)
J Vasc Surg 47:1141-1149, 2008

Objective.—It has been suggested that endovascular aneurysm repair (EVAR) in concert with serial contrast-enhanced computed tomography (CT) surveillance adversely impacts renal function. Our primary objectives were to assess serial renal function in patients undergoing EVAR and open repair (OR) and to evaluate the relative effects of method of repair on renal function.

Methods.—A thorough retrospective chart review was performed on 223 consecutive patients (103 EVAR, 120 OR) who underwent abdominal aortic aneurysm (AAA) repair. Demographics, pertinent risk factors, CT scan number, morbidity, and mortality were recorded in a database. Baseline, 30- and 90-day, and most recent glomerular filtration rate (GFR) were calculated. Mean GFR changes and renal function decline (using

Chronic Kidney Disease [CKD] staging and Kaplan-Meier plot) were determined. EVAR and OR patients were compared. CKD prevalence (≥stage 3, National Kidney Foundation) was determined before repair and in longitudinal follow-up. Observed-expected (OE) ratios for CKD were calculated for EVAR and OR patients by comparing observed CKD prevalence with the expected, age-adjusted prevalence.

Results.—The only baseline difference between EVAR and OR cohorts was female gender (4% vs 12%, $P = .029$). Thirty-day GFR was significantly reduced in OR patients ($P = .047$), but it recovered and there were no differences in mean GFR at a mean follow-up of 23.2 months. However, 18% to 39% of patients in the EVAR and OR groups developed significant renal function decline over time depending on its definition. OE ratios for CKD prevalence were greater in AAA patients at baseline (OE 1.28-3.23, depending upon age group). During follow-up, the prevalence and severity of CKD increased regardless of method of repair (OE 1.8-9.0). Deterioration of renal function was independently associated with age >70 years in all patients (RR 2.92) and performance of EVAR compared with OR (RR 3.5) during long-term follow-up.

Conclusions.—Compared with EVAR, OR was associated with a significant but transient fall in GFR at 30 days. Renal function decline after AAA repair was common, regardless of method, especially in patients >70 years of age. However, the renal function decline was significantly greater by Kaplan-Meier analysis in EVAR than OR patients during long-term follow-up. More aggressive strategies to monitor and preserve renal function after AAA repair are warranted.

▶ This retrospective, non-randomized study evaluated the effect of types of aneurysm repair (open vs endovascular) on renal function over time, utilizing surrogate markers of glomerular filtration rate (GFR) and chronic kidney disease (CKD) stage. The authors are to be commended in presenting a well-conceived, logical, and evidence-based approach for this assessment.

The authors appropriately observe that the baseline incidence of CKD is higher in patients with abdominal aortic aneurysms than in age-matched controls. Furthermore, a significant difference was identified in the incidence of long-term renal function decline for endovascular aneurysm repair (EVAR) compared with patients undergoing open repair. The authors attributed this decline in renal function in the EVAR group to the ongoing administration of contrast associated with routine follow up. This topic is of significant interest and defines a well-structured method for surveillance of renal function over time. However, these observations may become irrelevant, as various methods of follow-up imaging that do not use iodinated contrast become available.

B. W. Starnes, MD

Zenith abdominal aortic aneurysm endovascular graft

Greenberg RK, Chuter TAM, Cambria RP, et al (Cleveland Clinic Foundation, OH; Univ of San Francisco, CA; Massachusetts Gen Hosp, Boston, MA; et al)
J Vasc Surg 48:1-9, 2008

Purpose.—The safety and efficacy of the Zenith (Cook Inc, Bloomington, Ind) endovascular graft was assessed based on the United States multicenter trial through 5 years of follow-up.

Methods.—Between 2000 and 2003, the pivotal study enrolled patients to open surgery (control) or the Zenith endovascular graft (endovascular). A separate continued access study arm enrolled endovascular patients using the same inclusion/exclusion criteria. Both studies were designed for 2-year follow-up, and the pivotal endovascular patients had the option of extending the study follow-up through 5 years. All endovascular patients were stratified by physiologic risk into high-risk and standard-risk groups to assess overall mortality, rupture, conversion, endoleaks, secondary interventions, and sac enlargement. The entire endovascular cohort was pooled to assess device integrity, limb occlusion, component separation, and migration. The suboptimal endovascular result (SER) was established as an end point to assess late adverse outcomes. Statistical analyses included Kaplan-Meier estimations and Cox regression to assess factors contributing to sac enlargement and SER.

Results.—The study enrolled 739 endovascular patients (352 pivotal, 387 continued access); 158 patients in the pivotal study reconsented to be followed up for 5 years. For the patients at standard and high risk at 5 years, the respective survival estimate was 83% and 61%, aneurysm-related death was 2% and 4%, and freedom from rupture was 100% and 99.6%, respectively. Cumulative risk of conversion, limb occlusion, migration >10 mm, or component separation was ≤3% at 5 years. Cumulative risk of late endoleak was 12% to 15%, representing the primary indication for secondary interventions which occurred in 20% of standard-risk patients and 25% of high-risk patients through 5 years. Sac enlargement was very rare and associated with advanced age and larger aneurysms. SER was predicted by advanced age and internal iliac artery occlusion.

Conclusion.—These middle- and long-term data support long-term durability of the Zenith endovascular graft. Risk of aneurysm-related death or rupture was exceptionally low, and complications of migration, limb occlusion, and device integrity issues were uncommon. Incidence of late endoleaks and association of endoleaks with sac growth underscore the need for long-term follow-up of patients treated with endovascular grafts, although the sequelae of such events are unknown.

▶ The article presents middle- and long-term data that supports the efficacy and durability of the Zenith endovascular graft. There is really not much new here with regard to insights for aortic endografting. It is now quite clear that a good quality endovascular graft with good surveillance results in minimal numbers of ruptures and small numbers of open conversions. There is also very low risk of migration, graft limb thrombosis, component separation, or loss of integrity of the graft material. Unfortunately, although 736 patients had successful implantation of the Zenith graft in the context of the study, the 5-year results are based on only 158 patients, which seriously reduces the power of the statistical analysis. Nevertheless, there are no obvious red flags here. Although some may view the accumulated data somewhat differently, to my eye, based on the available long-term data, the Gore and the Cook endovascular aneurysm grafts have emerged as the grafts of choice for endovascular infrarenal aortic aneurysm repair.

G. L. Moneta, MD

The Powerlink system for endovascular abdominal aortic aneurysm repair: Six-year results

Wang GJ, Carpenter JP (Univ of Pennsylvania School of Med, Philadelphia, PA)
J Vasc Surg 48:535-545, 2008

Objective.—We compared the results of endovascular repair using the Powerlink endovascular graft with conventional open abdominal aortic aneurysm repair through a 6-year follow-up period.

Methods.—Two hundred fifty-eight patients with abdominal aortic aneurysms were prospectively enrolled in a multicenter trial and underwent endovascular repair (N = 192) or conventional open surgery (N = 66). All endovascular repairs were approached through a surgically exposed femoral artery and a percutaneously accessed femoral artery. Study endpoints included all-cause mortality and morbidity. Follow-up imaging consisted of contrast-enhanced CT scans and plain abdominal x-rays at 1, 6, 12 months, and annually postoperatively.

Results.—Technical success was achieved in 97.9% of test patients, with four failed insertions (three early conversions because of deployment issues, one access failure). Mean follow-up was 4.1 ± 1.7 years (test group) and 3.1 ± 1.9 years (control group). Perioperative morbidity and mortality were significantly reduced in the test group compared with the control group ($P < .05$). At 6 years, all-cause mortality and morbidity was no different in the Powerlink group compared with the open repair group. There were no reported stent fractures, graft disruptions, or aneurysm ruptures. Core laboratory-reported endoleaks included proximal or distal type I (n = 1) and type I/II (n = 3), with no type III or type IV endoleaks. One explant (0.5%) was undertaken to resolve a refractory type I endoleak. A total of 37 secondary procedures were performed in 26 patients to treat site-reported endoleak (n = 26; 7 for type I and 19 for type II), graft limb occlusion (n = 7), native artery occlusion (n = 3), or endograft migration (n = 1). A reduction in mean aneurysm sac diameters and volumes has been noted at every follow-up interval.

Conclusion.—Consistent with other reports, perioperative morbidity and mortality were significantly reduced in the endovascular group compared with the open repair group. Six-year follow-up of patients treated with the Powerlink system demonstrates the continued safety and efficacy of its treatment of abdominal aortic aneurysm.

▶ The data indicate that the Powerlink system is effective in the endovascular repair of abdominal aortic aneurysms. The device has some potential theoretic advantages. Although complete percutaneous placement of aortic endografts has been reported, most surgeons continue to use femoral artery cut-downs for groin access. The contralateral limb of the Powerlink system requires only a 9F sheath and, therefore, can routinely be placed percutaneously. The device is deployed on top of the aortic bifurcation. It is essentially built from the bottom-up rather than the top-down. Deployment of the device on top of the aortic bifurcation theoretically allows for fixation separate from the infrarenal aortic and iliac artery seal zones. It should be noted that the aneurysms treated with the Powerlink system in this study were relatively small with a mean diameter of 5.1 cm with aneurysms as small as 4 cm included in the study. There is a suggestion from multiple groups that treatment of larger aortic aneurysms may be associated with more complications using the endovascular aneurysm repair (EVAR) technique. I suspect this graft will be like all the others. It will have its advocates and its detractors. The data suggest that the Powerlink system, in the short-term and intermediate-term, is unlikely to be substantially better or worse than other commercially available aortic endografts. Surgeons should use whatever graft appears most applicable to their patient and most consistent with their personal experience.

G. L. Moneta, MD

What is the clinical utility of a 6-month computed tomography in the follow-up of endovascular aneurysm repair patients?
Go MR, Barbato JE, Rhee RY, et al (Univ of Pittsburgh Med Ctr, PA)
J Vasc Surg 47:1181-1187, 2008

Objective.—A drawback of endovascular aneurysm repair (EVAR) is the need for ongoing surveillance. Follow-up schedules including 1-, 6-, and 12-month computed tomography (CT) established by regulatory trials have been carried into clinical practice without critical assessment. The utility of a 6-month CT, with its associated radiation exposure and contrast toxicity, obtained after a normal result at 1-month CT has not been established.

Methods.—All EVAR patients from 1996 to 2004 at one institution with complete local 1-year follow-up were reviewed for clinically significant CT findings at 1, 6, and 12 months. Before 2000, all patients underwent 1-, 6-, and 12-month CT. In 2000, a policy of omitting the 6-month CT in patients who had a normal result on the 1-month scan was adopted.

Results.—During the study period, 573 patients underwent EVAR, and 376 patients who had complete local 1-year follow-up were included in this review. All had a 1-month CT scan and the result was abnormal in 40 (10.6%): five had type 1 leaks (1.3%), 34 had type 2 leaks (9.0%), and one had a type 3 leak (0.3%); all were followed with 6-month CT. The 1-month CT scan result was normal for 336 (89.4%) patients. Of these, group I (130 patients, 67 treated after 2000) underwent routine 6-month CT, with only two abnormalities noted (1.5%); both were type 2 endoleaks not associated with sac growth. No 6-month CT in this group demonstrated findings warranting intervention. The 6-month CT was omitted in group II (206 patients, all treated after 2000), and follow-up was only at 1 year. In this group, no patient's management would have been altered by findings on a 6-month CT. No patient in either group experienced aneurysm sac growth by 1 year. Clinical complications occurred in three group I patients (2.3%): seroma, limb occlusion, and main body thrombosis. Only one group II patient (0.5%) experienced a complication ≤1 year, a limb occlusion at 9 months.

Conclusions.—After EVAR, a 6-month CT after a normal 1-month CT result does not identify any clinically significant findings warranting intervention and can be omitted safely from the follow-up schedule.

▶ The answer to the question posed in the title of this article is "not much," provided things were okay at 1 month. There is certainly a need to simply follow-up patients with endovascular aneurysm repair. Not everyone is as likely to be as organized as the Pittsburgh group, but everyone who performs endovascular aneurysm repair should have a specific protocol for follow-up of these patients. The data are sufficiently convincing that the recommendations of the authors should be widely accepted.

G. L. Moneta, MD

The trifurcated endograft technique for hypogastric preservation during endovascular aneurysm repair
Minion DJ, Xenos E, Sorial E, et al (Univ of Kentucky Med Ctr, Lexington, KY)
J Vasc Surg 47:658-661, 2008

Bilateral common iliac artery involvement remains a significant challenge for endovascular aneurysm repair. We describe a technique to overcome this obstacle that we have termed the trifurcated endograft. The technique involves the deployment of a second bifurcated endoprosthesis into an iliac limb to create a three-limbed graft. The third limb is then used as the origin for an extension into one hypogastric artery (Fig 1).

▶ Data on branched endografts to preserve hypogastric arteries during repair of combined aortic and iliac aneurysms are available from outside the United States. Early data using the Zenith endograft system have demonstrated that

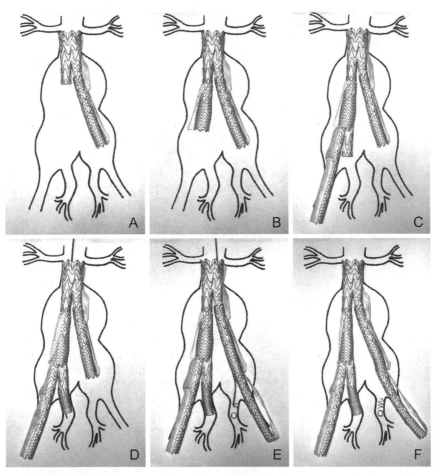

FIGURE 1.—Steps in the creation of the trifurcated endograft. See text for details. (Reprinted from Minion DJ, Xenos E, Sorial E, et al. The trifurcated endograft technique for hypogastric preservation during endovascular aneurysm repair. *J Vasc Surg.* 2008;47:658-661, with permission from The society for Vascular Surgery.)

this technique is feasible and can produce encouraging results. The authors of this study point out that trifurcated endografts are, in essence, branched endografts. Their technique is a bit of a Rube Goldberg approach (Fig 1). It does, however, have the advantage for United States physicians of using endograft components that are readily available in the United States. Potential disadvantages of the technique are the need for a large enough aortic diameter to accommodate 3 limbs of an endoprosthesis. There must also be a certain minimum length (16.5 cm) from the lowest renal artery through the hypogastric artery to be preserved. The need for brachial access is also a disadvantage and the authors cleverly don't tell us how long the procedure takes or how much it costs. By my count, at least 6 Excluder components are needed to complete the procedure; 2 of which are main body grafts. This is a nice check for Gore but a nightmare for the hospital administrator operating under the constraints of the DRG system.

G. L. Moneta, MD

Branched devices for thoracoabdominal aneurysm repair: Early experience
Ferreira M, Lanziotti L, Monteiro M (Serviço Integrado de Técnicas Endovasculares (SITE, Endovascular Techniques Integrated Service), Rio de Janeiro-RJ, Brazil)
J Vasc Surg 48:30S-36S, 2008

Objective.—This study reports the initial clinical results and experience with the planning of branched stent grafts in high-risk patients with thoracoabdominal aortic aneurysms (TAAAs).

Methods.—High-risk patients with TAAAs were considered for this study. Based on evaluation with computed tomography angiography (CTA), 21 custom-made branched stent grafts were designed for the selected patients. Two patients had associated bilateral aneurysms of the common iliac arteries, so an iliac branched device was also used.

Results.—Between August 2006 and April 2008, 23 patients (10 women, 13 men) were selected to undergo endovascular TAAA repair. Mean age was 72 years old. Two patients were excluded after 1-mm-slice CTA analysis. Eleven patients have underdone TAAA repair so far. The mean follow-up period at present is 8 months (range, 18 days-21 months). Overall technical success was accomplished in all 11 patients. Two renal artery branches occluded. Operative times varied from 3 to 8 hours. Mean contrast volume was 193 mL (range, 48-420 mL). Eight patients required a stay of ≤4 days at the intensive care unit. Three patients died. Two deaths were procedurally related: one patient died of myocardial infarction, and the other had ischemic cerebellar stroke and died 3 months later of pulmonary sepsis. The third patient was readmitted 3 days after hospital discharge and died of alcoholic pancreatitis. One man had permanent paraplegia. Two women had transitory paraparesis. Striking hematologic and systemic inflammatory abnormalities were observed.

Conclusion.—Increasing reports on stent graft technology indicate that this procedure might become a reality in the future for endovascular treatment of complex aneurysms in all aortic segments. Branched stent grafts seem to be feasible and can be offered as an effective alternative to most patients with TAAAs, especially for those who are currently excluded from open surgical procedures.

▶ This interesting report on the early experience of branched endografting provides a small amount of data on 11 high-risk patients undergoing purely endovascular repair of thoracoabdominal aortic aneurysms. Although the experience is small, the results are impressive with a 100% technical success rate and no type-1 or -3 endoleaks or limb occlusions. Of the 43 target visceral arteries approached, only 2 occluded in the follow-up period.

The authors make a strong argument for the mere feasibility of this approach in this high-risk population, but the risks of significant morbidity and mortality in this patient population remain high. Perhaps, the most important aspect of this article is the description that the origin of branch vessels from planned branched endografting is somewhat predictable, a fact that will be extremely important for the future development of branch-endograft technology.

B. W. Starnes, MD

9 Visceral and Renal Artery Disease

Renal Stenting for Incidentally Discovered Renal Artery Stenosis: Is There any Outcome Benefit?

Suliman A, Imhoff L, Greenberg JI, et al (Univ of California, San Diego)
Ann Vasc Surg 22:525-533, 2008

We evaluated whether there was a clinical outcome benefit in patients incidentally discovered to have high-grade renal artery stenosis (RAS) and treated with percutaneous transluminal renal angioplasty and stenting (PTRAS) at the time of angiogram for another indicated procedure. A retrospective chart review was performed on all patients undergoing renal arteriography over 4 years at our academic tertiary-care referral center. Review of catheterization reports was used to identify patients diagnosed with high-grade RAS (reduction of $\geq 70\%$ luminal diameter by arteriogram). Patients treated with PTRAS were identified. Baseline and postprocedure blood pressure (BP, an average of at least three independent measurements), glomerular filtration rate, serum creatinine, and antihypertensive medication regimen were compared for 12 months of follow-up. Over 4 years, 124 patients underwent renal arteriography and 78 (63%) were diagnosed with high-grade RAS. Fifty-eight patients (74% of those with high-grade RAS) received PTRAS. Patients treated with PTRAS had similar baseline characteristics to those with high-grade RAS with no intervention, with the exception of lower diastolic BP (DBP; 74 ± 11.2 vs. 80 ± 14.2 mm Hg, $p = 0.04$) and a higher proportion of hyperlipidemia (78 vs. 55%, $p = 0.05$). Thirty-eight out of 58 PTRAS patients (66%) received sufficient follow-up to assess outcomes. When baseline and postprocedure variables were compared in PTRAS patients with 12-month follow-up, there was a reduction in systolic BP (SBP, 153 ± 20.8 vs. 136 ± 27.2 mm Hg, $p = 0.01$) and mean arterial pressure (MAP, 103 ± 11.2 vs. 95 ± 14 mm Hg, $p = 0.04$). When these patients were stratified by those with an increase, decrease, or no change in postprocedure antihypertensive medications, significant reductions in SBP, MAP, and DBP were noted only in the patient population that also had an increase in the number of antihypertensive medications. No differences in renal insufficiency were detected. Patients with high-grade RAS incidentally discovered during arteriography performed for extrarenal disease and treated with PTRAS have a modest reduction in BP, which is significant only in those patients with an increased number of antihypertensive medications postprocedure. Caution must be taken in stenting patients with incidental RAS as outcome benefit may be minimal when compared to medical management only.

▶ In recent years, use of renal artery stents for treatment of renal artery stenosis has exploded. Beyond a few specific clinical situations such as bilateral high-grade stenosis with recurrent pulmonary edema, there is little data to support the liberal use of stents to treat stenotic renal arteries. The use of renal artery stenting and so-called drive-by procedures by numerous practitioners recently led the Center for Medicare Services (CMS) to reconsider payment for renal artery stents. Payment was preserved for these procedures, but just barely. This article does not help the cause of the renal artery stenters. Although it is a retrospective study with incomplete data, it is certainly not a testimonial to the efficacy of renal artery stents in patients with previously unsuspected renal artery stenosis. The only parameter that improved in the stented patient is blood pressure, and that only improved if there was an increase in anti-hypertensive medications! These data clearly do not support routine practice of renal angioplasty and stenting for incidentally discovered lesions. The management of such lesions remains highly controversial.

G. L. Moneta, MD

Embolic Protection and Platelet Inhibition During Renal Artery Stenting

Cooper CJ, Haller ST, Colyer W, et al (Univ of Toledo, OH; et al)
Circulation 117:2752-2760, 2008

Background.—Preservation of renal function is an important objective of renal artery stent procedures. Although atheroembolization can cause renal dysfunction during renal stent procedures, whether adjunctive use of embolic protection devices or glycoprotein IIb/IIIa inhibitors improves renal function is unknown.

Methods and Results.—One hundred patients undergoing renal artery stenting at 7 centers were randomly assigned to an open-label embolic protection device, Angioguard, or double-blind use of a platelet glycoprotein IIb/IIIa inhibitor, abciximab, in a 2×2 factorial design. The main effects of treatments and their interaction were assessed on percentage change in Modification in Diet in Renal Disease–derived glomerular filtration rate from baseline to 1 month using centrally analyzed creatinine. Filter devices were analyzed for the presence of platelet-rich thrombus. With stenting alone, stenting and embolic protection, and stenting with abciximab alone, glomerular filtration rate declined ($P<0.05$), but with combination therapy, it did not decline and was superior to the other allocations in the 2×2 design ($P<0.01$). The main effects of treatment demonstrated no overall improvement in glomerular filtration rate; although abciximab was superior to placebo ($0\pm27\%$ versus $-10\pm20\%$;

$P<0.05$), embolic protection was not $(-1\pm28\%$ versus $-10\pm20\%$; $P=0.08$). An interaction was observed between abciximab and embolic protection ($P<0.05$), favoring combination treatment. Abciximab reduced the occurrence of platelet-rich emboli in the filters from 42% to 7% ($P<0.01$).

Conclusions.—Renal artery stenting alone, stenting with embolic protection, and stenting with abciximab were associated with a decline in glomerular filtration rate. An unanticipated interaction between Angioguard and abciximab was seen, with combination therapy better than no treatment or either treatment alone.

▶ Atheroembolization can result in renal dysfunction as a result of renal artery stenting procedures. The lack of efficacy of the embolic protection device in improving glomerular filtration rate (GFR) after renal artery stenting despite capturing debris suggests that emboli from before or after filter deployment or alternative mechanisms to renal injury offset the efficacy of the embolic protection device when used in isolation. Abciximab may work by decreasing emboli to the kidney before deployment of the filter device or perhaps reducing adverse effects of platelet activation in ischemia-induced renal dysfunction. It is important to keep in mind that the end points used in this study are merely surrogate end points for the more clinically important end points of long-term blood pressure control and renal preservation. Whether the use of embolic protection devices and platelet IIb-IIIa inhibitors favorably influence these more important clinical parameters after renal artery stenting is yet to be determined.

G. L. Moneta, MD

Efficacy of protected renal artery primary stenting in the solitary functioning kidney
Klonaris C, Katsargyris A, Alexandrou A, et al (Athens Univ Med School, Greece)
J Vasc Surg 48:1414-1422, 2008

Background.—Significant renal artery stenosis (RAS) in a solitary functioning kidney (SFK) represents one of the most acceptable indications for renal revascularization. Percutaneous transluminal renal artery stenting (PTRAS) is increasingly being used as a first line treatment for renal revascularization, associated with renal function improvement or stabilization in the majority of the patients with solitary kidneys, but also with deterioration in up to 38% of the cases. Atheroembolism during PTRAS has been postulated as a potential cause for this acute renal function worsening. The aim of this study was to report on the feasibility, safety, and early outcomes of PTRAS in a series of patients with SFK using distal embolic protection (DEP).

Methods.—All PTRAS procedures in SFKs performed under DEP between June 2002 and September 2007 were reviewed. Renal function,

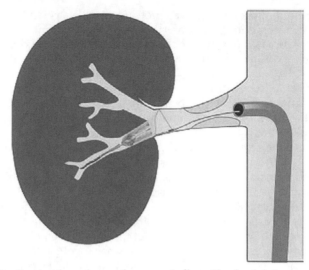

FIGURE 3.—Drawing shows the use of an eccentric filter with a beveled ring in order to provide complete renal protection in cases of short main renal artery; the tip of the filter is anchored distally in one renal artery branch, while the proximal beveled part of the basket remains in the main renal artery protecting both renal artery divisions. (Reprinted from Klonaris C, Katsargyris A, Alexandrou A, et al. Efficacy of protected renal artery primary stenting in the solitary functioning kidney. *J Vasc Surg.* 2008;48:1414-1422, with permission from The Society for Vascular Surgery.)

blood pressure, and the number of anti-hypertensive medications were assessed pre- and post-intervention. Renal function improvement and deterioration were defined as a 20% increase and decrease in serum creatinine, respectively, compared with preoperative values. Primary and primary assisted patency rates were also calculated. Statistical differences between values before and after intervention were determined by the Student t test and statistical significance was taken at $P < .05$.

Results.—Protected PTRAS was performed in 14 patients with a SFK (9 men, 6 women, mean age 65.6 ± 6.8 years). All patients were hypertensive and had varying degrees of azotemia. Mean pre-intervention stenosis degree was 86.8% ± 7.8%. Immediate technical success was obtained in 100% of the patients. Renal function was cured (7.1%), improved (50%), or stabilized (42.9%) in all 14 (100%) patients after the procedure and no deterioration was noticed in any patient at 6-month follow-up. Pre- and postintervention serum creatinine levels were 3.01 ± 1.15 mg/dL and 2.16 ± 0.68 mg/dL, respectively, ($P = .02$). Hypertension was improved in 6 (42.9%) patients and stabilized in the remaining 8 (57.1%). Primary patency was 100% and 90% at 1 and 3 years, respectively, while primary assisted patency remained 100% for the whole follow-up period (mean, 31.8 ± 19.4 months).

Conclusion.—These findings suggest that in patients with a SFK, protected PTRAS represents a safe and effective treatment for halting the progression of renal dysfunction to renal loss and warrants further investigation (Fig 3).

▶ Stenting of the renal artery for atherosclerotic disease is currently under a bit of pressure. The Center for Medicare Services (CMS) recently reviewed the funding policy for renal artery stents and barely agreed to continue funding renal artery stents for atherosclerotic disease. It makes sense, although it may not be true, that certain patients are more likely to benefit from renal artery stenting than others. Certainly the individual with a single functioning kidney, similar to the subjects in this study, might be one of those types of patients. While the goal of renal artery stenting is to improve or stabilize renal function, it can be associated with deterioration of renal function as well.

The idea of using embolic protective devices to enhance the efficacy of renal artery stenting is catching on. If any group is potentially going to benefit, it would be the individual with the single functioning kidney. There are, however, no approved devices for embolic protection for stenting the renal artery. Current devices are approved for use in coronary saphenous vein grafts, and in conjunction with carotid artery stenting. Ideally, the protective device for renal artery stenting would have a low profile and high flexibility, with increased guidewire strength to minimize the need for distal anchoring and to facilitate stent advancement over an ostial lesion. In addition, devices should have relatively large ring diameters to provide complete vessel wall opposition in patients with larger renal arteries (Fig 3).

This article should be viewed as a description of a technique rather than proof of efficacy. The results here were good and seem promising, but there was a small cohort of patients, and even a few adverse events could significantly shift the perception of benefit that is implied in this article. In addition, the authors did not compare their patients with a randomized group of patients with single functioning kidneys undergoing renal artery stenting without distal embolic protection. Nevertheless, the results here are good enough that, in a patient with favorable anatomy and a single functioning kidney, the interventionist should consider the use of an embolic protection device if renal artery stenting is chosen for therapy.

G. L. Moneta, MD

Operative mortality for renal artery bypass in the United States: Results from the National Inpatient Sample
Modrall JG, Rosero EB, Smith ST, et al (Univ of Texas Southwestern Med Ctr, Dallas, TX)
J Vasc Surg 48:317-322, 2008

Background.—The mortality rate for renal artery bypass grafting (RABG) is reported to be 0% to 4% for patients with renovascular hypertension and 4% to 7% for patients with ischemic nephropathy. However, these data come from high-volume referral centers known for their expertise in treating these conditions. Because of the relative infrequency of these operations in most vascular surgery practices, the nationwide outcomes for RABG are not known. The purpose of this study was to define the operative mortality rate for RABG in the United States and to identify risk factors for perioperative mortality.

Methods.—The National Inpatient Sample was analyzed to identify patients undergoing RABG for the years 2000 to 2004. Categoric data were analyzed using χ^2 and the Cochran-Armitage trend tests. Multivariate logistic regression analyses were performed to identify risk factors for perioperative mortality after RABG.

Results.—During the study period, 6608 patients underwent RABG, representing a frequency of 3.51 operations per 100,000 discharges. More than two-thirds were performed at teaching hospitals (4564 vs 2,044; $P < .0001$). The frequency of RABG decreased by 30.7% between 2000 and 2004 (4.28 vs 2.96 RABGs per 100,000 discharges; P for trend $< .0001$). The in-hospital mortality for RABG was 10.0%. On univariate analysis, in-hospital mortality after RABG varied with increasing age, race, region of the country, and a preoperative history of chronic renal failure, congestive heart failure, or chronic lung disease. Logistic regression models identified advanced age (odds ratio [OR] 1.57; 95% confidence interval [CI], 1.44-1.72], female gender (OR, 1.20; 95% CI, 1.02-1.41), and a history of chronic renal failure (OR, 2.21; 95% CI, 1.75-2.78), congestive heart failure (OR, 1.94; 95% CI, 1.44-2.62), or chronic lung disease (OR, 1.40; 95% CI, 1.18-1.67) as independent markers of risk-adjusted, in-hospital mortality ($P < .0001$ for each of these five variables).

Conclusions.—Nationwide in-hospital mortality after RABG is higher than predicted by prior reports from high-volume referral centers. Advanced age, female gender, and a history of chronic renal failure, congestive heart failure, or chronic lung disease were predictive of perioperative death. For the typical vascular practice, these data may provide a rationale for lower risk alternatives, such as renal artery stenting or referral to high-volume referral centers for RABG.

▶ The National Inpatient Sample Database is the largest all-payer inpatient database in the United States. It represents more than 1000 hospitals with > 38 million discharges annually and included 32 to 37 states from 2000-2004. The numbers presented here, therefore, are reasonably representative of what is actually out there. The reported 10% mortality rate for renal artery bypass in this article is indeed sobering. It is particularly sobering when 1 considers that high volume centers, perhaps performing most of the renal artery bypasses, have reported much less mortality rates for renal artery bypass for both hypertension and ischemic nephropathy. The implication is that, in low volume centers, the mortality rate for renal artery bypass may actually be significantly > 10%. As with many other complex surgical procedures, the data argue strongly for regionalization of complex procedures to those institutions and surgeons who perform high volumes of those procedures.

G. L. Moneta, MD

Outcomes after endarterectomy for chronic mesenteric ischemia

Mell MW, Acher CW, Hoch JR, et al (Univ of Wisconsin School of Med and Public Health, Madison)

J Vasc Surg 48:1132-1138, 2008

Objectives.—A retrospective study was performed to identify optimal factors affecting outcomes after open revascularization for chronic mesenteric ischemia.

Methods.—All patients who underwent open surgery for chronic mesenteric ischemia from 1987 to 2006 were reviewed. Patients with acute mesenteric ischemia or median arcuate ligament syndrome were excluded. Mortality, recurrent stenosis, and symptomatic recurrence were analyzed using logistic regression, and univariate and multivariate analysis.

Results.—We identified 80 patients (69% women, 31% men). Mean age was 64 years (range, 31-86 years). Acute-on-chronic symptoms were present in 26%. Presenting symptoms included postprandial pain (91%), weight loss (69%), and food fear and diarrhea (25%). Preoperative imaging demonstrated severe (>70%) stenosis of the superior mesenteric artery in 75 patients (24 occluded), the celiac axis in 63 (20 occluded), and the inferior mesenteric artery in 53 (20 occluded). Multivessel disease was present in 72 patients (90%), and 40 (50%) underwent multivessel reconstruction. Revascularization was achieved by endarterectomy in 37 patients, mesenteric bypass in 29, and combined procedures in 14. Concurrent aortic reconstruction was required in 13 patients (16%). Three hospital deaths occurred (3.8%). Mean follow-up was 3.8 years (range, 0-17.2 years). One- and 5-year survival was 92.2% and 64.5%. Mortality was associated with age ($P = .019$) and renal insufficiency ($P = .007$), but not by clinical presentation. Symptom-free survival was 89.7% and 82.1% at 1 and 5 years, respectively. Symptoms requiring reintervention occurred in nine patients (11%) at a mean of 29 months (range, 5-127 months). Multivariate analysis showed that freedom from recurrent symptoms correlated with endarterectomy for revascularization (5.2% vs 27.6%; hazard ratio, 0.20; 95% confidence interval, 0.04-0.92; $P = .02$).

Conclusion.—For open surgical candidates, endarterectomy appears to provide the most durable long-term symptom relief in patients with chronic mesenteric ischemia (Fig 3).

▶ There are many approaches to revascularization of the splanchnic vessels. These include antegrade bypass, retrograde bypass, bypass to both the celiac and superior mesenteric artery, and bypass to the superior mesenteric artery alone. An additional approach, although not used nearly as frequently as bypass, is endarterectomy of the visceral aortic segment and visceral vessels.

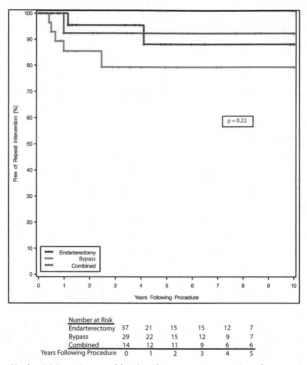

FIGURE 3.—Kaplan-Meier estimates of freedom from repeat intervention after open repair for mesenteric ischemia with endarterectomy *(blue line)*, bypass *(red line)*, and combined procedures *(green line)*. (Reprinted from Mell MW, Acher CW, Hoch JR, et al. Outcomes after endarterectomy for chronic mesenteric ischemia. *J Vasc Surg.* 2008;48:1132-1138, with permission from the Society for Vascular Surgery.)

This approach has the advantage of providing an all autogenous reconstruction with excellent freedom from repeat intervention (Fig 3). The operation, however, is more technically difficult than a bypass procedure and in most cases will require a longer period of visceral ischemia than a bypass procedure. This is a procedure that I recommend to be performed only by experienced visceral artery surgeons who can operate efficiently. It is not for the slow surgeon who only performs an occasional mesenteric artery revascularization.

G. L. Moneta, MD

Isolated spontaneous dissection of the splanchnic arteries

Takayama T, Miyata T, Shirakawa M, et al (The Univ of Tokyo, Japan; Fujieda Municipal Gen Hosp, Shizuoka)
J Vasc Surg 48:329-333, 2008

Objectives.—Isolated dissection of a splanchnic artery, including the celiac artery, superior mesenteric artery (SMA), and inferior mesenteric artery, and their branches, is a relatively rare condition. This study was conducted to define the characteristics of patients with splanchnic artery dissection and the clinical course of isolated splanchnic artery dissection.

Methods.—The records of 19 patients were reviewed to survey demographic data, the location of dissection, symptoms, diagnostic modalities, treatment, and long-term outcome.

Results.—The locations of dissection were the superior mesenteric artery (SMA) in 11 patients, celiac artery in 3, both celiac artery and SMA in 2, and common hepatic artery, celiac artery to splenic artery, and celiac artery to proper hepatic artery in 1 each. In all but one with systemic sclerosis and Sjögren syndrome, the underlying cause of dissection was unclear. There were 12 asymptomatic and seven symptomatic patients. All cases were diagnosed by computed tomography. Surgical treatment was performed in one patient with a large aneurysm of the common hepatic artery, and the remaining 18 patients were followed-up conservatively. The mean follow-up duration was 20.9 ± 25.4 months (range, 2-116 months). No expansion or progression of the false lumen was observed in these patients.

Conclusion.—Patients with spontaneous dissection of the splanchnic arteries are often asymptomatic, and in this series, none developed significant end organ ischemia. Most patients with this rare condition can be managed expectantly with clinical follow-up including computed tomography imaging to assess aneurysm formation.

▶ Spontaneous dissection of a splanchnic artery is increasingly recognized. Although still a relatively rare condition, the wide availability of advanced CT imaging has led to increased recognition of this problem in both symptomatic and asymptomatic patients. This is the largest series of splanchnic artery dissections that I am aware of. There are a number of things to be emphasized. First of all, many of the patients are asymptomatic and remain asymptomatic. Follow-up with CT scanning is appropriate and, at least in the short-term, expansion or progression of the false lumen is distinctly uncommon. Overall, it appears that in the absence of gut-threatening ischemia, splanchnic artery dissection can and should be managed conservatively with repeat CT scans. Longer follow-up will be required to know at what point such dissections can be truly considered "stable."

G. L. Moneta, MD

Epidemiology, risk and prognostic factors in mesenteric venous thrombosis
Acosta S, Alhadad A, Svensson P, et al (Malmö Univ Hosp, Sweden)
Br J Surg 95:1245-1251, 2008

Background.—Epidemiological reports on risk and prognostic factors in patients with mesenteric venous thrombosis (MVT) are scarce.

Methods.—Patients with MVT were identified through the inpatient and autopsy registry between 2000 and 2006 at Malmö University Hospital.

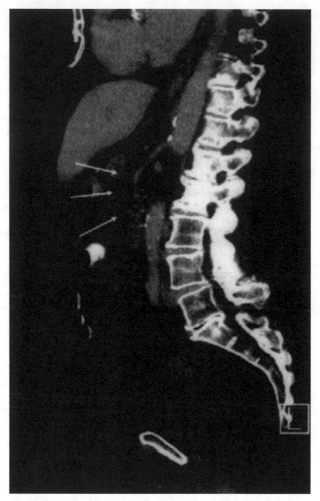

FIGURE 1.—Multidetector row computed tomogram of the abdomen in portal venous phase. Multi-planar reconstruction in sagittal view, showing thrombosis in the superior mesentric vein (arrow). (Reprinted from Acosta S, Alhadad A, Svensson P, et al. Epidemiology, risk and prognostic factors in mesenteric venous thrombosis. *Br J Surg.* 2008;95:1245-1251. Permission is granted by John Wiley & Sons Ltd on behalf of the BJSS Ltd.)

Results.—Fifty-one patients had MVT, diagnosed at autopsy in six. The highest incidence (11·3 per 100 000 person-years) was in the age category 70–79 years. Activated protein C resistance was present in 13 of 29 patients tested. D-dimer at admission was raised in all five patients tested. Multidetector row computed tomography (CT) in the portal venous phase was diagnostic in all 20 patients investigated, of whom 19 were managed conservatively. The median length of resected bowel in 12 patients who had surgery was 0.6 (range 0.1–2.2) m. The overall 30-day mortality rate was 20 per cent; intestinal infarction ($P = 0.046$), treatment on a non-surgical ward ($P = 0.001$) and CT not done ($P = 0.022$) were associated with increased mortality. Cancer was independently associated with long-term mortality: hazard ratio 4.03, 95 per cent confidence interval 1.03 to 15.85; $P = 0.046$.

Conclusion.—Portal venous phase CT appeared sensitive in diagnosing MVT. As activated protein C resistance was a strong risk factor, lifelong anticoagulation should be considered (Fig 1).

▶ Mesenteric venous thrombosis (MVT), at least symptomatic MVT, occurs infrequently. The diagnosis is difficult, as symptoms are generally nonspecific. Mortality rates can be high. The authors' data are consistent with what one would suspect. CT scanning with a venous phase works well for diagnosis (Fig 1), and many of these patients will have a hypercoagulable state with, at least in this study, factor V Leiden mutation identified as the most prevalent abnormality. The study highlights the current standard-of-care for patients with possible MVT—a CT scan for diagnosis, anticoagulation for most patients, bowel resection for those with peritonitis, and an aggressive evaluation for hypercoagulable state with likely long-term anticoagulation. Long-term prognosis is largely related to the presence of malignancy.

G. L. Moneta, MD

Superficial venous thrombosis: Prevalence of common genetic risk factors and their role on spreading to deep veins
Milio G, Siragusa S, Minà C, et al (Univ of Palermo, Italy)
Thromb Res 123:194-199, 2008

Introduction.—Superficial venous thrombosis (SVT) has been considered for a long time a limited clinical condition with a low importance, but this approach has changed in recent years, when several studies demonstrated spreading to deep veins occurring from 7.3 to 44%, with high prevalence of pulmonary embolism.

Materials and Methods.—To evaluate the prevalence of genetic risk factors for VTE in patients suffering from SVT on both normal and varicose vein, and to understand their role on spreading to deep veins, we studied 107 patients with SVT, without other risk factors. Ultrasound examination was performed, and the presence of FV Leiden, Prothrombin G20210A mutation, and MTHFR C677T mutation was researched.

Results.—In the patients where SVT occurred in normal veins, the presence of FV Leiden was 26.3% of the non-spreading and 60% of the spreading to deep veins SVT; Prothrombin mutation was found in 7.9% of the former case and in 20% of the latter; MTHFR C677T mutation was found respectively in 23.7% and 40%. In the patients with SVT on varicose veins, the presence of these factors was less evident (6.7%, 4.4% and 6.7% respectively), but their prevalence was considerably higher (35.7%, 7.4% and 21.4% respectively) in SVT spreading to deep veins than in non-spreading.

Conclusions.—Our data demonstrate the high prevalence of these mutations, especially FV Leiden and associations, in patients with SVT on normal veins and their role in the progression to deep vein system.

▶ Superficial venous thrombosis (SVT) that occurs in varicose veins is considered of low clinical relevance because of the generally favorable outcome. SVT occurring in so-called healthy veins represents only approximately 25% of all SVT. This type of SVT is generally considered of greater clinical relevance, as it has been associated with various neoplastic conditions. It is also known that SVT occurring in so-called healthy veins can progress into the deep system. Depending on the study, propagation into deep veins ranges approximately from 3% to 15%. It is also known that genetic abnormalities of coagulation can predispose to SVT. Less well studied is whether the presence of a genetic coagulation abnormality occurring in patients with SVT predisposes such patients to progression into the deep system. The article provides guidance as to which patients with SVT should undergo a thrombophilia evaluation. Although patients with SVT occurring in normal veins were previously recognized as having a reasonably high incidence of genetic coagulation abnormalities, this article points out that those patients who have SVT in varicose veins that extends into the deep system have a significant prevalence of genetic abnormalities as well. SVT patients appropriate for thrombophilia workup are those where the SVT occurs in normal veins and those with SVT in varicose veins that extend into the deep system.

G. L. Moneta, MD

10 Thoracic Aorta

Characterization of the inflammatory cells in ascending thoracic aortic aneurysms in patients with Marfan syndrome, familial thoracic aortic aneurysms, and sporadic aneurysms
He R, Guo D-C, Sun W, et al (Univ of Texas Med School at Houston; Baylor College of Medicine, Houston, TX)
J Thorac Cardiovasc Surg 136:922-929, 2008

Objective.—This study sought to characterize the inflammatory infiltrate in ascending thoracic aortic aneurysm in patients with Marfan syndrome, familial thoracic aortic aneurysm, or nonfamilial thoracic aortic aneurysm.

Background.—Thoracic aortic aneurysms are associated with a pathologic lesion termed "medial degeneration," which is described as a noninflammatory lesion. Thoracic aortic aneurysms are a complication of Marfan syndrome and can be inherited in an autosomal dominant manner of familial thoracic aortic aneurysm.

Methods.—Full aortic segments were collected from patients undergoing elective repair with Marfan syndrome (n = 5), familial thoracic aortic aneurysm (n = 6), and thoracic aortic aneurysms (n = 9), along with control aortas (n = 5). Immunohistochemistry staining was performed using antibodies directed against markers of lymphocytes and macrophages. Real-time polymerase chain reaction analysis was performed to quantify the expression level of the T-cell receptor β-chain variable region gene.

Results.—Immunohistochemistry of thoracic aortic aneurysm aortas demonstrated that the media and adventitia from Marfan syndrome, familial thoracic aortic aneurysm, and sporadic cases had increased numbers of T lymphocytes and macrophages when compared with control aortas. The number of T cells and macrophages in the aortic media of the aneurysm correlated inversely with the patient's age at the time of prophylactic surgical repair of the aorta. T-cell receptor profiling indicated a similar clonal nature of the T cells in the aortic wall in a majority of aneurysms, whether the patient had Marfan syndrome, familial thoracic aortic aneurysm, or sporadic disease.

Conclusion.—These results indicate that the infiltration of inflammatory cells contributes to the pathogenesis of thoracic aortic aneurysms. Superantigen-driven stimulation of T lymphocytes in the aortic tissues of patients with thoracic aortic aneurysms may contribute to the initial immune response.

▶ The etiologies of abdominal aortic aneurysms (AAA) and thoracic aortic aneurysms (TAA) are likely not the same. Although some TAAs are degenerative, as are AAAs, there are significant numbers of TAAs that affect a younger population and in which the primary pathology is some genetically influenced degeneration of the medial layer of the arterial wall. Histologically this is represented by loss of smooth muscle cells, increased accumulation of proteoglycans, and diminished numbers of and fragmentation of elastic fibers. Such patients have an inflammatory infiltrate in the aortic wall. In this study, the number of macrophages and inflammatory T-lymphocytes in the aortic media of the samples used in this study negatively correlated with the patient's age. This raises the possibility that inflammatory cells may contribute to disease progression and aortic expansion in patients with TAAs. An alternative explanation is that the inflammatory infiltrates correlate with aortic dilatation and parallel dilatation and corresponding pathologic changes, but in themselves do not contribute to disease progression. However, there was no correlation between aortic diameter and the number of inflammatory cells, implying that the inflammatory infiltrate is not simply a result of the aortic dilatation and irritation of the tissues from enlargement of the aorta. Clearly the biologic activity of the macrophages and T-cells present in the aortic media of patients with TAAs needs to be further characterized. The authors also point out that an immune-mediated aortitis may contribute to the spectrum of aortic diseases, perhaps linking patients with Takayasu's and the various subgroups of degenerative and genetically-related TAAs.

G. L. Moneta, MD

Degree of fusiform dilatation of the proximal descending aorta in type B acute aortic dissection can predict late aortic events
Marui A, Mochizuki T, Koyama T, et al (Akane-Foundation Tsuchiya General Hosp, Hiroshima, Japan; Shin-Katsushika Hosp, Tokyo, Japan; et al)
J Thorac Cardiovasc Surg 134:1163-1170, 2007

Objective.—Predicting the risk factors for late aortic events in patients with type B acute aortic dissection without complications may help to determine a therapeutic strategy for this disorder. We investigated whether late aortic events in type B acute aortic dissection can be predicted accurately by an index that expresses the degree of fusiform dilatation of the proximal descending aorta during the acute phase; this index can be calculated as follows: (maximum diameter of the proximal descending aorta)/ (diameter of the distal aortic arch + diameter of the descending aorta at the pulmonary artery level).

Methods.—Patients with type B acute aortic dissection without complications (n = 141) were retrospectively analyzed to determine the predictors of late aortic events; these include aortic dilatation, rupture, refractory pain, organ ischemia, rapid aortic enlargement, and rapid enlargement of ulcer-like projections.

Results.—The fusiform index in patients with late aortic events (0.59) was higher than that in patients without late aortic events (0.53, $P < .01$). Patients with a higher fusiform index exhibited aortic dilatation earlier than those with a lower fusiform index. By multivariate analysis, we conclude that the predominant independent predictors of late aortic events were a maximum aortic diameter of 40 mm or more, a patent false lumen, and a fusiform index of 0.64 or more (hazard ratios, 3.18, 2.64, and 2.73, respectively). The values of actuarial freedom from aortic events for patients with all 3 predictors at 1, 5, and 10 years were 22%, 17%, and 8%, respectively, whereas the values in those without these predictors were 97%, 94%, and 90%, respectively.

Conclusions.—The degree of fusiform dilatation of the proximal descending aorta, a patent false lumen, and a large aortic diameter can be predominant predictors of late aortic events in patients with type B acute aortic dissection. Patients with these predictors should be recommended to undergo early interventions (surgery or stent-graft implantation) or at least be closely followed up during the chronic phase before such events develop.

▶ This is another recent article trying to predict which patients with type B aortic dissection are most likely to require surgical intervention. It is very clear that most patients with type B aortic dissection are well managed, medically. This type of data should be of interest to those planning intervention trials for acute type B aortic dissection. A positive result, favoring intervention, is more likely if the correct patients are studied.

G. L. Moneta, MD

Outcomes and Survival in Surgical Treatment of Descending Thoracic Aorta With Acute Dissection

Bozinovski J, Coselli JS (The Texas Heart Inst, St. Luke's Episcopal Hosp, Houston; Bayor College of Medicine, Houston)
Ann Thorac Surg 85:965-971, 2008

Background.—Thoracic aortic replacement for acute DeBakey type III aortic dissection is associated with significant morbidity and mortality. We report the outcomes of 76 consecutive patients who underwent surgical repair of the descending thoracic aorta or the thoracoabdominal aorta for acute dissection.

Methods.—During a 16-year period (1989 to 2004), we identified 76 patients who underwent surgery for acute type III aortic dissection. The average patient age was 64.1 ± 12.3 years (range, 36 to 84), and 55 patients (72.4%) were male. Surgical adjuncts included hypothermic circulatory arrest (8 patients), left heart bypass (15 patients), and cerebro-spinal fluid drainage (5 patients). The mean aortic clamp time was 38.4 ± 17.3 minutes. Rupture was present in 17 patients (22.4%).

Results.—There was 1 intraoperative death. Operative mortality was 22.4% (17 patients), including 11 patients (14.5%) who died within 30 days of operation. Five patients (6.6%) had paraplegia, and 15 patients (19.7%) required hemodialysis, 7 temporarily. Cardiac complications occurred in 33 patients (43.4%), 2 patients (2.6%) were returned to the operating room for bleeding, and 10 patients (13.6%) required tracheostomy. The mean hospital stay was 26.0 ± 29.7 days. Rupture was not associated with increased risk of postoperative complications or operative mortality.

Conclusions.—In selected patients with emergent indications, operative intervention with open replacement of the descending thoracic aorta or thoracoabdominal aorta for acute dissection repair can be carried out with respectable mortality, morbidity, and survival rates.

▶ The article highlights why it is best to avoid operation in acute type B dissections. The data come from a center with acknowledged expertise in thoracic aortic surgery. Dr Coselli is among the most experienced thoracic aortic surgeons around. Despite all this, the mortality is high for repair of acute descending thoracic aortic dissections, and morbidity is also very high. Because mortality and morbidity rates were the same for patients with and without rupture, it is important to reassess indications for emergent or urgent open thoracic aortic repair in patients with acute type B dissection. We need better natural history data to know whether continued pain predicts rupture, or if a larger initial diameter of the dissection predicts actual rupture. One can also see this article as providing justification for endovascular repair of ruptured, or severely symptomatic, acute type B dissections. Given the results here, most centers will probably do better with endovascular repair, rather than open repair of an acute type B dissection.

G. L. Moneta, MD

Complicated acute type B aortic dissection: Midterm results of emergency endovascular stent–grafting

Verhoye JP, Miller DC, Sze D, et al (Stanford Univ School of Medicine, CA; et al)
J Thorac Cardiovasc Surg 136:424-430, 2008

Objective.—This study assessed midterm results of emergency endovascular stent–grafting for patients with life-threatening complications of acute type B aortic dissection.

Methods.—Between November 1996 and June 2004, 16 patients with complicated acute type B aortic dissections (mean age 57 years, range 16–88 years) underwent endovascular stent–grafting within 48 hours of presentation. Complications included contained rupture, hemothorax, refractory chest pain, and severe visceral or lower limb ischemia. Stent–graft types included custom-made first-generation endografts and second-generation commercial stent–grafts (Gore Excluder or TAG; W. L. Gore & Associates, Inc, Flagstaff, Ariz.). Follow-up was 100% complete, averaged 36 ± 36 months, and included postprocedural surveillance computed tomographic scans.

Results.—Early mortality was 25% ± 11% (70% confidence limit), with no late deaths. No new neurologic complications occurred. According to the latest scan, 4 patients (25%) had complete thrombosis of the false lumen; the lumen was partially thrombosed in 6 patients (38%). Distal aortic diameter was increased in only 1 patient. Actuarial survival at 1 and 5 years was 73% ± 11%; freedom from treatment failure (including aortic rupture, device fault, reintervention, aortic death, or sudden, unexplained late death) was 67% ± 14% at 5 years.

Conclusion.—With follow-up to 9 years, endovascular stent–grafting for patients with complicated acute type B aortic dissection conferred benefit. Consideration of emergency stent–grafting may improve the dismal outlook for these patients; future refinements in stent–graft design and technology and earlier diagnosis and intervention should be associated with improved results.

▶ Thoracic aortic pathologies are more varied and complex than those of the abdominal aorta. Thus far, stent grafts for use in the thoracic aorta in the United States are approved only for degenerative aneurysms of the descending thoracic aorta. However, as is obvious to everyone, this genie is out of the bottle and there is no getting it back in. I have seen, will continue to see, articles such as this reporting off-label use of thoracic aortic stent grafts. This particular study by very experienced and well-respected practitioners must be taken seriously. Of particular interest is that there were only 16 emergent repairs using stent grafts for life-threatening complications of an acute type-B aortic dissection over a period of 8 years in this high-volume center. Mortality was significant at 25% but likely would have been 100% without treatment and much higher than 25% with open repair. Particularly encouraging is that there were no late deaths, no new neurologic deficits following stent graft repair; there was only 1 proximal endoleak without enlargement of the false lumen, and the fact that late distal aortic enlargement occurred only in 1 of 12 survivors of the procedure. At least at Stanford emergency use of thoracic aortic stent grafts for life-threatening complications of acute type-B aortic dissection "saves lives and is effective to 5 years."

G. L. Moneta, MD

Aortic remodeling after endografting of thoracoabdominal aortic dissection

Rodriguez JA, Olsen DM, Lucas L, et al (Arizona Heart Inst and Hosp, Phoenix)
J Vasc Surg 47:1188-1194, 2008

Purpose.—This study assessed the clinical outcome, morphologic changes, and behavior of acute and chronic type B aortic dissections after endovascular repair and evaluated the extent of dissection and diameter changes in the true (TL), false (FL), and whole lumen (WL) during follow-up.

Methods.—From May 2000 to September 2006, preprocedural and follow-up computed tomography scans were evaluated in 106 patients. Indices of the TL (TLi) and FL (FLi) were calculated at the proximal (p), middle (m), and distal (d) third of the descending thoracic aorta by dividing the TL or FL diameter by the WL. Analyses were by paired t test and χ^2.

Results.—Stent grafts were used to treat 106 patients (mean age, 55 years, 70% men) with acute 59 (55.7%) and chronic 47 (44.3%) lesions. The entry site was successfully covered in 100 patients. The incidences of paraplegia and paresis were 2.8% and 1.0%. Mortality was 7.5% (8 patients), including two intraoperative deaths of contained ruptures. Seven (6.6%) early endoleaks occurred. At a mean follow-up of 15.6 months, TLi improved from 0.45 to 0.88 in the proximal third (p/3), from 0.42 to 0.81 in the middle third (m/3), and from 0.44 to 0.74 in the distal third (d/3), demonstrating expansion of the TL. Two patients had decrease in TL due to endoleak needing reintervention. The FLi decreased from 0.41 to 0.06 in p/3, from 0.44 to 0.10 in the m/3, and from 0.42 to 0.21 in the d/3, indicating FL shrinkage. Changes in the TLi and FLi were statistically significant. The decrease in the WL after repair was statistically significant in the proximal and middle aorta. Fourteen patients (13.2%) had increase in WL; seven required a second intervention. FL thrombosis occurred in 69 (65.1%). During follow-up, 36 (36.9%) patients had no retrograde flow, with complete shrinkage of the FL. The FL completely shrank in 28 patients (26.4%) despite retrograde flow. The FL increased in eight patients (7.5%); five needed reintervention. Thrombosis of FL was statistically significant with acute dissections and when dissection remained above the diaphragm (type IIIA; $P = .001$ and $P = .0133$).

Conclusion.—Remodeling changes were seen when the entry tear was covered. The fate of the FL was determined by persistent antegrade flow and the level of the retrograde flow. Endografting for thoracic type B dissection was successful and promoted positive aortic remodeling changes.

▶ This retrospective study of aortic remodeling after endovascular treatment of acute and chronic aortic dissection represents an analysis of changes over a brief follow-up interval for specific thoracic aortic diameter measurements in a heterogeneous population of patients presenting with this condition. The authors evaluated their experience with 106 patients presenting with acute or chronic type B aortic dissections. In brief, true lumen diameters were noted to increase in size, and false lumen diameters were noted to decrease in size over the follow-up interval (mean 15.6 months).

Most of the patients treated in this study were asymptomatic (n = 64, 60.4%), and of the symptomatic patients (n = 42, 39.6%), 8 patients (7.5%) had malperfusion and 21 (19.8%) had "intractable pain." The authors' approach to the endovascular management of type B dissections remains controversial and, because of the absence of long term follow-up and the relatively small number of patients, fails to convince the reader that this approach should be used for all patients presenting with this condition. The authors are, however, to be commended for their careful analysis of their own results. This evidence can be classified as grade 2B. The optimal treatment of acute and chronic type B aortic dissection remains uncertain, but these data would suggest that positive aortic remodeling could occur in a significant number of patients treated by endovascular means.

B. W. Starnes, MD

Early and midterm results after endovascular stent graft repair of penetrating aortic ulcers
Geisbüsch P, Kotelis D, Weber TF, et al (German Cancer Res Ctr, Heidelberg, Germany)
J Vasc Surg 48:1361-1368, 2008

Purpose.—To present early and midterm results after endovascular stent graft repair of patients with penetrating aortic ulcers (PAU).

Methods.—Between January 1997 and March 2008, a total of 202 patients received thoracic aortic endografting in our institution, 48 patients (32 men, median age 70 years, range, 48-89) with PAU. A retrospective analysis of these patients was performed. Thirty-one patients (65%) showed an acute aortic syndrome (8 contained rupture, 23 symptomatic). Follow-up scheme included postoperative computed tomography angiography prior to discharge, at 3, 6, and 12 months, and yearly thereafter. Mean follow-up was 31.3 months (1.3-112.6).

Results.—Technical success was achieved in 93.7%. Primary clinical success rate was 81.2%. In-hospital mortality was 14.6%. Perioperative mortality was significantly ($P = .036$) higher in patients with acute aortic syndrome compared to asymptomatic patients (22.5% vs 0%). Postoperative complications occurred in 15 patients (31%), including 2 patients with minor strokes and 6, respectively, 5 patients with cardiac and/or respiratory complications. Early endoleaks were observed in 9 patients (19%), late endoleaks in another 2 patients. Reintervention was necessary in 4 out of 48 patients (8.4%). The actuarial survival estimates at 1, 3, and 5 years were 78% ± 6%, 74% ± 7%, and 61% ± 10%, respectively.

There was no aortic-related death during follow-up. Cox regression showed age (hazard ratio [HR]; 1.08, $P = .036$) and a maximum aortic diameter >50 mm (HR, 4.92; $P = .021$) as independent predictors of death.

Conclusion.—Endovascular treatment of penetrating aortic ulcers is associated with a relevant morbidity and mortality rate in frequently highly comorbid patients. Midterm results could prove a sustained treatment success regarding actuarial survival and aortic-related death. Emergencies show a significantly worse outcome, but treatment is still warranted in these symptomatic patients.

▶ Penetrating aortic ulcers (PAU) are still a bit of an enigma. Symptomatic PAUs appear to have a poor natural history with reported rupture rates up to 40%.[1] Less data are available about asymptomatic PAUs, but current literature suggests that approximately 30% to 50% of PAUs will eventually develop a pseudoaneurysm. Because PAUs are generally short and relatively localized lesions (Fig 1 in the original article), they would seem to be ideal for treatment with thoracic endovascular devices. The authors' data suggest that treatment of PAUs is highly likely to be associated with technical success, but symptomatic patients had a relatively high mortality rate, in this series, 20%. Asymptomatic patients, in whom the natural history of PAUs is much less known, can be treated with a very low mortality rate, 0% in this series.

We really don't know what to do with an asymptomatic patient with a thoracic aortic ulcer. Until there is better natural history data, I am reluctant to recommend routine placement of thoracic endografts for asymptomatic PAUs. These authors have decided that they know best, and in their article advocate routine treatment of asymptomatic PAUs with thoracic endograft. I disagree with what is essentially a "ready-fire-aim" approach. We need better studies than this one by more patient-oriented rather than lesion-oriented doctors to determine which patients with asymptomatic PAUs are best treated with thoracic endografts, and which are best observed. This study says we can treat asymptomatic PAUs with thoracic endografts; it does not allow one to conclude they should be treated.

G. L. Moneta, MD

Reference

1. Vilacosta I, Roman JA. Acute Aortic Syndrome. *Heart.* 2001;85:365-368.

Outcome and Quality of Life After Surgical and Endovascular Treatment of Descending Aortic Lesions
Dick F, Hinder D, Immer FF, et al (Univ of Bern, Switzerland)
Ann Thorac Surg 85:1605-1613, 2008

Background.—Thoracic endovascular aortic repair (TEVAR) represents an attractive alternative to open aortic repair (OAR). The aim of this study was to assess outcome and quality of life in patients treated either by TEVAR or OAR for diseased descending thoracic aorta.

Methods.—A post hoc analysis of a prospectively collected consecutive series of 136 patients presenting with surgical diseases of the descending aorta between January 2001 and December 2005 was conducted. Fourteen patients were excluded because of involvement of the ascending aorta. Assessed treatment cohorts were TEVAR (n = 52) and OAR (n = 70). Mean follow-up was 34 ± 18 months. End points were perioperative and late mortality rates and long-term quality of life as assessed by the Short Form Health Survey (SF-36) and Hospital Anxiety and Depression Score questionnaires.

Results.—Mean age was significantly higher in TEVAR patients (69 ± 10 years versus 62 ± 15 years; $p = 0.002$). Perioperative mortality rates were 9% (OAR) and 8% (TEVAR), respectively ($p = 0.254$). Accordingly, cumulative long-term mortality rates were similar in both cohorts. Overall quality-of-life scores were 93 (63–110, OAR) and 83 (60–112, TEVAR), respectively. Normal quality-of-life scores range from 85 to 115. Anxiety and depression scores were not increased after open surgery.

Conclusions.—Thoracic endovascular aortic repair and OAR both provide excellent long-term results in treatment of thoracic aortic disease.

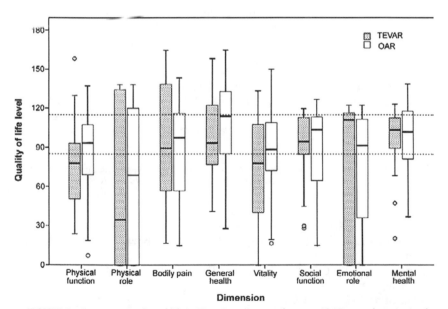

FIGURE 2.—Long-term quality of life in 75 patients 3 years after open (OAR; open boxes) or endovascular (TEVAR; stippled boxes) repair of descending thoracic aortic disease as assessed by the Short Form 36 Health Survey questionnaire. Data are corrected for age and sex. Boxes show the interquartile range (25% to 75%) with the horizontal line in the middle representing the median. Dotted horizontal lines delineate normal range of quality of life (ie, between 85 and 115 points) as assessed in an age-corrected and sex-corrected standard population (n = 8,930). Values less than this range reflect a significant impairment in the assessed aspect. No statistically significant differences were found between treatment cohorts by nonparametric testing. (Reprinted from Dick F, Hinder D, Immer FF, et al. Outcome and quality of life after surgical and endovascular treatment of descending aortic lesions. *Ann Thorac Surg.* 2008;85:1605-1612, with permission from The Society of Thoracic Surgeons.)

Long-term quality of life, however, is reduced after thoracic aortic repair. Interestingly, TEVAR patients did not score higher in overall quality of life despite all advantages of minimized access trauma. Similarly, anxiety and depression scores are not reduced by TEVAR, possibly reflecting a certain caution against the new technology (Fig 2).

▶ The results of this study are a bit surprising. It is one of the first to assess quality of life following either open or endovascular thoracic aortic repair. The patients were not randomized and the demographics of the thoracic endo-vascular aortic repair (TEVAR) versus open aortic repair (OAR) groups suggest a selection bias favoring entry into the TEVAR arm for patients > 65 years of age and for those with disease confined to the thorax and those presenting with an emergency situation. These differences in the baseline characteristics of the patients led the authors to compare their quality of life (QoL) results with an age- and sex-adjusted standard population rather than comparing the OAR patients directly with the TEVAR patients. Surprisingly, QoL scores in the OAR patients were within the normal range. Those of the TEVAR were lower compared with the normalized population (Fig 2). The DREAM trial assessed QoL after endovascular abdominal aortic aneurysm repair and also found poor long-term QoL after endovascular abdominal aortic aneurysm repair.[1] We do not know if the patients in the current study treated with TEVAR and OAR had similar preoperative QoL scores, and there may be some selection bias, in that patients with higher levels of pre-existing depression and anxiety may be offered the less invasive procedure. One thing is becoming increasingly clear: While TEVAR clearly has some advantages with respect to open thoracic aortic repair, underlying comorbidities in patients with thoracic aortic disease make it rare to truly hit a "home run" in patients with thoracic aortic pathology.

G. L. Moneta, MD

Reference

1. Blankensteijn JD, de Jong SE, Prinssen M, et al. Two-year outcomes after conventional or endovascular repair of abdominal aortic aneurysms. *N Engl J Med.* 2005; 352:2398-2405.

Population-based outcomes of open descending thoracic aortic aneurysm repair
Schermerhorn ML, Giles KA, Hamdan AD, et al (Beth Israel Deaconess Med Ctr, Boston, MA)
J Vasc Surg 48:821-827, 2008

Objective.—To evaluate national outcomes after open repair of descending thoracic aortic aneurysm (DTA).

Methods.—The DTA repairs were identified from the NIS database from 1988-2003 by ICD9 codes for thoracic vascular resection and replacement (38.45) and a diagnosis of intact (441.1) or ruptured

(441.2) thoracic aortic aneurysm; excluding thoraco-abdominal aneurysm, abdominal aortic aneurysm repair, cardioplegia, hypothermia, cardiac surgery, or aorta to carotid or subclavian bypass. Demographics and comorbidities were noted. Outcomes included in-hospital mortality, length of stay, and complications. Annual hospital surgical volume terciles (high, medium, and low) were quantified for the series and patients assigned accordingly. Outcomes were compared between intact and ruptured aneurysm characteristics as well as annual hospital volume. Predictors of peri-operative mortality were analyzed by multivariate logistic regression.

Results.—A total of 2549 DTA repairs were identified (1976 intact, 573 ruptured). Mortality was 18% overall; 10% for intact (age <65 6.2%, 65-74 11.3%, ≥75 17.6%, $P < .001$), 45% for ruptured (age <65 33.3%, 65-74 47.1%, ≥75 52.4%, $P < .001$). Mortality decreased over the 15-year time-period ($P < .0001$). Mortality after intact repair was lower at a high volume hospital (HVH) (8%) than a low volume hospital (LVH) (13%) or medium volume hospital (MVH) (12%). Hospital volume tercile did not predict rupture mortality. Complications after intact DTA repair were coded in 42%; including respiratory (13%), cardiac (11%), acute renal failure (8%), stroke (3%), and neurologic (non-stroke) (2%). Complications were coded in 49% after ruptured DTA repair including respiratory (13%), cardiac (13%), acute renal failure (20%), stroke (3%), and neuro (non-stroke) (2%). Predictors of mortality (for all DTA repairs) were (odd ratio [OR], 95% confidence interval [CI]): age 65-74 vs age <65 (1.8, 1.4-2.4), age ≥75 vs age <65 (2.7, 2.0-3.6), rupture (6.3, 5.1-7.9), and LVH or MVH vs HVH (1.3, 1.1-1.7).

Conclusion.—Mortality after open repair of DTA is high and complications are common. Mortality is dependent upon age, rupture status, and hospital surgical volume. Results of endovascular DTA repair should be compared using similar population-based data.

▶ These authors identified nationwide trends in repair of these complex aneurysms and compared the results with the few comprehensive reports from selected centers of excellence. Their findings were not surprising per se, but reinforced the concept that hospital surgical volume will influence the results. The authors acknowledge the limitations associated with use of the nationwide database, in particular the potential influence of coding variability among institutions, limiting their ability to accurately identify comorbid conditions, complications, and possibly the primary diagnoses and procedures.

M. T. Watkins, MD

Pivotal results of the Medtronic Vascular Talent Thoracic Stent Graft System: The VALOR Trial

Fairman RM, Criado F, Farber M, et al (Hosp of the Univ of Pennsylvania, Philadelphia, PA; Union Memorial Hosp, Baltimore, MD; Univ of North Carolina, Chapel Hill, NC; et al)
J Vasc Surg 48:546-554, 2008

Objective.—This report summarizes the 30-day and 12-month results of endovascular treatment using the Medtronic Vascular Talent Thoracic Stent Graft System (Medtronic Vascular, Santa Rosa, Calif) for patients with thoracic aortic aneurysms (TAA) who are considered candidates for open surgical repair.

Methods.—The study was a prospective, nonrandomized, multicenter, pivotal trial conducted at 38 sites. Enrollment occurred between December 2003 and June 2005. Standard follow-up interval examinations were prescribed at 1 month, 6 months, 1 year, and annually thereafter. These endovascular results were compared with retrospective open surgical data from three centers of excellence.

Results.—The Evaluation of the Medtronic Vascular Talent Thoracic Stent Graft System for the Treatment of Thoracic Aortic Aneurysms (VALOR) trial enrolled 195 patients, and 189 were identified as retrospective open surgical subjects. Compared with the open surgery group, the VALOR test group had similar age and sex distributions, but had a smaller TAA size. Patients received a mean number of 2.7 ± 1.3 stent graft components. The diameters of 25% of the proximal stent graft components implanted were <26 mm or >40 mm. Left subclavian artery revascularization was performed before the initial stent graft procedure in 5.2% of patients. Iliac conduits were used in 21.1% of patients. In 33.5% of patients, the bare spring segment of the most proximally implanted device was in zones 1 or 2 of the aortic arch. In 194 patients (99.5%), vessel access and stent graft deployment were successful at the intended site. The 30-day VALOR results included perioperative mortality, 2.1%; major adverse advents, 41%; incidence of paraplegia, 1.5%; paraparesis, 7.2%; and stroke, 3.6%. The 12-month VALOR results included all-cause mortality, 16.1%; aneurysm-related mortality, 3.1%; conversion to open surgery, 0.5%; target aneurysm rupture, 0.5%; stent graft migration >10 mm, 3.9%; endoleak (12.2%), stent graft patency, 100%; stable or decreasing aneurysm diameter, 91.5%; and loss of stent graft integrity, four patients. No deployment-related events or perforation of the aorta by a graft component occurred. The Talent Thoracic Stent Graft showed statistically superior performance with respect to acute procedural outcomes ($P < .001$), 30-day major adverse events (41% vs 84.4%, $P < .001$), perioperative mortality (2% vs 8%, $P < .01$), and 12-month aneurysm-related mortality (3.1% vs 11.6%, $P < .002$) vs open surgery.

Conclusions.—The pivotal VALOR 12-month trial results demonstrate that the Medtronic Talent Thoracic Stent Graft System is a safe and effective endovascular therapy as an alternative to open surgery in patients with TAA who were considered candidates for open surgical repair.

▶ The Talent Thoracic Stent Graft System is Medtronic's entry into the competition for the thoracic aortic endograft market. Results are reasonably compatible with the already approved Gore TAG device. The Talent system offers wider ranges of available sizes than the Gore system. Of the patients in this study, 25% had grafts implanted with diameters < 24 mm or > 40 mm. The largest size grafts require larger introducing systems. Most of the delivery systems in this study were 24 or 25 French. Iliac artery conduits were required in 21% of the cases. The Talent system also has shorter available components necessitating a mean of 2.7 ± 1.3 devices per patient treated (range, 1-7 devices). There were, however, no type 3 (junctional) endoleaks detected at 12 months of follow-up. The device has a bare-spring segment proximally with nearly one third of the devices being implanted such that the bare-spring segment traversed the left subclavian or left common carotid artery. There were no strokes associated with the bare-spring segment residing in zone 1 or zone 2 of the aorta. Overall, the graft appears to be reasonably safe and effective for the limited follow-up currently available.

G. L. Moneta, MD

Hybrid procedures for thoracoabdominal aortic aneurysms and chronic aortic dissections – A single center experience in 28 patients
Böckler D, Kotelis D, Geisbüsch P, et al (Ruprecht-Karls Univ, Heidelberg, Germany; German Cancer Ctr, Heidelberg)
J Vasc Surg 47:724-732, 2008

Objective.—We report our 6-year experience with the visceral hybrid procedure for high-risk patients with thoracoabdominal aortic aneurysms (TAAA) and chronic expanding aortic dissections (CEAD).

Methods.—Hybrid procedure includes debranching of the visceral and renal arteries followed by endovascular exclusion of the aneurysm. A series of 28 patients (20 male, mean age 66 years) were treated between January 2001 and July 2007. Sixteen patients had TAAAs type I-III, one type IV, four thoracoabdominal placque ruptures, and seven patients CEAD. Patients were treated for asymptomatic, symptomatic, and ruptured aortic pathologies in 20, and 4 patients, respectively. Two patients had Marfan's syndrome; 61% had previous infrarenal aortic surgery. The infrarenal aorta was the distal landing zone in 70%. In elective cases, simultaneous approach (n = 9, group I) and staged approach (n = 11, group II) were performed. Mean follow-up is 22 months (range 0.1-78).

Results.—Primary technical success was achieved in 89%. All stent grafts were implanted in the entire thoracoabdominal aorta. Additionally, three patients had previous complete arch vessel revascularization. Left subclavian artery was intentionally covered in three patients (11%). Thirty-day mortality rate was 14.3% (4/28). One patient had a rupture before the staged endovascular procedure and died. Overall survival rate at 3 years was 70%, in group I 80%, and in group II 60% (P = .234). Type I endoleak rate was 8%. Permanent paraplegia rate was 11%. Three patients required long-term dialysis (11%). Peripheral graft occlusion rate was 11% at 30 days. Gut infarction with consecutive bowel resection occurred in two patients. There was no significant difference between group I and II regarding paraplegia and complications.

Conclusions.—Early results of visceral hybrid repair for high-risk patients with complex and extended TAAAs and CEADs are encouraging in a selected group of high risk patients in whom open repair is hazardous and branched endografts are not yet optional.

▶ It seems that every couple of months someone else presents their little puddle of patients that are treated using the so-called hybrid approach to the thoracoabdominal aorta. This is one of the larger series, and the article is well written and illustrated. The message, however, is the same as previous articles. These procedures are possible and, given the patient population, have acceptable, although reasonably high, morbidity and mortality rates. It is, however, not possible to compare hybrid and standard approaches with thoracoabdominal aorta repair. The patients are too different, and the number of patients treated with the hybrid approach was relatively small. I don't think this approach shows replace standard thoracoabdominal repair in a standard or good risk patient. I also don't think this approach should be adopted by surgeons wishing to dabble on the fringes of thoracoabdominal aortic surgery.

G. L. Moneta, MD

Visceral aortic patch aneurysm after thoracoabdominal aortic repair: Conventional vs hybrid treatment

Tshomba Y, Bertoglio L, Marone EM, et al (Università Vita-Salute San Raffaele, Milan, Italy)
J Vasc Surg 48:1083-1091, 2008

Objective.—Visceral aortic patch (VAP) aneurysm repair following thoracoabdominal aortic aneurysm (TAAA) open treatment carries high morbidity and mortality rates. The aim of this study is to compare the outcomes of our series of patients who underwent redo VAP aneurysm open surgery (conventional group) with a selected group of high-risk patients who underwent, in the same time period from 2001-2007, an alternative hybrid surgical and endovascular approach (hybrid group).

Methods.—Conventional group: Twelve patients (11 males, median age 71.5 years, range, 65 to 77 years) underwent VAP aneurysm (median maximum diameter 62 mm, range, 52 to 75 mm) repair with re-inclusion technique via redo thoracophrenolaparotomy or bilateral subcostal laparotomy. Reimplantation of a single undersized VAP or separate revascularization of one or more visceral arteries was performed. *Hybrid group*: Seven patients (5 males, median age 70 years, range, 63 to 78 years) defined as at high risk for conventional surgery having American Society of Anesthesiology (ASA) class 3 or 4 associated with a preoperative forced expiratory volume in 1 second (FEV1) <50% or an ejection fraction <40%, underwent VAP aneurysm (median maximum diameter 73 mm, range, 62 to 84 mm) repair via median laparotomy, visceral arteries rerouting, and VAP aneurysm exclusion using commercially available thoracic aortic endografts.

Results.—Conventional group: Perioperative mortality was 16.7% and major morbidity 33.3%. One perioperative anuria was successfully treated with bilateral renal artery stenting. No paraplegia or paraparesis were observed. At a median follow-up of 2.3 years (range, 1.6-7 years), we observed one case of peri-graft fluid collection with sepsis at postoperative day 46 requiring surgical drainage and prolonged antibiotic therapy and one case of renal failure at day 68 requiring permanent hemodialysis. *Hybrid group:* perioperative mortality was 14.3% and major morbidity 28.6% with one case of transient delayed paraplegia. At a median follow-up of 1.9 years (range, 0.3-6.8 years), we observed one case of late pancreatitis (46 days postoperatively) resolved with pharmacologic treatment and one death due to an acute visceral grafts thrombosis (78 days postoperatively). We did not observe other procedure-related deaths or complications, VAP aneurysm growth, endoleak, and endograft migration.

*Conclusion.—*Hybrid repair is clearly a feasible alternative to simple observation for patients unfit for redo VAP aneurysm open surgery.

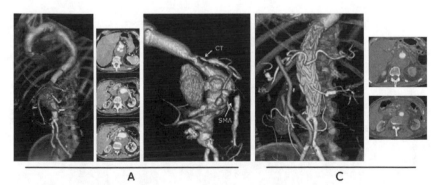

A   C

FIGURE 2.—A, Preoperative angioCT of a patient with previous type III thoracoabdominal aortic aneurysm (TAAA) open repair with a 79 mm VAP aneurysm. Please note the complete displacement of visceral arteries origin with a stenosis at the origin of the celiac trunk (CT) and the superior mesenteric artery (SMA). C, Postoperative CT scan demonstrates complete exclusion with a Valiant stent-graft (blue) of the VAP aneurysm without endoleak and patency of the retrograde revascularization of visceral arteries (red). For interpretation of the references to color in this figure legend, the reader is referred to web version of this article. (Reprinted from Tshomba Y, Bertoglio L, Marone EM, et al. Visceral aortic patch aneurysm after thoracoabdominal aortic repair: conventional vs hybrid treatment. *J Vasc Surg.* 2008;48:1083-1091, with permission from the Society for Vascular Surgery.)

However, despite our promising early results, new mid-term specific procedure-related complications have been observed and a widespread use of this technique should be currently limited until longer-term follow-up is available (Fig 2A and C).

▶ A complication of open thoracoabdominal aneurysm repair that employs a visceral artery inclusion patch is subsequent aneurysmal dilation of the patch. Traditionally, aneurysms of the visceral aortic patch following thoracoabdominal aneurysm repair have been repaired with a redo of the inclusion patch. Recently, a few reports in the literature have begun to appear where visceral aortic patch aneurysms (VAPs) are subject to repair with a hybrid approach similar to the hybrid approach for repair of primary thoracoabdominal aneurysms. The hybrid technique for repair of VAPs is appealing (Fig 2A and C). It would seem a procedure that does not involve clamping of the aorta and has only limited periods of controlled ischemia of the abdominal organs that would provide excellent outcome with little morbidity. Unfortunately, the data reported here also indicate that there is significant morbidity using a hybrid approach to repair VAPs. This relatively large report, the largest so far in the literature, reports 12 cases of conventional repair of VAPs and 7 cases of hybrid repair of VAPs. Although the number of patients is small in each group, morbidity and mortality were still significant. The hybrid approach for repair of VAPs is difficult for the patients but likely less technically demanding for the surgeon. Therefore, ultimately, the likelihood of an acceptable result is probably improved with the hybrid approach for repair of VAPs. Obviously, longer periods of follow-up will be required to determine whether such repairs are durable.

G. L. Moneta, MD

11 Leg Ischemia

Incident Physical Disability in People with Lower Extremity Peripheral Arterial Disease: The Role of Cardiovascular Disease
Brach JS, Solomon C, Naydeck BL, et al (School of Health and Rehabilitation Sciences; Univ of Pittsburgh, PA; Univ of Washington, Seattle; et al)
J Am Geriatr Soc 56:1037-1044, 2008

Objectives.—To evaluate the risk of incident physical disability and the decline in gait speed over a 6-year follow-up associated with a low ankle-arm index (AAI) in older adults.

Design.—Observational cohort study.

Setting.—Forsyth County, North Carolina; Sacramento County, California; Washington County, Maryland; and Allegheny County, Pennsylvania.

Participants.—Four thousand seven hundred five older adults, 58% women and 17.6% black, participating in the Cardiovascular Health Study.

Measurements.—AAI was measured in 1992/93 (baseline). Self-reported mobility, activity of daily living (ADL), and instrumental activity of daily living (IADL) disability and gait speed were recorded at baseline and at 1-year intervals over 6 years of follow-up. Mobility disability was defined as any difficulty walking half a mile and ADL and IADL disability was defined as any difficulty with 11 specific ADL and IADL tasks. Individuals with mobility, ADL, or IADL disability at baseline were excluded from the respective incident disability analyses.

Results.—Lower baseline AAI values were associated with increased risk of mobility disability and ADL/IADL disability. Clinical cardiovascular disease (CVD), diabetes mellitus, and interim CVD events partially explained these associations for mobility disability and clinical CVD and diabetes mellitus partially explained these associations for ADL and IADL disability. Individuals with an AAI less than 0.9 had on average a mean decrease in gait speed of 0.02 m/s per year, or a decline of 0.12 m/s over the 6-year follow-up. Prevalent CVD partly explained this decrease but interim CVD events did not further attenuate it.

Conclusion.—Low AAI serves as marker of future disability risk. Reduction of disability risk in patients with a low AAI should consider cardiovascular comorbidity and the prevention of additional disabling CVD events.

▶ There is an association between peripheral arterial disease (PAD) and function in people with clinically diagnosed PAD. The authors sought to determine, in this study, whether nondisabled community-dwelling older adults with a decreased ankle/brachial index (ABI) were at increased risk for development of new disability. Their conclusion that a low ABI serves as a marker of future disability seems justified by their data. This study has some weaknesses in that disability in the subjects is based primarily on self-reporting. This may both systematically underestimate or overestimate disability, with underestimation of disability being more likely in my opinion. In addition, most of the patients in this study had mild PAD, and the results likely cannot be applied to patients with more severe decreases of the ABI. Nevertheless, it does appear that asymptomatic PAD, although a well-recognized risk for death from cardiovascular disease, is also a significant risk factor for future disability in asymptomatic patients with detectable PAD on the basis of a lowered ABI.

G. L. Moneta, MD

Asymptomatic Peripheral Arterial Disease Is Associated With More Adverse Lower Extremity Characteristics Than Intermittent Claudication
McDermott MM, Guralnik JM, Ferrucci L, et al (Northwestern Univ, Chicago, IL; Natl Inst on Aging, Bethesda, MD; et al)
Circulation 117:2484-2491, 2008

Background.—This study assessed functional performance, calf muscle characteristics, peripheral nerve function, and quality of life in asymptomatic persons with peripheral arterial disease (PAD).

Methods and Results.—PAD participants (n=465) had an ankle brachial index <0.90. Non-PAD participants (n=292) had an ankle brachial index of 0.90 to 1.30. PAD participants were categorized into leg symptom groups including intermittent claudication (n=215) and always asymptomatic (participants who never experienced exertional leg pain, even during the 6-minute walk; n=72). Calf muscle was measured with computed tomography. Analyses were adjusted for age, sex, race, ankle brachial index, comorbidities, and other confounders. Compared with participants with intermittent claudication, always asymptomatic PAD participants had smaller calf muscle area (4935 versus 5592 mm^2; $P<0.001$), higher calf muscle percent fat (16.10% versus 9.45%; $P<0.001$), poorer 6-minute walk performance (966 versus 1129 ft; $P=0.0002$), slower usual-paced walking speed ($P=0.0019$), slower fast-paced walking speed ($P<0.001$), and a poorer Short-Form 36 Physical Functioning score ($P=0.016$). Compared with an age-matched, sedentary, non-PAD cohort, always asymptomatic PAD participants had smaller calf muscle area (5061 versus 5895 mm^2; $P=0.009$), poorer 6-minute walk performance (1126 versus 1452 ft; $P<0.001$), and poorer Walking Impairment Questionnaire speed scores (40.87 versus 57.78; $P=0.001$).

Conclusions.—Persons with PAD who never experience exertional leg symptoms have poorer functional performance, poorer quality of life, and more adverse calf muscle characteristics compared with persons with intermittent claudication and a sedentary, asymptomatic, age-matched group of non-PAD persons.

▶ The asymptomatic patient with peripheral arterial disease (PAD) is coming under increasing scrutiny. Dr McDermott and her group from Northwestern University are the undisputed leaders in this field. Their research is always well analyzed and well presented, although occasionally a bit repetitive. This study, however, breaks new ground in examining anatomic characteristics of subgroups of patients with PAD. The study does have a number of limitations that are acknowledged by the authors. These include the fact that most of the patients were recruited not from the community at large but from vascular laboratories. This makes generalization of the data to a community setting uncertain. The large majority of patients approached to be in the study declined, and we do not know how these individuals compared with those who consented to be in the study. The data are also cross sectional; therefore, any associations between variables cannot be construed as casual but rather as mere associations with uncertain natural histories. Nevertheless, isn't it fascinating that patients with always asymptomatic PAD have quantifiable adverse calf muscle characteristics compared with sedentary, asymptomatic age-matched non-PAD subjects and symptomatic PAD subjects? We can always count on Dr McDermott's research to be both interesting and a bit controversial. This undoubtedly is only the first of a number of studies that will be forthcoming from this group on the consequences of always-symptomatic PAD.

G. L. Moneta, MD

Risk attitudes to treatment among patients with severe intermittent claudication
Letterstål A, Forsberg C, Olofsson P, et al (Karolinska Inst, Sweden)
J Vasc Surg 47:988-994, 2008

Objectives.—To determine claudication patients' risk attitude to invasive treatment and whether this treatment is cost effective.

Methods.—Quality of life and health state utility status of 50 consecutive patients with severe intermittent claudication was assessed and compared with ankle-brachial pressure index values (ABPI) and results from treadmill tests before and after endovascular or open revascularization. Health utility scores were then calculated and used in a cost-utility analysis.

Results.—Before surgery, patients were assigned a utility score of 0.51 (EQ-5D index) for their disease, and the standard gamble (SG) and time trade-off (TTO) median scores were 0.88 and 0.70, respectively. Before treatment, a weak correlation ($r = 0.43$, $P < .001$) between having a high risk perception of treatment and patients' walking distance were observed, where patients able to walk short distances accepted a higher risk. After treatment, ABI ($P = .003$) and walking distance ($P = .002$) improved significantly as well the physical components of the quality of life instruments ($P < .001$). The surgical treatment generated an improvement in quality of life expressed in QALYs equivalent to 0.17. With an estimated survival of 5 years, it adds up to a value of 0.85, corresponding to a sum of 51,000 US$ gained.

Conclusions.—Patients with severe intermittent claudication are risk-seeking when it comes to surgical treatment and their risk attitude is correlated to their walking ability and quality of life. The incremental QALYs gained by treatment are achieved at a reasonable cost and revascularization appears to be cost effective.

▶ Using quality of life and health state utility assessment, patients are seemingly more willing to accept risk if benefit can be achieved with direct correlation to walking ability and quality of life. While it may be easier for patients with severe claudication to perceive benefit because they can better relate to the disability caused by their claudication, perception of risk is more difficult to determine because patients may not have had direct experience with the specific risks. Therefore, patients may be more willing to accept these perceived risks based on the more concrete anticipation of benefit. As vascular specialists, we should not only present a balanced perspective of benefit and risk before treatment for severe claudication, but we should also consider patients' perception of these benefits and risks in our clinical decision making and informed patient discussions.

M. A. Passman, MD

Treadmill Exercise and Resistance Training in Patients With Peripheral Arterial Disease With and Without Intermittent Claudication: A Randomized Controlled Trial
McDermott MM, Ades P, Guralnik JM, et al (Northwestern Univ Feinberg School of Medicine, Chicago, IL; Univ of Vermont, Burlington; Laboratory of Epidemiology, Demography, and Biometry, Bethesda, MD; et al)
JAMA 301:165-174, 2009

Context.—Neither supervised treadmill exercise nor strength training for patients with peripheral arterial disease (PAD) without intermittent claudication have been established as beneficial.

Objective.—To determine whether supervised treadmill exercise or lower extremity resistance training improve functional performance of patients with PAD with or without claudication.

Design, Setting, and Participants.—Randomized controlled clinical trial performed at an urban academic medical center between April 1, 2004, and August 8, 2008, involving 156 patients with PAD who were randomly assigned to supervised treadmill exercise, to lower extremity resistance training, or to a control group.

Main Outcome Measures.—Six-minute walk performance and the short physical performance battery. Secondary outcomes were brachial artery flow-mediated dilation, treadmill walking performance, the Walking Impairment Questionnaire, and the 36-Item Short Form Health Survey physical functioning (SF-36 PF) score.

Results.—For the 6-minute walk, those in the supervised treadmill exercise group increased their distance walked by 35.9 m (95% confidence interval [CI], 15.3-56.5 m; $P < .001$) compared with the control group, whereas those in the resistance training group increased their distance walked by 12.4 m (95% CI, -8.42 to 33.3 m; $P = .24$) compared with the control group. Neither exercise group improved its short physical performance battery scores. For brachial artery flow-mediated dilation, those in the treadmill group had a mean improvement of 1.53% (95% CI, 0.35%-2.70%; $P = .02$) compared with the control group. The treadmill group had greater increases in maximal treadmill walking time (3.44 minutes; 95% CI, 2.05-4.84 minutes; $P < .001$); walking impairment distance score (10.7; 95% CI, 1.56-19.9; $P = .02$); and SF-36 PF score (7.5; 95% CI, 0.00-15.0; $P = .02$) than the control group. The resistance training group had greater increases in maximal treadmill walking time (1.90 minutes; 95% CI, 0.49-3.31 minutes; $P = .009$); walking impairment scores for distance (6.92; 95% CI, 1.07-12.8; $P = .02$) and stair climbing (10.4; 95% CI, 0.00-20.8; $P = .03$); and SF-36 PF score (7.5; 95% CI, 0.0-15.0; $P = .04$) than the control group.

Conclusions.—Supervised treadmill training improved 6-minute walk performance, treadmill walking performance, brachial artery flow-mediated dilation, and quality of life but did not improve the short physical performance battery scores of PAD participants with and without intermittent claudication. Lower extremity resistance training improved functional performance measured by treadmill walking, quality of life, and stair climbing ability.

Trial Registration.—clinicaltrials.gov Identifier: NCT00106327.

▶ It is known that treadmill exercise training under supervised conditions improves walking performance in patients with peripheral arterial disease (PAD) and intermittent claudication. The effect of treadmill training on patients with PAD who do not have symptoms of claudication is unknown. Also, it is unknown whether lower extremity resistance (strength) training in patients with PAD provides additional benefits. It is known that adults with PAD have smaller calf muscle area and diminished strength of their legs than those patients without PAD, and that these muscle characteristics are associated with greater functional impairment. This randomized trial was designed to address 2 questions. The first was to determine whether supervised exercise training on a treadmill improved functional performance in patients with PAD with and without classic symptoms of claudication. The second objective was to determine whether lower extremity strength training improved functional performance in patients with PAD with and without symptoms of claudication.

The study indicated that patients with PAD without symptoms of claudication should be treated with supervised treadmill exercise to improve function and, as suggested by improvements in brachial artery flow-mediated dilatation, improve underlying endothelial dysfunction that may contribute to atherosclerosis. Supervised treadmill exercise produces greater increases in 6-minute walk performance than resistance training. Resistance training, however, also produced potentially clinical improvements on quality-of-life measures and stair-climbing ability. In effect, it is becoming increasingly clear that patients with PAD, whether or not they are symptomatic, should be treated essentially as low level, deconditioned athletes. Benefits can be measured from both resistance and nonresistance training that may, over time, reduce the accelerated functional decline associated with PAD.

G. L. Moneta, MD

Functional assessment at the buttock level of the effect of aortobifemoral bypass surgery
Jaquinandi V, Picquet J, Saumet J-L, et al (Université d'Angers, France; Univ Hosp of Angers, France; et al)
Ann Surg 247:869-876, 2008

Background.—Little is known about the prevalence of proximal (hip, buttock, lower back) claudication after aortobifemoral bypass (AF2B) grafting and its hemodynamic effects at the buttock level.

Methods.—Forty-eight patients performed a treadmill test before and within 6 months after AF2B. The San Diego Claudication Questionnaire and the chest-corrected decrease from rest of transcutaneous oxygen pressure on buttocks were used to study exercise-induced proximal claudication and regional pelvic blood flow impairment. A decrease from rest of transcutaneous oxygen pressure value <-15 mm Hg was used to indicate regional blood flow impairment (RBFI).

Results.—Patients had the following characteristics: 39 were men and 9 were women, 60 ± 9 years, lowest ankle-to-brachial index (ABI) of 0.55 ± 0.18 and maximal walking distance (MWD) on treadmill of 188 ± 192 m at inclusion. ABI and MWD were significantly improved after surgery at 0.83 ± 0.19 and 518 ± 359 m ($P < 0.0001$). Unilateral or bilateral RBFI at the buttocks was found in 39 versus 29 patients before and after AF2B, respectively. Proximal claudication with underlying RBFI on one or both sides on treadmill were observed in 29 patients before AF2B, and in 9 of 26 (41%) versus 6 of 22 (23%) patients in end-to-end versus end-to-side proximal aorto-graft anastomosis of the AF2B, respectively ($P < 0.05$).

Conclusion.—A significant increase in MWD and ABI, but little improvement of proximal perfusion is observed after surgery, a finding that is expected from the absence of hypogastric artery revascularization. The prevalence of proximal claudication and proximal blood flow impairment is higher in case of end-to-end when compared with end-to-side proximal aorto-graft anastomosis, confirming the role of collaterals such as lumbar arteries in the buttock circulation during exercise in patients suffering from peripheral arterial disease. Proximal claudication on treadmill early after surgery affects almost one third of the patients and must not be underestimated among patients receiving AF2B. Attempts at hypogastric artery revascularization, if possible, might be preferable to decrease the risk of proximal claudication after AF2B.

▶ There is little known about proximal claudication following aortobifemoral bypass grafting. Only a few studies have focused on the prevalence of proximal (hip, buttock, lower back) claudication after surgical repair for aortoiliac occlusive disease. Even when buttock claudication is reported, objective measurements for assessment of arterial insufficiency in the hypogastric territory have been rarely presented. The use of such objective measurements to determine reasonable pelvic blood flow impairment in patients following aortobifemoral bypass grafting is what makes this study unique and interesting. It was not surprising that aortobifemoral bypass grafting did not uniformly improve thigh and buttock claudication. After all, the hypogastric arteries are generally not revascularized in these procedures. It is important for physicians to realize that claudication may not completely improve and their patients should understand this before undergoing aortofemoral grafting. The authors' suggestion, that when technically possible, end-to-side rather than end-to-end aortic anastomoses should be used to maximize pelvic blood flow, does seem reasonable.

G. L. Moneta, MD

Long-term results of a multicenter randomized study on direct versus crossover bypass for unilateral iliac artery occlusive disease
Ricco J-B, Probst H, on behalf of the French University Surgeons Association (Univ Hosp of Poitiers, France; Univ Hosp, CHUV, Lausanne)
J Vasc Surg 47:45-54, 2008

Objective.—To compare late patency after direct and crossover bypass in good-risk patients with unilateral iliac occlusive disease not amenable to angioplasty.

Methods.—Between May 1986 and March 1991, 143 patients with unilateral iliac artery occlusive disease and disabling claudication were randomized into two surgical treatment groups, ie, crossover bypass (n = 74) or direct bypass (n = 69). The size of the patient population was calculated to allow detection of a possible 20% difference in patency in favor of direct bypass with a one-sided alpha risk of 0.05 and a beta risk of 0.10. Patients underwent yearly follow-up examinations using color flow duplex scanning with ankle-brachial systolic pressure index measurement. Digital angiography was performed if hemodynamic abnormalities were noted. Median follow-up was 7.4 years. Primary endpoints were primary patency and assisted primary patency estimated by the

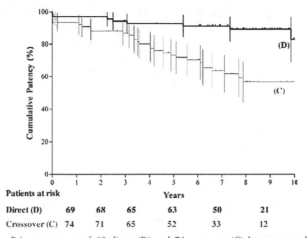

FIGURE 2.—Primary patency of 69 direct (D) and 74 crossover (C) bypass procedures analyzed according to the Kaplan-Meier method. The number of patients at risk in each group at various intervals is indicated at the bottom of the figure. Results are expressed as percentage with 95% confidence interval (95% CI). Primary patency rates at 5 and 10 years were 71.8 ± 10% and 55.6 ± 12%, respectively in the crossover bypass group compared with 92.7 ± 6% and 82.9 ± 13%, respectively in the direct bypass group ($P =.001$, hazard ratio: 4.1 with 95% CI: 1.8 to 6.7). (Reprinted from Ricco J-B, Probst H, Long-term results of a multicenter randomized study on direct versus crossover bypass for unilateral iliac artery occlusive disease. *J Vasc Surg.* 2008;47:45-54, with permission from The Society for Vascular Surgery.)

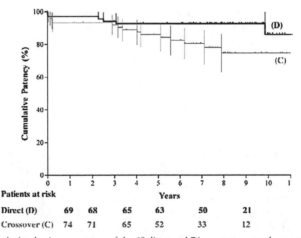

FIGURE 3.—Assisted primary patency of the 69 direct and 74 crossover procedures analyzed according to the Kaplan-Meier method. The number of patients at risk in each group at various intervals is indicated at the bottom of the figure. Results are expressed as percentage with 95% confidence interval (95% CI). Assisted primary patency rates at 5 and 10 years were 84.3% and 74.8%, respectively in the crossover bypass group and 92.7% vs 86.1%, respectively in the direct bypass group ($P =.04$, hazard ratio: 2.5 with 95% CI: 1.1 to 5.8). (Reprinted from Ricco J-B, Probst H, Long-term results of a multicenter randomized study on direct versus crossover bypass for unilateral iliac artery occlusive disease. *J Vasc Surg.* 2008;47:45-54, with permission from The Society for Vascular Surgery.)

Kaplan-Meier method with 95% confidence interval. Secondary endpoints were secondary patency and postoperative mortality and morbidity.

Results.—Cardiovascular risk factors, preoperative symptoms, iliac lesions TASC class (C in 87 [61%] patients and D in 56 [39%] patients), and superficial femoral artery (SFA) run-off were comparable in the two treatment groups. One patient in the direct bypass group died postoperatively. Primary patency at 5 years was higher in the direct bypass group than in the crossover bypass group (92.7 ± 6.1% vs 73.2 ± 10%, $P = .001$). Assisted primary patency and secondary patency at 5 years were also higher after direct bypass than crossover bypass (92.7 ± 6.1% vs 84.3 ± 8.5%, $P = .04$ and 97.0 ± 3.0% vs 89.8 ± 7.1%, $P = .03$, respectively). Patency at 5 years after crossover bypass was significantly higher in patients presenting no or low-grade SFA stenosis than in patients presenting high-grade ($\geq 50\%$) stenosis or occlusion of the SFA (74.0 ± 12% vs 62.5 ± 19%, $P = .04$). In both treatment groups, patency was comparable using polytetrafluoroethylene (PTFE) and polyester grafts. Overall survival was 59.5 ± 12% at 10 years.

Conclusion.—This study showed that late patency was higher after direct bypass than crossover bypass in good-risk patients with unilateral iliac occlusive disease not amenable to angioplasty. Crossover bypass should be reserved for high-risk patients with unilateral iliac occlusion not amenable to percutaneous recanalization (Figs 2 and 3).

▶ This well-conducted randomized study showed that primary patency, assisted primary patency, and secondary patency were significantly better after direct bypass than after femoral-femoral bypass for unilateral iliac occlusive disease not amendable to percutaneous revascularization in reasonable risk patients (Figs 2 and 3). The study incorporated progression of disease in the donor artery as an end of primary patency. This is reasonable, as progression of atherosclerosis in the donor artery is a well-established cause of failure of a femoral-femoral bypass. I think this study will do a great service to vascular surgeons everywhere if it helps to limit the use of femoral-femoral bypass—an operation that seems like a good idea but, in my opinion, has an unacceptable failure and infection rate.

G. L. Moneta, MD

The management of severe aortoiliac occlusive disease: Endovascular therapy rivals open reconstruction
Kashyap VS, Pavkov ML, Bena JF, et al (The Cleveland Clinic, OH)
J Vasc Surg 48:1451-1457, 2008

Objective.—Aortobifemoral bypass (ABF) grafting has been the traditional treatment for extensive aortoiliac occlusive disease (AIOD). This retrospective study compared the outcomes and durability of recanalization, percutaneous transluminal angioplasty, and stenting (R/PTAS) vs ABF for severe AIOD.

Methods.—Between 1998 and 2004, 86 patients (161 limbs) underwent ABF (n = 75) or iliofemoral bypass (n = 11), and 83 patients (127 limbs) underwent R/PTAS. All patients had severe symptomatic AIOD (claudication, 53%; rest pain, 28%; tissue loss, 12%; acute limb ischemia, 7%). The analyses excluded patients treated for aneurysms, extra-anatomic procedures, and endovascular treatment of iliac stenoses. Original angiographic imaging, medical records, and noninvasive testing were reviewed. Kaplan-Meier estimates for patency and survival were calculated and univariate analyses performed. Mortality was verified by the Social Security database.

Results.—The ABF patients were younger than the R/PTAS patients (60 vs 65 years; $P = .003$) and had higher rates of hyperlipidemia ($P = .009$) and smoking ($P < .001$). All other clinical variables, including cardiac status, diabetes, symptoms at presentation, TransAtlantic Inter-Society Consensus stratification, and presence of poor outflow were similar between the two groups. Patients underwent ABF with general anesthesia (96%), often with concomitant treatment of femoral or infrainguinal disease (61% endarterectomy, profundaplasty, or distal bypass). Technical success was universal, with marked improvement in ankle-brachial indices (0.48 to 0.84, $P < .001$). Patients underwent R/PTAS with local anesthesia/sedation (78%), with a 96% technical success rate and similar hemodynamic improvement (0.36 to 0.82, $P < .001$). At the time of R/PTAS, 21% of patients underwent femoral endarterectomy/profundaplasty or bypass (n = 5) for concomitant infrainguinal disease. Limb-based primary patency at 3 years was significantly higher for ABF than for R/PTAS (93% vs 74%, $P = .002$). Secondary patency rates (97% vs 95%), limb salvage (98% vs. 98%), and long-term survival (80% vs 80%) were similar. Diabetes mellitus and the requirement of distal bypass were associated with decreased patency ($P < .001$). Critical limb ischemia at presentation (tissue loss, hazard ratio [HR], 8.1; $P < .001$), poor outflow (HR, 2; $P = .023$), and renal failure (HR, 2.5; $P = .02$) were associated with decreased survival.

Conclusion.—R/PTAS is a suitable, less invasive alternative to ABF for the treatment of severe AIOD. Repair of the concomitant femoral occlusive disease is often needed regardless of open or endovascular treatment. Infrainguinal disease negatively affects the durability of the procedure and patient survival.

▶ Iliac stenoses are treated preferentially using endovascular techniques. Such techniques provide high technical success, low morbidity, and very reasonable long-term durability. This article uses a traditional, but not very scientifically valid, technique of concurrent, but not randomized, controls to try and compare the efficacy of endovascular therapy and open operation for severe aortoiliac occlusive disease. However, as can be seen from the abstract, the patients treated with aortofemoral bypass grafting were not the same as those treated with endovascular techniques. Despite the authors' attempts to justify the comparability of the 2 groups, the use of concurrent, but nonrandomized, controls makes comparisons between the 2 techniques essentially worthless. What is of value here is the fact that both techniques seem to work well in the patients selected for the individual procedure. It is important to note that the excellent results in the patients treated with transluminal techniques may be related, in part, to the authors' willingness to perform open inguinal and infrainguinal procedures such as femoral endarterectomy or infrainguinal bypass concurrently with endovascular treatment of aortoiliac disease.

G. L. Moneta, MD

Female gender and oral anticoagulants are associated with wound complications in lower extremity vein bypass: An analysis of 1404 operations for critical limb ischemia
Nguyen LL, Brahmanandam S, Bandyk DF, et al (Brigham and Women's Hosp, Harvard Med School, Boston, MA)
J Vasc Surg 46:1191-1197, 2007

Background.—Infrainguinal bypass (IB) surgery is an effective means of improving arterial circulation to the lower extremity for patients with critical limb ischemia (CLI). However, wound complications (WC) of the surgical incision following IB can impart significant morbidity.

Methods.—A retrospective analysis of WC from the 1404 patients enrolled in a multicenter clinical trial of vein bypass grafting for CLI was performed. Univariate and multivariable regression models were used to determine WC predictors and associated outcomes, including graft patency, limb salvage, quality of life (QoL), resource utilization (RU), and mortality.

Results.—A total of 543 (39%) patients developed a reported WC within 30 days of surgery, with infections (284, 52%) and hematoma/hemorrhage (121, 22%) being the most common type. Postoperative anticoagulation (odds ratio [OR], 1.554; 95% confidence interval [CI] 1.202 to 2.009; $P = .0008$) and female gender (OR, 1.376; 95% CI, 1.076 to 1.757; $P = .0108$) were independent factors associated with WC. Primary, primary-assisted, and secondary graft patency rates were not influenced by the presence of WC; though, patients with WC were at increased risk for limb loss (hazard ratio [HR], 1.511; 95% CI 1.096 to 2.079; $P = .0116$) and higher mortality (HR, 1.449; 95% CI 1.098 to 1.912; $P = .0089$). WC was not significantly associated with lower QoL at 3 months (4.67 vs 4.79, $P = .1947$) and 12 months (5.02 vs 5.13, $P = .2806$). However, the subset of patients with serious WC (SWC) demonstrated significantly lower QoL at 3 months compared with patients without WC, (4.43 vs 4.79, respectively, $P = .0166$), though this difference was not seen at 12 months (4.94 vs 5.13, $P = .2411$). Patients with WC had higher RU than patients who did not have WC. Mean index length of hospital stay (LOS) was 2.3 days longer, mean cumulative 1-year LOS was 8.1 days longer, and mean number of hospitalizations was 0.5 occurrences greater for patients with WC compared with patients without WC (all $P < .0001$).

Conclusions.—WC is a frequent complication of IB for CLI, associated with increased risk for major amputation, mortality, and greater RU. Further detailed investigation into the link between female gender and oral anticoagulation use with WC may help identify causes of WC and perhaps prevent or lessen their occurrence.

▶ The Prevent III trial continues to be the source of interesting data, applicable to patients undergoing vein bypass for critical lower extremity ischemia. It is not surprising that anticoagulation is associated with increased wound complications; hematomas are never good, but reasons why female gender should increase such a risk is unknown. The authors note that weight was not associated with wound complications, but the distribution of weight may be different in males and females undergoing leg bypass for critical limb ischemia. Women may have more fat, as a percentage of their total body mass, compared with males. The incidence of wound complications in this study (39%) was at the high end of what was previously reported for patients undergoing leg bypass for critical ischemia, and it probably reflects the prospective data collection and the strict definition of wound complication used in the trial. Serious wound complications, however, were only 11%, and only 1 graft became infected with none exposed. Quality of life was not affected at 1 year but was adversely impacted early, postoperatively, by wound complications. Despite this, wound problems remain a vexing problem after leg bypass surgery; however, it must be kept in mind that ischemic wounds require longer to heal, compared with the surgical wounds in patients with critical limb ischemia. Decreasing surgical wound complications is only part of the problem with wound problems in patients with critical limb ischemia.

G. L. Moneta, MD

Factors associated with early failure of infrainguinal lower extremity arterial bypass
Singh N, Sidawy AN, DeZee KJ, et al (Georgetown Univ Hosp, Washington, DC)
J Vasc Surg 47:556-561, 2008

Objectives.—We analyzed the Veterans Affairs (VA) National Surgical Quality Improvement Program (NSQIP), a large clinical database, to investigate which factors, other than technical, were associated with a higher incidence of early graft failure in infrainguinal bypass.

Methods.—Data are prospectively collected in NSQIP from 123 participating VA Medical Centers. All patients from 1995 to 2003 in the NSQIP database who underwent infrainguinal arterial bypass were identified by Current Procedural Terminology (CPT) codes (CPT is a registered trademark of the American Medical Association, Chicago, Ill, Copyright 2007). Data for 30-day graft failure were evaluated by univariate analysis, and multivariate logistic regression was used to control for possible confounders.

Results.—The NSQIP database identified 14,788 patients who underwent infrainguinal lower extremity arterial bypasses during the study period, and 723 acute graft failures (4.9%) occurred. On multivariate analysis, compared with patients aged >70 years, patient ages of <50 and 51 to 60 years were significantly associated with early graft failure (odds ratio [OR], 2.2; 95% confidence interval [CI], 1.6-3.0; $P < .001$; OR, 1.4; 95% CI, 1.2-1.6, $P < .001$; respectively); age range of 61 to 70 years was not significantly associated with early graft failure. African American race was also associated with early graft failure, and diabetes mellitus had a negative association with early graft failure (OR, 1.4; 95% CI, 1.3-1.5; $P < .001$; OR, 0.72; 95% CI, 0.58-0.89; P = .002; respectively). Although smoking was a significant factor for acute graft failure on univariate analysis, it was not significant on multivariate analysis. Multivariate analysis of the type of procedure performed revealed that femoral to popliteal bypass with vein or prosthetic graft was associated with better early graft patency than any of the tibial vessel bypass procedures except for popliteal to tibial bypass with autogenous vein.

Conclusion.—These data suggest that factors other than technique have an effect on the 30-day graft failure rates of infrainguinal bypasses. These results help the vascular surgeon to predict more accurately early bypass failure rates while planning the procedure and counseling patients about its prognosis.

▶ I am beginning to think there are now more articles providing a relatively droll analysis of large multi-institutional databases than there are fleas on a North Carolina dog in August. Articles such as this are interesting in that they can tell us how frequently a procedure is being done and how often certain hard endpoints, such as death or graft failure, are reached within a specified time period. To try and extrapolate explanations for events observed are beyond the attended usage of such databases. Associations can be observed but causation cannot be determined. The observed associations in this article are expected. The observations that young patients, those with African American heritage and nondiabetics have higher early graft failure rates are not surprising in that they have been highlighted in numerous previous reports. It is also not an epiphany to most of us that femoropopliteal bypass does better than femorotibial bypass. I am growing a bit weary of these large database studies. They will, however, undoubtedly continue as long as program committees and journal editors are impressed by large numbers. If you have enough time and a computer, you can now produce high-profile surgical "research" without ever going to the bench or to the operating room!

G. L. Moneta, MD

Disparity in Outcomes of Surgical Revascularization for Limb Salvage: Race and Gender are Synergistic Determinants of Vein Graft Failure and Limb Loss

Nguyen LL, Hevelone N, Rogers SO, et al (Brigham and Women's Hosp, Boston, MA; et al)

Circulation 119:123-130, 2009

Background.—Vein bypass surgery is an effective therapy for athero-sclerotic occlusive disease in the coronary and peripheral circulations; however, long-term results are limited by progressive attrition of graft patency. Failure of vein bypass grafts in patients with critical limb ischemia results in morbidity, limb loss, and additional resource use. Although technical factors are known to be critical to the success of surgical revascularization, patient-specific risk factors are not well defined. In particular, the relationship of race/ethnicity and gender to the outcomes of peripheral bypass surgery has been controversial.

Methods and Results.—We analyzed the Project of Ex Vivo Vein Graft Engineering via Transfection III (PREVENT III) randomized trial database, which included 1404 lower extremity vein graft operations performed exclusively for critical limb ischemia at 83 North American centers. Trial design included intensive ultrasound surveillance of the bypass graft and clinical follow-up to 1 year. Multivariable modeling (Cox proportional hazards and propensity score) was used to examine the relationships of demographic variables to clinical end points, including perioperative (30-day) events and 1-year outcomes (vein graft patency, limb salvage, and patient survival). Final propensity score models adjusted for 16 covariates (including type of institution, technical factors, selected comorbidities, and adjunctive medications) to examine the associations between race, gender, and outcomes. Among the 249 black patients enrolled in PREVENT III, 118 were women and 131 were men. Black men were at increased risk for early graft failure (hazard ratio [HR], 2.832 for 30-day failure; 95% confidence interval [CI], 1.393 to 5.759; $P = 0.0004$), even when the analysis was restricted to exclude high-risk venous conduits. Black patients experienced reduced secondary patency (HR, 1.49; 95% CI, 1.08 to 2.06; $P = 0.016$) and limb salvage (HR, 2.02; 95% CI, 1.27 to 3.20; $P = 0.003$) at 1 year. Propensity score models demonstrate that black women were the most disadvantaged, with an increased risk for loss of graft patency (HR, 2.02 for secondary patency; 95% CI, 1.27 to 3.20; $P = 0.003$) and major amputation (HR, 2.38; 95% CI, 1.18 to 4.83; $P = 0.016$) at 1 year. Perioperative mortality and 1-year mortality were similar across race/gender groups.

Conclusions.—Black race and female gender are risk factors for adverse outcomes after vein bypass surgery for limb salvage. Graft failure and limb loss are more common events in black patients, with black women being a particularly high-risk group. These data suggest the possibility of an altered biological response to vein grafting in this population; however, further studies are needed to determine the mechanisms underlying these observed disparities in outcome.

▶ This article represents another of the many interesting post hoc analyses derived from the Project of Ex Vivo Vein Graft Engineering via Transfection III (PREVENT III) trial. PREVENT III was a multi-center clinical trial of patients undergoing vein bypass for critical limb ischemia.[1] The PREVENT III database represents the largest prospective cohort of surgically treated critical limb ischemic patients. The database includes 1404 lower extremity vein graft operations performed for critical limb ischemia at 83 North American centers. The patients had intensive ultrasound surveillance of the bypass graft and clinical follow-up for up to 1 year. This particular analysis was designed to examine the interactions of race and gender as they affect graft patency, limb salvage, and mortality. It has been previously suggested that African-Americans and women have poorer results with vascular surgery. Therefore, it is not surprising that the study found particularly poor results for African-American women. The authors suggest that the data raise the possibility of an altered response to vein bypass surgery in that particular subgroup. It is certainly not obvious as to what this biologic response would be. Nevertheless, the clinical implication is that African American women undergoing vein graft bypass surgery are a particularly high-risk group that may benefit from very aggressive postoperative surveillance and medical management.

G. L. Moneta, MD

Reference

1. Conte MS, Bandyk DF, Clowes AW, et al. Results of PREVENT III: a multicenter, randomized trial of edifoligide for the prevention of vein graft failure in lower extremity bypass surgery. *J Vasc Surg.* 2006;43:742-751.

Prospective 2-Years Follow-up Quality of Life Study after Infrageniculate Bypass Surgery for Limb Salvage: Lasting Improvements Only in Non-diabetic Patients
Engelhardt M, Bruijnen H, Scharmer C, et al (Military Hosp Ulm, Germany; Zentralklinikum Augsburg, Germany; et al)
Eur J Vasc Endovasc Surg 36:63-70, 2008

Objectives.—To assess health-related quality of life (HRQoL) up to 24 months after successful infrageniculate bypass surgery for limb-threatening ischaemia.

Methods.—89 patients with infrageniculate bypass surgery for limb-salvage were studied. HRQoL was assessed using the Short Form (SF)-36v1 questionnaire before, 6, 12, and 24 months after revascularisation.

Results.—47 patients (53%) with intact limb and functioning graft were assessed after 24 months, 27 patients (30%) died, further 7 required secondary amputation, 3 suffered irremediable graft occlusion, and 4 were lost to follow-up. The 24-months HRQoL-values were significantly improved in 4 domains: physical functioning ($p < 0.01$), bodily pain ($p < 0.01$), mental health ($p = 0.04$), and social functioning ($p = 0.01$). Except for baseline-values, HRQoL remained inferior in diabetics compared to non-diabetics throughout follow-up. Maximum improvement of HRQoL was delayed in diabetics (12 months vs 6 months) and less pronounced. After 24 months non-diabetic patients maintained improvement in 5 domains and diabetic patients only in bodily pain.

Conclusions.—Improvement in HRQoL is sustained for more than 12 months after successful infrageniculate bypass surgery. Therefore, an aggressive approach towards revascularisation seems to be justified from the patient's perspective. However, this benefit in quality of life is less in diabetic patients, despite similar limb-salvage rates.

▶ While improved quality of life seems sustained at 2 years for patients undergoing infrageniculate bypass for chronic limb-threatening ischemia is promising on the surface, these observations should be tempered by the small sample size, lack of a control group, evaluation of time intervals, and quality of life parameters paralleling the excellent bypass graft patency and limb salvage rates reported at 2 years. While the improved quality of life parameters noted at 6 months seem to be maintained at 2 years, most of the impact of bypass operation on quality of life that occurs < 6 months is missed by the study design questionnaire intervals. Furthermore, these reported quality of life outcomes in the absence of a control group including either quality of life in patients with chronic limb ischemia and no revascularization options, and/or those treated with endovascular options, can only be interpreted in that context.

M. A. Passman, MD

Major Lower Extremity Amputation after Multiple Revascularizations: Was It Worth It?

Reed AB, Delvecchio C, Giglia JS (Univ of Cincinnati, OH)
Ann Vasc Surg 22:335-340, 2008

Lower extremity revascularization is often described as excessively lesion-centric, with insufficient focus on the patient. We investigated patients' perspectives of multiple procedures for limb salvage that culminated in major lower extremity amputation. A prospective vascular surgery database was queried from January 2000 to December 2005 for patients who had undergone below-knee (BKA) or above-knee (AKA) amputation after failed lower extremity revascularization. Patients were surveyed via telephone by a vascular nurse regarding thoughts on undergoing multiple procedures for limb salvage, involvement in decision making, functional status (work, meal preparation, shopping, driving), use of prosthesis, and independence. The Social Security Death Index was utilized to verify patient survival. Amputations for infection were excluded. Seventy-eight patients underwent AKA or BKA after failed revascularization. Forty-six patients (59%) were alive at 5 years. Thirteen patients were lost to follow-up, leaving 33 available for survey. A total of 142 lower extremity revascularizations (median = 4/patient) were performed on these patients including 94 surgical bypasses (median = 3/patient) and 48 percutaneous interventions (median =1/patient). Eighty-five percent (28 of 33 patients) of amputees surveyed would do everything to save the leg if faced with a similar scenario, regardless of the number of procedures. Fifty-four percent (18/33) of patients actively used a prosthesis, and 91% (30/33) resided at home. In retrospect, patients are willing to undergo multiple revascularizations—percutaneous or open—to attempt limb salvage even if the eventual result is major amputation. Independence and functional status appear to be obtainable in a majority of patients. Patient-oriented outcomes are necessary to guide revascularization, whether it is by a percutaneous or open technique.

▶ Both lesion-specific and patient-specific outcomes are important in the assessment of treatments for lower extremity arterial occlusive disease. In particular, lower extremity revascularization is often described as lesion centric, with excessive focus on treatment of the lesion and inadequate assessment of patient quality of life. In this study, the authors sought to investigate patients' perspectives of multiple procedures for limb salvage that eventually culminated in a major lower extremity amputation. Their conclusion, that patients are willing to undergo multiple revascularizations in an attempt to salvage a limb even if the eventual result is amputation, fits with my clinical experience. Patients who lose limbs and who have undergone multiple attempts at revascularization are justifiably discouraged, but the possibility of limb salvage is a strong motivator. The weakness of this study is that only survivors who appeared to be doing reasonably well were available for participation in the survey that formed the basis of the authors' conclusions. In addition, only 33 of the 78 patients who underwent above-knee (AK) or below-knee (BK) amputation after failed revascularization were actually surveyed. The attitudes of the patients who were lost to follow-up or who did not survive are crucial to the validity of the authors' conclusion and limit the general applicability of this study.

G. L. Moneta, MD

Preservation for Future Use of the Autologous Saphenous Vein During Femoro-Popliteal Bypass Surgery Is Inexpedient
Dirven M, Scharn DM, Blankensteijn JD, et al (Radboud Univ Med Ctr, Nijmegen, The Netherlands)
Eur J Vasc Endovasc Surg 36:420-423, 2008

Purpose.—To investigate the usefulness of greater saphenous vein preservation for future vascular reconstructions during femoro-popliteal bypass surgery.

Design.—Post-hoc analysis of data acquired in a randomized multi-centre clinical trial comparing two different vascular prostheses (*Clinical-Trials.gov ID: NCT 00523263*).

Patients and methods.—The true frequency of ipsilateral saphenous vein use in subsequent femoro-popliteal and coronary bypass surgery was investigated through case-record analysis with a median follow-up of 60 months in 100 consecutive patients, that received a prosthetic femoro-popliteal bypass between 1996 and 2001.

Results.—An ipsilateral secondary femoro-popliteal bypass was performed in 11 patients (11%) at a mean interval of 34 months (range 1–96). The ipsilateral saphenous vein was applied for these procedures in 8 cases (8%). The cumulative probability of receiving a subsequent bypass was 8% at 3 years and 10% at 5 years follow-up respectively. One patient (1%) underwent CABG at 8 years follow-up with the use of ipsilateral lower leg saphenous vein segments only.

Conclusion.—Preservation of the greater saphenous vein in supragenicular femoro-popliteal bypass surgery is not a valid argument for application of prosthetic material (Fig1).

▶ I could not agree more with the authors' data (Fig 1) and the concluding statement in the abstract. The save-the-vein argument has, seemingly forever,

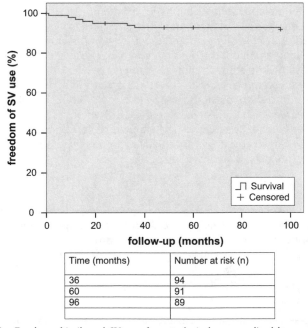

Time (months)	Number at risk (n)
36	94
60	91
96	89

FIGURE 1.—Freedom of ipsilateral SV use after prosthetic femoro-popliteal bypass (Kaplan-Meier analysis). (Reprinted from Dirven M, Scharn DM, Blankensteijn JD, et al. Preservation for future use of the autologous saphenous vein during femoro-popliteal bypass surgery is inexpedient. *Eur J Vasc Endovasc Surg.* 2008;36:420-423, with permission from Elsevier.)

generally been fostered by well-meaning but ill-informed surgeons and, perhaps, now by less well-meaning individuals who are only capable of offering catheter-based therapies for peripheral artery occlusive disease. The subject has been addressed in various other iterations over the years and the conclusions are basically the same—the save-the-vein argument is basically horse byprod-uct (marginally politically correct terminology). Unless it is crystal clear that the ipsilateral saphenous vein will be needed for an additional operation that has already been identified and scheduled, the ipsilateral saphenous vein should be used for the current operation. Conduit quality drives the outcomes of infrainguinal reconstructions. Use the best conduit available for the operation that needs to be done now. Arterial surgery is all about the present and is not about the future. Many of these patients have a very limited future.

G. L. Moneta, MD

Revascularization to an isolated ("blind") popliteal artery segment: A viable procedure for critical limb ischemia
Ballotta E, Da Giau G, Gruppo M, et al (Univ of Padua, School of Medicine, Italy)
Surgery 145:426-434, 2009

Background.—The purpose of this study was to analyze our experience of bypass procedures to an isolated ("blind") popliteal artery segment (IPAS) to revascularize the perigeniculate arteries in patients with critical limb ischemia (CLI), to establish whether such revascularizations could yield acceptable results in terms of patency and limb salvage (LS) rates.

Methods.—Over a decade, 347 above-knee arterial revascularizations were performed in 293 patients and in 51 (14.7%) of these the outflow vessels were the perigeniculate arteries arising from an IPAS, through a reversed saphenous vein or spliced veins ($n = 30$, 58.8%; group I) or poly-tetrafluoroethylene ($n = 21$, 41.2%; group II) prosthetic grafts. Patency, LS, and survival rates were assessed using Kaplan-Meier life-table analysis. A complete follow-up (range, 0.1–10.4 years; mean, 5.6 years) was obtained in 49 patients.

Results.—The IPAS was chosen as the last resort in 39 patients (76.5%) because no other infrapopliteal artery was identified as being available at angiography; in 12 patients (23.5%) it was chosen because of an invasive foot infection or ischemic necrosis overlying the dorsalis pedis or the posterior tibial arteries. The study series was mainly male, with signifi-cantly more younger patients in group I (72 ± 1 years vs 74 ± 5 years, $P = .037$). Group I had a statistically higher incidence of diabetes mellitus (76.6% vs 47.6%, $P = .033$), insulin dependence (56.7% vs 28.6%, $P = .047$) and history of smoking (80% vs 47.6%, $P = .016$) than group II. None of the patients died in the perioperative period. There were 3 early graft failures (2 in group I), prompting 3 major amputations. Kaplan-Meier analysis identified 5-year patency and LS rates of

51.4 ± 9.6% and 90 ± 4.3%, respectively, in the series as a whole, and the 2 groups had comparable 5-year patency, LS and survival rates.

Conclusion.—Revascularizations to an IPAS can be performed with acceptable results in terms of patency and LS rates, even when there is no infrapopliteal runoff vessel. Finding perigeniculate arteries arising from an IPAS with no tibio-peroneal vessel reconstitution at arteriography does not justify a pessimistic attitude to the performance of such revascularizations for LS.

▶ In 1967 Mannick et al reported limb salvage could be achieved in patients with critical limb ischemia with bypass to an isolated popliteal segment. Since that time, qualifications and modifications of the technique have been reported. Veith et al suggested that if the popliteal artery was 7 cm long with significant collateralization, and there was at least 1 patent infrapopliteal runoff artery distally in the calf, that acceptable patency and limb salvage rates could also be achieved with use of a synthetic conduit, particularly when the above-knee popliteal artery served as the anastomotic site.

This article serves to remind us that bypass to an isolated popliteal segment can be a viable alternative in selected patients with critical limb ischemia. It is interesting that polytetrafluoroethylene (PTFE) performed as well as vein grafts in this series, although the patients in this retrospective series were demographically not matched. It should be pointed out that there is a fairly large discrepancy between secondary patency and limb salvage in this series. The authors did not detail the extent of tissue loss present in the patients, only that most of the tissue loss involved only the toes or the forefoot. There are very few hind foot lesions treated in this series. Without greater detail of the degree of ischemic necrosis present, this series does not really justify the use of isolated popliteal segment bypass to treat major foot necrosis or hind foot lesions. Certainly, the relative absence of hind foot lesions in this series suggests some selection of more favorable patients for isolated popliteal segment bypass. The article would have been strengthened by a description of whether or not the authors chose to perform primary amputation in some patients in whom an isolated popliteal segment bypass would have been possible, but was felt imprudent because of the extent of foot necrosis. There is often also much to be learned from the patients who are not treated.

G. L. Moneta, MD

Bypass to the Perigeniculate Collateral Arteries: Mid-term Results
de Latour B, Nourissat G, Duprey A, et al (Service de Chirurgie Cardiovasculaire, Hôpital Nord St Etienne, Cedex, France)
Eur J Vasc Endovasc Surg 35:473-479, 2008

Purpose.—The purpose of this report is to present mid-term results of infrainguinal revascularizations using either the highest genicular artery or medial sural artery as the distal anastomosis site.

Material and Methods.—Between 1996 and 2005, a total of 59 bypass procedures to perigeniculate collateral arteries were performed in 57 patients (14 women, 43 men) with a mean age of 74. Fifty five patients presented with critical ischemia (tissue loss in 28 and rest pain in 27). Four patients presented with intermittent claudication. Mean ankle brachial index was 0.48. The distal anastomosis site was the highest genicular artery in 18 patients, medial sural artery in 37 cases, highest genicular and/or medial sural artery and/or tibial artery in sequential fashion in four cases. The proximal anastomosis was to the common femoral artery in 26 cases and superficial femoral artery in 33.

Results.—There were two deaths during the immediate postoperative period. Mean follow-up duration was 35 months (range 1–108 months). One patient was lost to follow-up. Six patients required major amputation. At 3 years, primary patency was 65 ± 7%, secondary patency was 70 ± 7%, limb salvage and survival rate were 90 ± 4% and 64 ± 7%, respectively.

Conclusion.—Bypass to perigeniculate collateral arteries provides acceptable patency and limb salvage rates.

▶ Bypass to geniculate arteries is seldom performed. The authors' results, however, argue that this procedure should be considered more often. Limb salvage rates were excellent, and the mean ankle/brachial index (ABI) at 3 months, postprocedure, was 0.75 for the entire population. In patients who did not have diabetes, the ABI improved from a mean of 0.38-0.63. The authors indicate that bypass to a geniculate artery can be considered under the following circumstances: (1) The diameter of the geniculate artery is approximately the same as that of the distal leg arteries; (2) There is arteriographic visualization of the whole vessel, with no evidence of distal stenosis or disease; (3) There is good distal runoff to one, or several, lower leg arteries with satisfactory perfusion of the ischemic foot. When vein is limited, this procedure may have advantages for splicing multiple pieces of vein to reach a more distal target or using a prosthetic bypass to a distal tibial artery.

G. L. Moneta, MD

Angioplasty for Diabetic Patients with Failing Bypass Graft or Residual Critical Ischemia after Bypass Graft
Faglia E, Clerici G, Clerissi J, et al (IRCCS Multimedica, Milan, Italy; et al)
Eur J Vasc Endovasc Surg 36:331-338, 2008

Objective.—To evaluate the efficacy of peripheral angioplasty (PTA) in the treatment of diabetic patients with previous peripheral bypass graft and recurrent critical limb ischemia (CLI).

Methods.—Between January and December 2006, 293 diabetic patients presenting with critical limb ischemia (CLI) according to the TASC 2000 criteria were admitted to our footcare centre. Among these patients, 32 of them had previously undergone bypass grafting: femoropopliteal in 26 patients, femoroposterior tibial in 3 patients, femoroperoneal in the remaining 3. All these patients underwent angiography and, whenever possible, a concomitant PTA procedure.

Results.—Six patients presented with stenosis at the distal anastomosis, 2 with stenosis at the proximal anastomosis and in 5 patients both the distal and proximal anastomosis were stenosed. In 12 patients the graft was completely occluded. In 7 patients the graft appeared patent but all the infrapopliteal arteries were occluded. The average time interval between bypass and subsequent hospital admission because of CLI was 6.3 ± 4.2 months for patients with patent grafts and 20.5 ± 12.0 months for those with failing grafts ($p = 0.004$).

A successful PTA was performed in 25 patients (78.1%). In all patients with patent grafts, PTA recanalized one infrapopliteal artery. Recanalization of the graft was obtained in all 13 patients with non-occluded graft. Recanalization of superficial femoral artery occlusion by means of PTA was obtained in 5 out of the 12 patients in whom the graft was completely occluded. Five patients underwent major amputation within 30 days and 3 further patients during the follow-up period. Patients were followed up until December 31 2007, with a mean follow-up of 1.89 ± 0.27 years. Restenosis occurred in 7 (28.0%) of the 25 patients in whom a successful PTA was performed. In 5 of these 7 patients, PTA was repeated successfully. In 2 patients in whom a further PTA was not feasible a major amputation was performed. At the end of the follow-up period the cumulative primary patency rate was 72%, the assisted patency rate was 92%.

Conclusions.—PTA is an effective method for revascularizing secondary obstructions in patients with graft failure (and no possibility of a redo graft). PTA also is effective in at least one subgenicular artery in patients with diabetes with inadequate run-off after femoropopliteal bypass grafting.

▶ The authors are clearly aggressive in using percutaneous techniques in patients with previous, but for various reasons ineffective, infra-inguinal bypass grafts. There are too many categories of patients with too small of numbers in each group to make any definitive statements. However, of interest is the concept of using percutaneous angioplasty of distal vessels as an adjunct to a more proximal bypass graft with a goal of improving progressive late distal disease or coexisting distal disease present at the time of the bypass graft. The latter is perhaps particularly applicable to patients with a limited quantity of optimal vein at the time of the original bypass. Also note that percutaneous angioplasty with short-term success can be performed as a bailout procedure in a few patients with occluded grafts. Whether this is preferable to a new bypass is unknown but should at least be given some consideration, although long-term success, at least in terms of graft patency, will likely be uncommon with such procedures.

G. L. Moneta, MD

The Adjuvant Benefit of Angioplasty in Patients with Mild to Moderate Intermittent Claudication (MIMIC) Managed by Supervised Exercise, Smoking Cessation Advice and Best Medical Therapy: Results from Two Randomised Trials for Stenotic Femoropopliteal and Aortoiliac Arterial Disease

The MIMIC Trial Participants (Imperial College London, UK)

Eur J Vasc Endovasc Surg 36:680-688, 2008

Background.—Uncertainty exists on whether there is adjuvant benefit of percutaneous transluminal angioplasty (PTA) over supervised exercise and best medical therapy in the treatment of intermittent claudication.

Methods.—Patients with symptoms of stable mild to moderate intermittent claudication (MIMIC) were randomised in two multi-centre trials, for femoropopliteal and aortoiliac arterial disease, to receive either PTA or no PTA against a background of supervised exercise and best medical therapy and followed up for 24 months. Initial claudication distance (ICD) and absolute walking distance (AWD) on treadmill were compared between randomised groups adjusting for the corresponding measure at baseline. Secondary outcomes included ankle-brachial pressure index (ABPI) and quality of life.

Findings.—A total of 93 patients were randomised into the femoropopliteal trial (48 into PTA) and 34 into the aortoiliac trial (19 to PTA). The mean (standard deviation, SD) age was 66(9) years for the femoropopliteal trial (63% male) and 63(9) for the aortoiliac trial (65% male). At 24 months, there were significant improvements in both AWD and ICD in the PTA groups for both trials. The adjusted AWD was 38% greater in the PTA group for the femoropopliteal trial (95%; CI 1–90) ($p = 0.04$) and 78% greater in the PTA group for the aortoiliac trial (95%; CI 0–216) ($p = 0.05$). Further benefits were demonstrated for ABPI but not for quality of life.

Interpretation.—PTA confers adjuvant benefit over supervised exercise and best medical therapy in terms of walking distances and ABPI 24 months after PTA in patients with stable mild to moderate intermittent claudication.

▶ Most trials comparing percutaneous transluminal angioplasty (PTA) to supervised exercise/best medical treatment for mild to moderate claudication have shown initial improvement favoring PTA, with more sustainable improvement for the latter. Surprisingly, this randomized study showed the opposite with PTA for both aortoiliac and femoropopliteal disease conferring benefit in terms of walking distance and ankle-brachial pressure indices sustainable at 24 months. Part of this sustained improvement likely reflects the prerequisite of supervised exercise/best medical therapy in the PTA group both before and after the procedure. There are some generalizability issues given the strict inclusion/exclusion criteria and problems with enrollment criteria reflected by the sample size numbers (1401 screened for participation, 144 determined to be eligible, 127 consented), and intent-to-treat/crossover issues with some participants in the supervised exercise/best medical therapy group ending up with PTA. There is also no additional analysis of the impact of PTA failure on outcome parameters.

M. A. Passman, MD

Contemporary outcomes after superficial femoral artery angioplasty and stenting: The influence of TASC classification and runoff score
Ihnat DM, Duong ST, Taylor ZC, et al (Univ of Arizona Health Science Ctr; et al)
J Vasc Surg 47:967-974, 2008

Objective.—A recent randomized trial suggested nitinol self-expanding stents (SES) were associated with reduced restenosis rates compared with simple percutaneous transluminal angioplasty (PTA). We evaluated our results with superficial femoral artery (SFA) SES to determine whether TransAtlantic InterSociety Consensus (TASC) classification, indication for intervention, patient risk factors, or Society of Vascular Surgery (SVS) runoff score correlated with patency and clinical outcome, and to evaluate if bare nitinol stents or expanded polytetrafluoroethylene (ePTFE) covered stent placement adversely impacts the tibial artery runoff.

Methods.—A total of 109 consecutive SFA stenting procedures (95 patients) at two university-affiliated hospitals from 2003 to 2006 were identified. Medical records, angiographic, and noninvasive studies were reviewed in detail. Patient demographics and risk factors were recorded. Procedural angiograms were classified according to TASC Criteria (I-2000 and II-2007 versions) and SVS runoff scores were determined in every patient; primary, primary-assisted, secondary patency, and limb salvage rates were calculated. Cox proportional hazard model was used to determine if indication, TASC classification, runoff score, and comorbidities affected outcome.

Results.—Seventy-one patients (65%) underwent SES for claudication and 38 patients (35%) for critical limb ischemia (CLI). Average treatment length was 15.7 cm, average runoff score was 4.6. Overall 36-month primary, primary-assisted, and secondary rates were 52%, 64%, and 59%, respectively. Limb salvage was 75% in CLI patients. No limbs were lost following interventions in claudicants (mean follow-up 16 months). In 24 patients with stent occlusion, 15 underwent endovascular revision, only five (33%) ultimately remained patent (15.8 months after reintervention). In contrast, all nine reinterventions for in-stent stenosis remained patent (17.8 months). Of 24 patients who underwent 37 endovascular revisions for either occlusion or stenosis, eight (35%) had worsening of their runoff score (4.1 to 6.4). By Cox proportional hazards analysis, hypertension (hazard ratio [HR] 0.35), TASC D lesions (HR 5.5), and runoff score > 5 (HR 2.6) significantly affected primary patency.

Conclusions.—Self-expanding stents produce acceptable outcomes for treatment of SFA disease. Poorer patency rates are associated with TASC D lesions and poor initial runoff score; HTN was associated with improved patency rates. Stent occlusion and in-stent stenosis were not entirely benign; one-third of patients had deterioration of their tibial artery runoff. Future studies of SFA interventions need to stratify TASC classification and runoff score. Further evaluation of the long-term effects of SFA stenting on tibial runoff is needed.

▶ This is, for the most part, a pretty standard series of superficial femoral artery (SFA) stents with the usual conclusion. TransAtlantic InterSociety Consensus (TASC) D lesions are associated with poorer outcomes, but overall self expanding stents produce "acceptable" outcomes for treatment of SFA disease. The unique finding in this report, however, is the observed deterioration in runoff in one third of the patients with failed stents. The authors felt that the reduction in runoff was the equivalent of going from 2-vessel to 1-vessel runoff. The clinical significance of this is unknown as the follow-up was short. We also do not know if runoff deterioration occurs in those who maintain stent patency as these patients did not have follow-up angiograms. What is becoming increasingly clear is that endovascular interventions, whether they are in the SFA, the carotid, or the renal artery, can produce problems downstream. Most of these problems, however, are not clinically significant in the short term. Long-term data are obviously needed.

G. L. Moneta, MD

Cost-effectiveness of endovascular revascularization compared to supervised hospital-based exercise training in patients with intermittent claudication: A randomized controlled trial
Spronk S, Bosch JL, den Hoed PT, et al (Erasmus Med Ctr, Rotterdam, The Netherlands; Ikazia Hosp, Rotterdam, The Netherlands; et al)
J Vasc Surg 48:1472-1480, 2008

Background.—The optimal first-line treatment for intermittent claudication is currently unclear.

Objective.—To compare the cost-effectiveness of endovascular revascularization vs supervised hospital-based exercise in patients with intermittent claudication during a 12-month follow-up period.

Design.—Randomized controlled trial with patient recruitment between September 2002-September 2006 and a 12-month follow-up per patient.

Setting.—A large community hospital.

Participants.—Patients with symptoms of intermittent claudication due to an iliac or femoro-popliteal arterial lesion (293) who fulfilled the inclusion criteria (151) were recruited. Excluded were, for example, patients with lesions unsuitable for revascularization (iliac or femoropopliteal TASC-type D and some TASC type-B/C).

Intervention.—Participants were randomly assigned to endovascular revascularization (76 patients) or supervised hospital-based exercise (75 patients).

Measurements.—Mean improvement of health-related quality-of-life and functional capacity over a 12-month period, cumulative 12-month costs, and incremental costs per quality-adjusted life year (QALY) were assessed from the societal perspective.

Results.—In the endovascular revascularization group, 73% (55 patients) had iliac disease vs 27% (20 patients) femoral disease. Stents were used in 46/71 iliac lesions (34 patients) and in 20/40 femoral lesions (16 patients). In the supervised hospital-based exercise group, 68% (51 patients) had iliac disease vs 32% (24 patients) with femoral disease. There was a non-significant difference in the adjusted 6- and 12-month EuroQol, rating scale, and SF36-physical functioning values between the treatment groups. The gain in total mean QALYs accumulated during 12 months, adjusted for baseline values, was not statistically different between the groups (mean difference revascularization versus exercise 0.01; 99% CI −0.05, 0.07; $P = .73$). The total mean cumulative costs per patient was significantly higher in the revascularization group (mean difference €2318; 99% CI €2130, € 2506; $P < .001$) and the incremental cost per QALY was 231 800 €/QALY adjusted for the baseline variables. One-way sensitivity analysis demonstrated improved effectiveness after revascularization (mean difference 0.03; CI 0.02, 0.05; $P < .001$), making the incremental costs 75 208 €/QALY.

Conclusion.—In conclusion, there was no significant difference in effectiveness between endovascular revascularization compared to supervised hospital-based exercise during 12-months follow-up, any gains with endovascular revascularization found were non-significant, and endovascular revascularization costs more than the generally accepted threshold willingness-to-pay value, which favors exercise.

▶ This was a randomized controlled trial comparing endovascular revascularization with supervised hospital-based exercise in patients with symptoms of intermittent claudication. The study was based on the assumption that there is an accepted threshold of so-called willingness-to-pay value of incremental cost per quality-adjusted life year (QALY) gain of €50 000 per QALY. This is the second study comparing quality of life and costs of intervention with exercise for treatment of intermittent claudication. The previous study[1] compared quality of life and costs for percutaneous transluminal angioplasty, bypass surgery, or exercise decision analysis combined with data from cohort studies. The findings were similar to this article. QALYs increased only slightly with vascular intervention, and the gain in QALYs obtained through vascular intervention was at a high cost of approximately $311 000 per QALY; remarkably similar to the €231 800 per QALY for vascular intervention demonstrated in this article (€230 000 equals approximately $330 000).

Overall, using a willingness-to-pay value of €50 000 per QALY, revascularization was an optimal first-line treatment in 5% of "bootstrap" samples (Fig 2A in the original article) and in close to 10% of samples in the sensitivity analysis (Fig 2B in the original article). (Bootstrapping is a statistical technique that can be used for constructing hypothesis tests. It allows one to gather alternative versions of a single statistic, which ordinarily are calculated from 1 sample. A classic example is that if one is interested in the height of people worldwide, obviously it is possible only to sample a part of the population. With bootstrapping, you randomly extract a new sample of a specific number of heights out of the data where each person can be selected many times. This creates a large number of data sets and provides an estimate of the distribution of the particular statistic. The idea is to create alternative versions of data that may have additional or different samples obtained. Sensitivity analysis allows one to apportion, qualitatively or quantitatively, the variation in a mathematical model to different sources of variation in the input of the model. By combining both bootstrapping and sensitivity analysis, it is possible to determine potential variations in the results of the study based on probability of different samples obtained from a larger population or variations in the inputs to the model. The basic point is to try and validate results of the model with respect to potential variations of the samples used to derive the model, theoretically making the model applicable to the population at large.) Those readers less inclined to this sort of sophisticated statistical analysis are asked to look at Table 3 in the original article, in which maximum pain-free walking distance and maximum walking distance at 6 months and 12 months were compared with those randomized to endovascular revascularization versus hospital-based exercise. The bottom line: There is no significant difference. It appears that when a patient can be treated with exercise, they will do as well or better than a patient treated with an endovascular intervention. Of course, the data in this trial apply only to those patients who are capable of a supervised exercise program. The data do not apply to those patients who are realistically incapable of an exercise program.

G. L. Moneta, MD

Reference

1. de Vries SO, Visser K, de Vries JA, Wong JB, Donaldson MC, Hunink MG, et al. Intermittent claudication: cost-effectiveness of revascularization versus exercise therapy. *Radiology.* 2002;222:25-36.

Comparison of Results of Subintimal Angioplasty and Percutaneous Transluminal Angioplasty in Superficial Femoral Artery Occlusions

Antusevas A, Aleksynas N, Kaupas RS, et al (Kaunas Univ of Medicine, Lithuania)

Eur J Vasc Endovasc Surg 36:101-106, 2008

Objectives.—To report results of subintimal angioplasty (SA) of superficial femoral artery occlusions and to compare these results with percutaneous transluminal angioplasty (PTA) of similar lesions.

184 / Vascular Surgery

Design.—Prospective study.

Patients.—In the period from June 2002 to August 2006, 73 SA procedures were performed in 71 patients and 75 PTA procedures were performed in 75 patients.

Methods.—All cases treated with SA or PTA for superficial femoral artery occlusions were prospectively registered and reviewed. Assessments of comorbidities, indication for procedure, run-off, occlusion length, calcification of the artery and graft patency were recorded.

Results.—The technical success rate of SA was 87.7% versus 81.3% for PTA. Primary patency rates in the SA group at 1, 6, 12, 24 months were respectively 84.9 ± 4.2, 71.2 ± 5.1, 68.5 ± 5.3 and 65.8 ± 5.2%; in the PTA group – 81.3 ± 4.4, 45.3 ± 5.7, 42.7 ± 5.6 and 38.7 ± 5.5% respectively. At the same time-points primary assisted patency rates were in SA group 84.9 ± 4.2, 83.6 ± 4.2, 71.2 ± 5.2 and 68.5 ± 5.3%; and in the PTA group 81.3 ± 4.4, 62.5 ± 5.5, 44 ± 5.6 and 42.7 ± 5.6%. Calcification was associated with SA failure. There were no amputations in the follow up of either SA or PTA procedures.

Conclusion.—Results from subintimal angioplasty of superficial femoral artery occlusions was superior to the results of PTA (Fig 2).

▶ This was a single-center nonrandomized study, and the small number of procedures in each group (subintimal angioplasty, 73; transluminal angioplasty, 75)

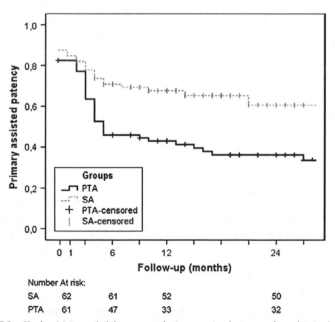

FIGURE 2.—Kaplan-Meier probability curves of primary assisted patency after subintimal angioplasty and percutaneous transluminal angioplasty. (Reprinted from Antusevas A, Aleksynas N, Kaupas RS, et al. Comparison of results of subintimal angioplasty and percutaneous transluminal angioplasty in superficial femoral artery occlusions. *Eur J Vasc Endovasc Surg.* 2008;36:101-106, with permission from Elsevier.)

makes generalized conclusions difficult. The authors' results are, however, in some respects consistent with other reports. For example, like others, they found calcification limited the technical success of subintimal angioplasty. However, in this study lesion length, distal runoff, and smoking were not associated with primary or primary-assisted patency—a finding different from some previous reports. The study was not randomized, and conclusions about the relative merits of either procedure, however, really only apply to the author's institution and to no one else as the potential for treatment bias in a nonrandomized study is obviously huge. It is clear that at the author's institution subintimal angioplasty does provide superior results to transluminal angioplasty in the patients they treat (Fig 2). In my opinion, the results of either procedure are still not good enough for treatment of patients with claudication or patients with critical limb ischemia who are good operative candidates.

G. L. Moneta, MD

Efficacy of Cilostazol After Endovascular Therapy for Femoropopliteal Artery Disease in Patients With Intermittent Claudication
Soga Y, Yokoi H, Kawasaki T, et al (Kokura Memorial Hosp, Kitakyusyu, Japan; Shin-Koga Hosp, Kurume, Japan; et al)
J Am Coll Cardiol 53:48-53, 2009

Objectives.—The purpose of this study was to investigate whether cilostazol reduces restenosis and revascularization after endovascular therapy (EVT) for femoropopliteal lesions.

Background.—Cilostazol improves walking distance in patients with intermittent claudication and reduces restenosis after coronary intervention, but its efficacy remains unclear after EVT for femoropopliteal disease.

Methods.—This study was performed as a multicenter, randomized, open-label clinical trial. Eighty patients (mean age 70.7 ± 6.2 years, 84% men) with intermittent claudication due to a femoropopliteal lesion were randomly assigned to receive or not receive cilostazol in addition to aspirin. The primary end point was freedom from target vessel revascularization, and the secondary end points were the rate of restenosis and freedom from target lesion revascularization and major adverse cardiovascular events, defined as all-cause death, myocardial infarction, stroke, repeat revascularization, and leg amputation.

Results.—Clinical follow-up information was obtained in all patients. Patient, lesion, and procedural characteristics did not differ significantly between the 2 groups. Stenting was performed in 36 patients (cilostazol, 16; control, 20; p = 0.36). Freedom from target vessel revascularization at 2 years after EVT was significantly higher compared with the control group (84.6% vs. 62.2%, p = 0.04). The rate of restenosis was lower in the cilostazol group (43.6% vs. 70.3%, p = 0.02), and freedom from target lesion revascularization and major adverse cardiovascular events was higher in the cilostazol group (87.2% vs. 67.6%, p = 0.046, 76.8%

vs. 45.6%, p = 0.006, respectively). There was no major bleeding in either group during follow-up period.

Conclusions.—Cilostazol reduced restenosis and repeat revascularization after EVT in patients with intermittent claudication due to femoropopliteal disease (Figs 2 and 3).

▶ Catheter-based therapies of the femoropopliteal artery are evolving and may be improving. Patency rates, however, are still inferior to those of bypass grafting with failure of catheter-based procedures most often resulting from restenosis secondary to intimal hyperplasia.

Cilostazol is approved for treatment of intermittent claudication. In patients with coronary disease it may lower recurrent stenosis and repeat revascularization after coronary intervention.[1] This study focused on the antiplatelet effects of cilostazol. In fact, some consider cilostazol a stronger antiplatelet agent that aspirin, dipyridamole, or ticlopidine. There is also some suggestion that cilostazol can act as an inhibitor of neointimal hyperplasia through its antiplatelet effects. Of course, another reason why cilostazol may be associated with a decreased incidence of target vessel revascularization is its anticlaudicant effects independent of restenosis may also improve the patient's ability to walk, thus making the patient less likely to seek or agree to reintervention. While the effects of cilostazol on the results of interventions for peripheral arterial disease (PAD) are being investigated, the drug is not recommended as primary or secondary prevention for cardiovascular events in patients with PAD, or for those at risk for PAD. Based on the very limited data presented here (Figs 2 and 3), physicians may choose to use cilostazol to supplement traditional antiplatelet therapy in their PAD patients who have undergone

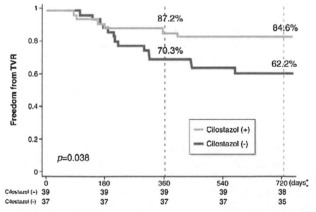

FIGURE 2.—Freedom From TVR. Freedom from target vessel revascularization (TVR) after 24 months was significantly higher in the cilostazol (+) group (**green line**) compared with the cilostazol (−) control group (**red line**) (84.6% vs. 62.2%, p = 0.038). For interpretation of the references to color in this figure legend, the reader is referred to web version of this article. (Reprinted from Soga Y, Yokoi H, Kawasaki T, et al. Efficacy of cilostazol after endovascular therapy for femoropopliteal artery disease in patients with intermittent claudication. *J Am Coll Cardiol.* 2009;53:48-53, with permission from the American College of Cardiology Foundation.)

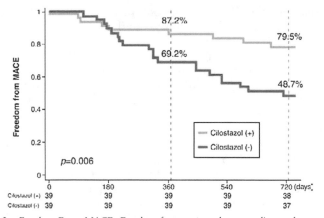

FIGURE 3.—Freedom From MACE. Freedom from major adverse cardiovascular events (MACE) after 24 months was significantly higher in the cilostazol (+) group (**green line**) compared with the cilostazol (−) control group (**red line**) (79.5% vs. 48.7%, p = 0.006). For interpretation of the references to color in this figure legend, the reader is referred to web version of this article. (Reprinted from Soga Y, Yokoi H, Kawasaki T, et al. Efficacy of cilostazol after endovascular therapy for femoropopliteal artery disease in patients with intermittent claudication. *J Am Coll Cardiol.* 2009;53:48-53, with permission from the American College of Cardiology Foundation.)

intervention, and can both afford and tolerate the drug. Cilostazol should not be used as a substitute for aspirin or clopidogrel.

G. L. Moneta, MD

Reference

1. Biondi-Zoccai GG, Lotrionte M, Anselmino M, et al. Systematic review and meta-analysis of randomized clinical trials appraising the impact of cilostazol after percutaneous coronary intervention. *Am Heart J.* 2008;155:1081-1089.

Cilostazol reduces restenosis after endovascular therapy in patients with femoropopliteal lesions

Iida O, Nanto S, Uematsu M, et al (Kansai Rosai Hosp, Hyogo; et al)
J Vasc Surg 48:144-149, 2008

Background.—Despite the recent development of endovascular therapy (EVT), a high incidence of restenosis remains as an unsolved issue in patients presenting with femoropopliteal lesions. We investigated whether cilostazol reduces restenosis after successful EVT for de novo femoropopliteal lesions.

Methods.—This study was designed as a prospective, randomized, open-label, blinded end point study in a single institution. Between March 2004 and June 2005, we randomized 127 patients who were successfully treated with EVT for de novo femoropopliteal lesions to receive cilostazol (200 mg/d, n = 63) or ticlopidine (200 mg/d, n = 64) in addition to aspirin (100 mg/d). Antiplatelet medications were started at least 1 week before EVT and were continued until the end of follow-up. Patency was defined by duplex ultrasound imaging with peak systolic velocity ratio >2.4.

Results.—There were no significant differences in the patients and lesion characteristics. Sixteen patients dropped out of the study protocol, six of whom were withdrawn due to adverse drug effects (cilostazol, n = 5; ticlopidine, n = 1; $P = .09$). Ten patients died (cilostazol, n = 4; ticlopidine, n = 6; $P = .53$) during the follow-up period. Patency rates at 12, 24, and 36 months were 87%, 82%, and 73% in the cilostazol group and 65%, 60%, and 51% in ticlopidine group by intention-to-treat analysis ($P = .013$) and were 87%, 82%, and 73% in the cilostazol group and 64%, 57%, and 48% in the ticlopidine group ($P = .0088$) by as-treated analysis. Freedom from target lesion revascularization and all adverse events (restenosis, amputation, and death) was significantly higher in cilostazol group than in ticlopidine group ($P = .036$, $P = .031$). No acute, subacute, or chronic thrombotic occlusion was encountered, and bleeding complication rates were similar between the two groups.

Conclusions.—Cilostazol significantly reduces restenosis after EVT in femoropopliteal lesions.

▶ Various adjunctive strategies have been proposed to improve patency rates with catheter-based interventions of the superficial femoral artery. These have included brachytherapy, sirolimus-eluting stents, nitinol stents, and others. The authors had previously reported a retrospective study suggesting that cilostazol could reduce restenosis following endovascular therapy of femoral popliteal disease.[1] In this study, all patients received aspirin before a catheter-based intervention in the femoral popliteal artery. They were then randomized to either triclopidine or cilostazol. Seventy-five percent of the patients treated were claudicants and about 75% had TASC C or D lesions. The results presented here suggest improvement in patency of endovascular reconstructions of femoral popliteal lesions at 2 years using cilostazol as an adjunct. Cilostazol has not previously been shown to be effective in improving patency of vascular reconstruction or as an effective drug in decreasing adverse cardiovascular events in patients at risk. Why cilostazol should be effective as an anti-intimal hyperplastic drug is unknown. It will be interesting to see if the results presented here can be duplicated in a blinded multi-institutional study.

G. L. Moneta, MD

Reference

1. Iida O, Nanto S, Uematsu M, et al. Cilostazol reduces target lesion revascularization after percutaneous transluminal angioplasty in the femoropopliteal artery. *Circ J.* 2005;69:1256-1259.

Local Delivery of Paclitaxel to Inhibit Restenosis during Angioplasty of the Leg

Tepe G, Zeller T, Albrecht T, et al (Radiologische Klinik, Diagnostische und Interventionelle Radiologie, Eberhard-Karls-Universität, Tübingen; Angiologie, Herz-Zentrum Bad Krozingen, Bad Krozingen; Radiologie, Charité, Universitätsmedizin, Berlin; et al)
N Engl J Med 358:689-699, 2008

Background.—Drug-eluting stents reduce restenosis in coronary arteries, but clinical trials have failed to prove their efficacy in peripheral arteries. We investigated the use of paclitaxel-coated angioplasty balloons and paclitaxel dissolved in the angiographic contrast medium during angioplasty of the leg.

Methods.—In a small, multicenter trial, we randomly assigned 154 patients with stenosis or occlusion of a femoropopliteal artery to treatment with standard balloon catheters coated with paclitaxel, uncoated balloons with paclitaxel dissolved in the contrast medium, or uncoated balloons without paclitaxel (control). The primary end point was late lumen loss at 6 months.

Results.—The mean ($\pm$SD) age of the patients was 68 ± 8 years, 24% were smokers, and 49% had diabetes. Twenty-seven percent of the lesions were total occlusions, and 36% were restenotic lesions. The mean lesion length was 7.4 ± 6.5 cm. There were no significant differences in baseline characteristics between the groups. There were no adverse events attributable to the paclitaxel-coated balloons. At 6 months, the mean late lumen loss was 1.7 ± 1.8 mm in the control group, as compared with 0.4 ± 1.2 mm ($P<0.001$) in the group treated with paclitaxel-coated balloons and 2.2 ± 1.6 mm ($P=0.11$) in the group treated with paclitaxel in the contrast medium. The rate of revascularization of target lesions at 6 months was 20 of 54 (37%) in the control group, 2 of 48 (4%) in the group treated with paclitaxel-coated balloons ($P<0.001$ vs. control), and 15 of 52 (29%) in the group treated with paclitaxel in the contrast medium ($P=0.41$ vs. control); at 24 months, the rates increased to 28 of 54 (52%), 7 of 48 (15%), and 21 of 52 (40%), respectively.

Conclusions.—Use of paclitaxel-coated angioplasty balloons during percutaneous treatment of femoropopliteal disease is associated with significant reductions in late lumen loss and target-lesion revascularization. No significant benefit is seen with the use of a paclitaxel-containing contrast medium.

▶ There is, obviously, an intense interest in extending the results of drug-eluting stents in the coronary circulation to the peripheral arteries. I cannot think of any reason why potentially drug-eluting stents in the peripheral arteries would not work; however, thus far, the data have been underwhelming. This is a different, but related, approach applying paclitaxel to the angioplasty balloon rather than the stent. The results seem almost too good to be believed. Nevertheless, based on animal data, they are not inconceivable. The investigators, however, were not fully blinded to the treatment arm of the individual patients. Some also served as consultants and received grant support from the industry sponsors or were involved in patent applications, with respect to the techniques used in the trial. Fully blinded studies with nonpotentially biased investigators will be required.

G. L. Moneta, MD

Midterm outcome predictors for lower extremity atherectomy procedures
Sarac TP, Altinel O, Bannazadeh M, et al (The Cleveland Clinic Lerner College of Medicine, OH)
J Vasc Surg 48:885-890, 2008

Purpose.—The performance of atherectomy devices has been variable. The purpose of this study was to evaluate our experience using the Silver-Hawk atherectomy (Fox Hollow Technologies, Redwood City, Calif) device for lower extremity procedures to determine predictors of midterm success.

Methods.—Records of all patients who underwent lower extremity atherectomy with the SilverHawk atherectomy catheter were reviewed. Patient demographics, vessel treated, number of vessels treated, lesion characteristics, and postoperative courses were analyzed. Cumulative patency rates, limb salvage, mortality, and factors associated with outcomes were determined using the Kaplan-Meier Method with Cox Proportional Hazards modeling.

Results.—Between January 2004 and January 2006, 167 vessels were atherectomized with the SilverHawk in 73 patients. There were 42 men and 31 women treated, and the mean age was 68.8 ± 13.8. Five patients had both legs treated for a total of 78 legs treated. Of the 78 legs intervened on, 25.6% (20/78) had 1 vessel treated, 51.3% (40/78) had 2 vessels treated, 11.5% (9/78) had 3 vessels treated, 9% (7/78) had 4 vessels treated, and 2.6% (2/78) had 5 vessels treated. A total of 78% (61/78) of patients had intermittent claudication, 71% (56/78) had rest pain, and 58% (45/78) had tissue loss. Adjunctive procedures were performed in 63 vessels in 33 patients (61 percutaneous transluminal angioplasty [PTA] and 2 PTA + stent). Eighty-four vessels treated were totally occluded and 83 stenotic. Cumulative 1-year primary, primary assisted, secondary patency, limb salvage, and survival rates with confidence intervals, respectively, are: 43% (30,57), 49% (36,63), 57% (43,71), 75% (57,92), and 90% (80,100). Multivariable analysis demonstrated tobacco use, renal disease, diabetes, and tissue loss are all predictors of patency loss, while only diabetes and tissue loss were associated with greater limb loss. There was no difference in patency rates irrespective of location of Trans Atlantic Inter-Societal Consensus (TASC) classification, vessel treated (femoral vs tibial), or degree of stenosis (occluded vs stenotic). Also, multiple vessels treated in the same patients had no affect on patency.

The mean ankle brachial index (ABI) pre-op was 0.57 ± 0.19, and this increased to 0.81 ± 0.21 ($P < .001$) at 30 days post-op.

Conclusion.—Lower extremity atherectomy procedures with the Silver-Hawk device are safe and effective means in improving symptoms. However, there is decreased durability and significant patency and limb loss over time. Diabetes, renal disease, tobacco use, and tissue loss are all associated with inferior outcomes.

▶ There have been several different reports on the use of SilverHawk atherectomy for lower extremity atherosclerotic occlusive disease. Aside from published observational reports from the Treating Peripherals with SilverHawk: Outcomes Collection (TALON) registry, while most studies suggest satisfactory early results, and mid- and long-term outcomes with SilverHawk atherectomy have been otherwise disappointing. This study is one of several in the growing body of literature to suggest that although use of the SilverHawk is safe and effective in reducing symptoms, there is decreased durability and significant patency and limb loss issues over time. This study also shows that patients with diabetes, renal failure, tobacco use, and tissue loss are more likely to experience these poorer outcomes. While SilverHawk atherectomy may be a consideration for those selected patients who are not satisfactory candidates for other interventional or open revascularization options, these other options, especially lower extremity bypass grafting, still offer better long-term outcomes and should be preferred when feasible.

M. A. Passman, MD

Do Current Outcomes Justify More Liberal Use of Revascularization for Vasculogenic Claudication? A Single Center Experience of 1,000 Consecutively Treated Limbs

Taylor SM, Kalbaugh CA, Healy MG, et al (Greenville Hosp System Univ Med Ctr, SC)
J Am Coll Surg 206:1053-1064, 2008

Background.—The purpose of this study was to reconsider current recommended treatment guidelines for vasculogenic claudication by examining the contemporary results of surgical intervention.

Study Design.—We performed a retrospective review of 1,000 consecutive limbs in 669 patients treated for medically refractory vasculogenic claudication and prospectively followed. Outcomes measured included procedural complication rates, reconstruction patency, limb salvage, maintenance of ambulatory status, maintenance of independent living status, survival, symptom resolution, and symptom recurrence.

Results.—Of the 1,000 limbs treated, endovascular therapy was used in 64.3% and open surgery in 35.7% of patients; aortoiliac occlusive disease was treated in 70.1% and infrainguinal disease in 29.9% of patients. The overall 30-day periprocedural complication rate was 7.5%, with no notable difference in complication rates when comparing types of treatment or levels of disease. Overall reconstruction primary patency rates were 87.7% and 70.8%; secondary patencies were 97.8% and 93.9%; limb salvage, 100% and 98.8%; and survivals, 95.4% and 76.9%, at 1 and 5 years, respectively. More than 96% of patients maintained independence and ambulatory ability at 5 years. Overall symptom resolution occurred in 78.8%, and symptom recurrence occurred in 18.1% of limbs treated, with slightly higher resolution and recurrence noted in patients treated with endovascular therapy.

Conclusions.—Contemporary treatment of vasculogenic claudication is safe, effective, and predominantly endovascular. These data support a more liberal use of revascularization for patients with claudication and suggest that current nonoperative treatment guidelines may be based more on surgical dogma than on achievable outcomes.

▶ You have to admire the fact that this group of surgeons keep track of what they do and try to report their results. Unfortunately, the way they report their results is not very useful. Patients were not stratified by degree of claudication, TransAtlantic InterSociety Consensus (TASC) lesions, pre- and post-hemodynamic status, or the occurrence of single or multilevel disease. We also have no idea about who was not treated. Nevertheless, it appears that if you are willing to spend a lot of money, you can treat a lot of patients with claudication, and you won't hurt many of them very much.

G. L. Moneta, MD

Outcomes of Combined Superficial Femoral Endovascular Revascularization and Popliteal to Distal Bypass for Patients with Tissue Loss
Lantis J, Jensen M, Benvenisty A, et al (St. Luke's-Roosevelt Hosp Ctr, NY)
Ann Vasc Surg 22:366-371, 2008

Over the last 5 years there has been a significant shift toward lower limb revascularization using endoluminal techniques. However, in many instances endoluminal techniques alone are unable to salvage limbs that exhibit tissue loss. Many of these patients do not have adequate conduit for a long leg bypass, while tibial angioplasty does not appear to restore adequate perfusion to heal many significant foot lesions, making combined procedures attractive. However, previously available data evaluating combined endoluminal and bypass procedures have been too anatomically heterogeneous to be easily applied to patients with infrainguinal disease and tissue loss. From January 2002 to December 2005, intraoperative superficial femoral artery (SFA) percutaneous transluminal angioplasty (PTA) with selective stenting combined with simultaneous popliteal to distal vein bypass was evaluated in 22 limbs of 22 patients with isolated infrainguinal disease and tissue loss. There were 12 men and 10 women, average age 69. All the patients were diabetic, all had tissue loss, and three had end-stage renal disease (ESRD). Four patients underwent common femoral endarterectomy at the time of the SFA PTA; all had the PTA performed first, with antegrade punctures and flow maintained. Fourteen patients had PTA without stenting, eight had self-expanding stents placed for residual stenosis or dissection. There were no failures, with three TASC A, 13 TASC B, and six TASC C lesions addressed. The origin of the bypass was the above-knee popliteal in eight patients and the below-knee popliteal in 14 patients. The target vessel was the dorsalis pedis in six patients, the posterior tibial at the malleolus in three, the proximal posterior tibial in five, the peroneal in five, and the anterior tibial in three. The conduit was greater saphenous vein in 16 cases, femoral vein in three cases, and arm vein in three cases. Follow-up ranged from 3 months to 4 years. The primary patency rate was 21/22 (95%), and the secondary patency rate was 22/22 (100%). There was one amputation for ongoing gangrene in an ESRD patient with a patent bypass, resulting in an early limb salvage rate of 95%. For patients with inadequate conduit and tissue loss secondary to multilevel infrainguinal disease, simultaneous angioplasty with selective stenting of the SFA followed by distal vein bypass is a viable long-term solution that allows for limb salvage. Simultaneous performance is not associated with increased morbidity and decreases overall hospital use.

▶ For patients with multilevel infrainguinal occlusive disease and inadequate conduit, the option of combined superficial femoral artery endovascular revascularization and a popliteal-to-distal bypass in this small series has reasonable short-term patency, but as a small sample size, long-term outcome remains uncertain. What is problematic in this analysis is that while each portion of the procedure has its own inherent patency issues, life-table methods used in this study are analyzed in a combined method. Whether combining these approaches has an additive effect (ie, the sum of the parts may or may not equal the whole) is not differentiated. While the combined endovascular and operative approach may have some advantages for selected patients with ischemic tissue loss and compromised conduit, traditional bypass options including spliced autogenous vein conduit, composite synthetic and vein graft, and infrainguinal synthetic grafts are still preferred in most situations.

M. A. Passman, MD

Improving limb salvage in critical ischemia with intermittent pneumatic compression: A controlled study with 18-month follow-up
Kavros SJ, Delis KT, Turner NS, et al (The Mayo Clinic, Rochester, MN)
J Vasc Surg 47:543-549, 2008

Background.—Intermittent pneumatic compression (IPC) is an effective method of leg inflow enhancement and amelioration of claudication in patients with peripheral arterial disease. This study evaluated the clinical efficacy of IPC in patients with chronic critical limb ischemia, tissue loss, and nonhealing wounds of the foot after limited foot surgery (toe or transmetatarsal amputation) on whom additional arterial revascularization had been exhausted.

Methods.—Performed in a community and multidisciplinary health care clinic (1998 through 2004), this retrospective study comprises 2 groups. Group 1 (IPC group) consisted of 24 consecutive patients, median age 70 years (interquartile range [IQR], 68.7-71.3) years, who received IPC for tissue loss and nonhealing amputation wounds of the foot attributable to critical limb ischemia in addition to wound care. Group 2 (control group) consisted of 24 consecutive patients, median age 69 years (IQR, 65.7-70.3 years), who received wound care for tissue loss and nonhealing amputation wounds of the foot due to critical limb ischemia, without use of IPC. Stringent exclusion criteria applied. Group allocation of patients depended solely on their willingness to undergo IPC therapy. Vascular assessment included determination of the resting ankle-brachial pressure index, transcutaneous oximetry ($TcPO_2$), duplex graft surveillance, and foot radiography. Outcome was considered favorable if complete healing and limb salvage occurred, and adverse if the patient had to undergo a below knee amputation subsequent to failure of wound healing. Follow-up was 18 months. Wound care consisted of weekly débridement and biologic dressings. IPC was delivered at an inflation pressure of 85 to 95 mm Hg, applied for 2 seconds with rapid rise (0.2 seconds), 3 cycles per minute; three 2-hourly sessions per day were requested. Compliance was closely monitored.

Results.—Baseline differences in demography, cardiovascular risk factors (diabetes mellitus, smoking, hypertension, dyslipidemia, renal impairment), and severity of peripheral arterial disease (ankle-brachial indices, $TcPO_2$, prior arterial reconstruction) were not significant. The types of local foot amputation that occurred in the two groups were not significantly different. In the control group, foot wounds failed to heal in 20 patients (83%) and they underwent a below knee amputation; the remaining four (17%, 95% confidence interval [CI], 0.59%-32.7%) had complete healing and limb salvage. In the IPC group, 14 patients (58%, 95% CI, 37.1%-79.6%) had complete foot wound healing and limb salvage, and 10 (42%) underwent below knee amputation for nonhealing foot wounds. Wound healing and limb salvage were significantly better in the IPC group ($P < .01$, χ^2). Compared with the IPC group, the odds ratio of limb loss in the control group was 7.0. On study completion, $TcPO_2$ on sitting was higher in the IPC group than in the control group ($P = .0038$).

Conclusion.—IPC used as an adjunct to wound care in patients with chronic critical limb ischemia and nonhealing amputation wounds/tissue loss improves the likelihood of wound healing and limb salvage when established treatment alternatives in current practice are lacking. This controlled study adds to the momentum of IPC clinical efficacy in critical limb ischemia set by previously published case series, compelling the pursuit of large scale multicentric level 1 studies to substantiate its actual clinical role, relative indications, and to enhance our insight into the pertinent physiologic mechanisms.

▶ There is a lot of flowery language in this article, but not a lot of real information. The study design actually precludes any definite endorsement of intermittent pneumatic compression (IPC) as a treatment for critical limb ischemia (CLI). There were small numbers of patients in each group, and 2 or 3 fewer amputations in the control group or 1 or 2 more amputations in the IPC group may well have rendered the differences in amputation rates insignificant between the 2 groups. There are, however, enough studies suggesting both anatomic and physiologic benefits of this therapy in patients with advanced peripheral vascular disease that IPC should be considered more than a fringe therapy offered only by physicians who don't know how to operate or dilate. A large majority of articles published on this subject, including this one, although insufficiently designed to determine the true use of this device have, in fact, suggested the benefit. The company that makes this device needs to step up to the plate and sponsor a proper multicenter randomized trial. It is a bit irresponsible not to do so.

G. L. Moneta, MD

Fifty percent area reduction after 4 weeks of treatment is a reliable indicator for healing—analysis of a single-center cohort of 704 diabetic patients
Coerper S, Beckert S, Küper MA, et al (Univ Hosp Tübingen, Germany; et al)
J Diabetes Complications 23:49-53, 2009

Introduction.—The aim of the study was to investigate whether an area reduction greater than 50% within the first 4 weeks of treatment is associated with a higher long-term probability of healing.

Patients and Methods.—We treated diabetic foot ulcers according to a comprehensive interdisciplinary wound care protocol. Follow-up was documented through a special wound documentation system. Data were entered into SPSS for statistical analysis to calculate the probability of healing according to the Kaplan–Meier method. Results were expressed as median (minimum–maximum), and the percentage of area reduction (PA) was defined as $[(area_{4\ weeks}/area_{baseline}) \times 100]/area_{baseline}$. Patients were divided into responders when PA reached at least 50% and nonresponders when PA was less than 50%. Healing was defined as PA = 100%.

Results.—In total, 704 patients were included into the analysis. Median time of follow-up was 71 (2–365) days. Wound duration was 31 (1–4018) days, and the initial wound size was calculated to be 1.18 (0.1–99) cm^2. In 27.8%, there was a positive probing to bone; in 64.5%, both pedal pulses were not palpable. Major amputation rate was 2.8% and minor amputation rate was 10.2%. The overall probability of healing was 35% after 12 weeks, 41% after 16 weeks, and 73% after 1 year. The surrogate visit (4 weeks) was performed after a median of 27 (14–42) days without a difference between responders and nonresponders. There were 334 (47%) responders and 370 (53%) nonresponders. Responders had a significantly higher probability of healing compared with nonresponders (12 weeks: 52.3% vs. 18.4%, $P=.0001$; 16 weeks: 46.7% vs. 26.5%, $P=.0001$; 1 year: 82.5% vs. 64.9%, $P=.0001$).

Conclusions.—The calculation of the percentage of area reduction after 4 weeks of treatment is a valid tool to estimate the probability of healing. In clinical practice, a reevaluation of the treatment schedule is recommended for wounds that do not reach 50% area reduction within the first 4 weeks of therapy.

▶ Diabetic foot wounds are common and treated by many different combinations of clinic and home visits and utilization of a wide range of local wound care products. There are both subjective and wound-based parameters to document healing, with the only objective wound-based parameters for healing being wound size and ultimate complete wound closure. The authors postulated that the pace of reduction of wound size during the course of treatment may be an indicator for complete healing response. In general, studies of diabetic foot wounds have evaluated healing rates after 12 to 24 weeks of care. There is interest in developing the so-called surrogate markers of wound healing at 12 to 16 weeks, and one of these potential surrogate markers is change in wound area after 4 weeks of treatment. The authors sought to investigate whether an area reduction greater than 50% within 4 weeks of treatment was associated with long-term probability of healing of a diabetic foot wound. The data suggest that diabetic foot wounds more prone to heal will exhibit a greater healing response early in the course of their treatment. The practical point is that if the wound has not decreased by 50% after 4 weeks, then an alternative form of wound therapy should be considered.

G. L. Moneta, MD

Outcomes of surgical management for popliteal artery aneurysms: An analysis of 583 cases

Johnson ON III, Slidell MB, Macsata RA, et al (Veterans Affairs Med Ctr, Houston, TX; et al)
J Vasc Surg 48:845-851, 2008

Background.—This study aimed to analyze outcomes of surgical management for popliteal artery aneurysms (PAA).

Methods.—This is a retrospective analysis of prospectively collected data regarding operations for PAA obtained from 123 United States Veterans Affairs Medical Centers as part of the National Surgical Quality Improvement Program. Univariate analyses and multivariate logistic regression were used to characterize 33 risk factors and their associations with 30-day morbidity and mortality. Survival and amputation rates, observed at one and two years after surgery, were subject to life-table and Cox regression analyses.

Results.—There were 583 operations for PAA in 537 patients during 1994-2005. Almost all were in men (99.8%) and median age was 69 years (range, 34 to 92 years). Most had multiple co-morbidities, 88% were ASA (American Society of Anesthesiologists) class 3 or 4, and 81% were current or past smokers (median pack-years = 50). Only 16% were diabetic. Serious complications occurred in 69 (11.8%) cases, of which 37 (6.3%) required arterial-specific reinterventions. Eight patients died within 30 days, a mortality of 1.4%. Risk factors associated with increased complications included: African-American race (odds ratio [OR] 2.8 [95% confidence interval 1.5-5.2], $P = .002$), emergency surgery (OR 3.8 [2.0-7.0], $P < .0001$), ASA 4 (OR 1.9 [1.1-3.5], $P = .04$), dependent functional status (OR 2.5 [1.4-4.7], $P = .004$), steroid use (OR 3.2 [1.2-8.7], $P = .03$), and need for intraoperative red blood cell transfusion of any quantity (OR 6.3 [3.5-11.2], $P < .0001$). Independent predictors for complications in the multivariate model were dependent functional status (adjusted OR 2.1 [1.1-4.3], $P = .049$) and intraoperative transfusion (adjusted OR 4.5 [2.3-8.9], $P = .0002$). Postoperative bleeding complications within 72 hours independently predicted early amputation (adjusted OR 25.5 [1.7-393], $P = .02$). Unadjusted patient survival was 92.6% at one year and 86.1% at two years. Limb salvage in surviving patients was 99.0% at 30 days, 97.6% at one year, and 96.2% at two years. Dependent preoperative functional status was the only factor predictive of worse two-year limb salvage (adjusted OR 4.6 [1.9-10.9], $P = .001$), but remained high at 88.2% versus 97.1% in independent patients.

Conclusions.—Surgical intervention for PAA is associated with low operative mortality and offers excellent two-year limb salvage, even in high-risk patients. Patients' preoperative functional status and perioperative blood transfusion requirements were the most predictive indicators of negative outcomes.

▶ While this study shows excellent outcomes from a large dataset of patients undergoing operative repair of popliteal aneurysms in Veterans Affairs Medical Centers entered into the National Surgical Quality Improvement Program (NSQIP), there are several limitations. Only surgical encounters for popliteal artery aneurysm were identified for the sample population, thereby limiting the dataset to only a subpopulation of all patients with popliteal aneurysms. Not included are patients with significant limb-threatening ischemia from popliteal aneurysm thrombosis who require primary amputation, and those who require ancillary procedures for limb preservation, such as thrombolysis and/ or thrombectomy, or endovascular repair. As an NSQIP-based review, further popliteal artery aneurysm–specific data are missing. That said, at best, this study shows that those selected patients with popliteal artery aneurysm who do require operative repair within the context of this dataset, in general, do well with low operative mortality and high limb salvage.

M. A. Passman, MD

12 Upper Extremity and Dialysis Access

The natural history of vascular access for hemodialysis: A single center study of 2,422 patients
Papanikolaou V, Papagiannis A, Vrochides D, et al (Aristotle Univ, Thessaloniki, Greece)
Surgery 145:272-279, 2009

Background.—Our objective is to provide provision of primary and secondary patency rates data and incidence of complications. Despite the publication of some review articles and small prospective trials about vascular accesses, controversy still exists regarding the choice of the outflow conduit and especially the choice of the fistula to be formed in secondary and tertiary access procedures.

Methods.—This is a retrospective study of 2,422 consecutive patients who underwent 3,685 vascular access procedures in a tertiary care hospital, including radial-cephalic (RCAVF), brachial-cephalic (BCAVF), brachial-basilic (BBAVF), and prosthetic graft (PTFE) fistulas. Maximum follow-up period was 20 years. Actuarial patency rates were obtained by Kaplan-Meier analysis.

Results.—The median primary patency (days) of the most common 1st choices for vascular access were 712 (95% CI: 606, 818), 1,009 (95% CI: 823, 1,195), and 384 (95% CI: 273, 945) days for RCAVF, BCAVF, and PTFE, respectively. The median secondary patency was 1809 days (95% CI: 1,692, 1,926) for the RCAVF. The median primary patency of BBAVF (2nd or 3rd choice for vascular access) was 1,582 days (95% CI: 415, 2,749). The cumulative incidence of clinically important complications for the patients who received a RCAVF, BCAVF, BBAVF, and u-PTFE was 0.25, 0.57, 0.33, and 0.61 per patient-year, respectively.

Conclusion.—We advocate maximal use of autogenous conduits, except probably the case of the older diabetic patient, in whom access at the antecubital fossa should be the first choice. BBAVF is an excellent fistula and should probably be constructed before prosthetic graft placement (Fig 1).

▶ The National Kidney Foundation Clinical Guidelines for Vascular Access (NKF/DOQI) recommend radial-cephalic arteriovenous fistulas and brachial-cephalic arteriovenous fistulas as the first and second choices for dialysis access. These are then followed by prosthetic grafts, brachial-basilic

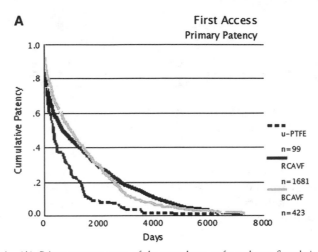

FIGURE 1.—(A), Primary patency rates of the procedures performed as a first choice for vascular access. Patency rate is shown in fractions and time in days. Notice that after 2000 days of function RCAVF patency is superior to BCAVF. (Reprinted from Papanikolaou V, Papagiannis A, Vrochides D, et al. The natural history of vascular access for hemodialysis: a single center study of 2,422 patients. *Surgery.* 2009;145:272-279.)

arteriovenous fistulas, and venous catheters as secondary choices. These recommendations have been verified by review articles and small prospective trials and small clinical series. This article represents a retrospective review of a very large dialysis access experience. The value of this study lies in the large number of patients and long period of follow-up. Otherwise, the conclusions are really not substantially different from those derived previously, although the superiority of long-term radial cephali versus brachial cephalic fistulas is a bit of new information (Fig 1A). There has, however, been some controversy as the use of prosthetic versus brachial-basilic fistulas as secondary or tertiary access procedures. This study would suggest that a brachial-basilic fistula is far superior to prosthetic access and that brachial-basilic arteriovenous fistula, although more technically demanding, should be the preferred secondary or tertiary access over a prosthetic fistula.

G. L. Moneta, MD

Arteriovenous Fistula Formation using Transposed Basilic Vein: Extensive Single Centre Experience

Harper SJF, Goncalves I, Doughman T, et al (Univ of Leicester, UK)
Eur J Vasc Endovasc Surg 36:237-241, 2008

Objectives.—The expanding haemodialysis population has lead to increased requirement for more complex vascular access. The aim of this study is to present the results of an extensive series of brachiobasilic arteriovenous fistulae.

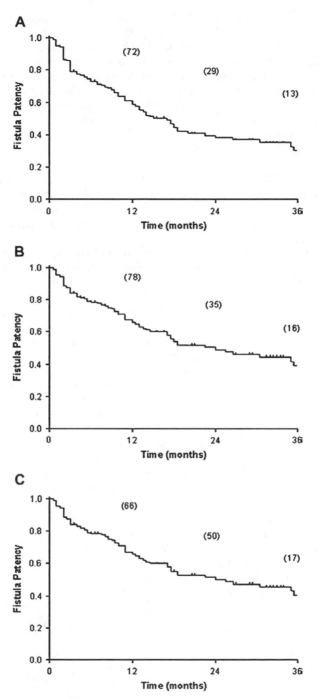

FIGURE 1.—Survival curve demonstrating fistula primary patency, assisted primary patency and secondary patency (number at risk in parentheses). (Reprinted from Harper SJF, Goncalves I, Doughman T, et al. Arteriovenous fistula formation using transposed basilic vein: extensive single centre experience. *Eur J Vasc Endovasc Surg.* 2008;36:237-241, with permission from Elsevier.)

Methods.—BBAVF were performed using single-stage vein transposition. A retrospective review of case notes was performed.

Results.—One hundred and sixty eight BBAVF were created in 144 patients. This was the first access procedure in only 30 cases and the fourth or fifth in 30. At 24 h, 165 fistulas (98%) were patent. One hundred and eleven fistulas (66%) were used for haemodialysis and 57 (34%) were never used, of which 39 (23%) were due to fistula failure. The cumulative secondary patency at 1, 2 and 3 years was 66%, 50% and 41% respectively. There were 201 complications in 119 patients (71%), including thrombosis (29%), arm oedema (17%), infection (13%) and arterial steal syndrome (11%). Ten angioplasties and 48 operative procedures were performed for complications. Pre-operative ipsilateral subclavian catheter had been placed in 62 cases (37%) and was associated with poor patency.

Conclusions.—BBAVF represents an important option for vascular access with acceptable patency rates, although complication rates remain significant (Fig 1).

▶ This is a large experience with basilic vein transposition for establishment of dialysis access. This article clearly outlines what to expect with these types of fistulas. The most important points are that the complication rate is significant and wound infection appears surprisingly common (13% in the perioperative period, and late wound infections in 12 patients as well). Seven fistulas required ligation for infection. Arm edema occurred in 17% and steal syndrome in 11%. Thirty-four percent of the fistulas were never used for dialysis either because of nonmaturation of the fistula, death before institution of dialysis, or fistula maturation. Three patients received a transplant before fistula usage. Secondary patency was about 40% at 3 years (Fig 1C), and when the fistula thrombosed, patency was re-established in only half these cases. Given all these problems, why do basilic vein transpositions when patency for basilic vein transpositions is not all that different from polytetrafluoroethylene (PTFE) grafts? Other studies also report high complication rates for basilic vein transposition between 47% and 71%. However, complication rates for PTFE grafts are likely, even higher, with reported rates between 60% and 100%. Re-operation rates are also likely lower for basilic vein transposition than PTFE grafts: 29% in this study versus 45% to 67% for PTFE grafts. Lower complication rates and lower re-operation rates favor basilic vein transposition over PTFE; patency probably is not all that better.

G. L. Moneta, MD

The brachial artery-brachial vein fistula: Expanding the possibilities for autogenous fistulae

Greenberg JI, May S, Suliman A, et al (Univ of California, San Diego)
J Vasc Surg 48:1245-1250, 2008

Objective.—The National Kidney Foundation Dialysis Outcomes and Quality Initiative recommends autogenous access for new dialysis procedures. The patient requiring hemodialysis with inadequate superficial arm veins represents a formidable challenge to the surgeon. Our objective is to describe results with an alternative access procedure, the autogenous brachial-brachial artery (ABBA) access in patients with inadequate superficial arm veins.

Methods.—One surgeon created 163 new dialysis accesses in 122 patients during 40 consecutive months at a university hospital. There was 97% patient follow-up. All patent but diminutive superficial arm veins as judged by preoperative ultrasound were explored. Arms with inadequate veins at exploration or arms with thrombosed veins on ultrasound received either prosthetic or ABBA procedures. Upper-arm access was often staged, involving a second "superficialization" procedure. This is a retrospective case series based on a comprehensive medical record review. Cox proportional hazards models were used to compare access patency for individual as well as multiple factors suspected or known to influence dialysis access outcomes. Society for Vascular Surgery reporting guidelines were used except where specifically noted and justified otherwise.

Results.—One hundred thirty-five autogenous and 28 prosthetic dialysis operations were performed. Primary patency for all access procedures at 12, 24, and 36 months was 58%, 50%, and 38%, respectively. Primary assisted patency for all access procedures at 12, 24, and 36 months was 97%, 91%, and 85%, respectively. Secondary patency at 12, 24, and 36 months was 99%, 97%, and 97%, respectively. Finally, functional patency at 12, 24, and 36 months was 71%, 67%, and 44.0%, respectively. Of the 122 patients, 70 patients received either ABBA or prosthetic access. ABBA out-performed prosthetic access in terms of primary patency (hazard ratio for prosthetic vs ABBA: 4.21 (95% confidence interval [CI]: 1.49, 11.91) and functional patency (hazard ratio for prosthetic vs ABBA: 6.27 95% CI: 1.24-31.72) in patients referred early. Functional patency was more likely to be compromised in elderly patients and in patients with hypercoagulable diagnoses.

Conclusions.—Autogenous brachial-brachial access for dialysis out-performed prosthetic access with respect to primary and functional patency in patients referred early without differences in overall complications (Fig 1).

▶ Use of the brachial vein in dialysis access is not new. In the days when prosthetic grafts were more common, the brachial vein often served as the outflow site for forearm loop grafts when no other vein was available in the antecubital fossa. As has been previously observed, and was also observed in this series,

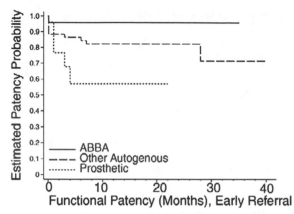

FIGURE 1.—Kaplan-Meier analysis of primary and functional access patency. (Reprinted from Greenberg JI, May S, Suliman A, et al. The brachial artery-brachial vein fistula: expanding the possibilities for autogenous fistulae. *J Vasc Surg.* 2008;48:1245-1250. Copyright 2008, with permission from The Society for Vascular Surgery.)

arm swelling is not a significant problem using the brachial vein for construction of an arterial-venous access.

The brachial artery-brachial vein fistula has functional patency that clearly exceeds that of prosthetic dialysis access. Two things are particularly noteworthy here. The first is that the authors advocate a 2-staged operation with initial construction of the arteriovenous anastomosis followed approximately 6 weeks later by transposition of the vein to the surface. I do not believe that this is necessary in all cases, and in fact in virtually every instance where I perform this operation I do it as a single-stage procedure.

The second point is that patients referred early for dialysis access had outstanding patency of their autogenous brachial artery-brachial vein fistula (Fig 1C). This is consistent with other reports suggesting that dialysis access patency is improved if the access can be placed before the patient needing dialysis.

G. L. Moneta, MD

Effect of Clopidogrel on Early Failure of Arteriovenous Fistulas for Hemodialysis: A Randomized Controlled Trial

Dember LM, Beck GJ, Allon M, et al (Boston Univ, MA; Cleveland Clinic Found, OH; Univ of Alabama at Birmingham; et al)
J Am Med Assoc 299:2164-2171, 2008

Context.—The arteriovenous fistula is the preferred type of vascular access for hemodialysis because of lower thrombosis and infection rates and lower health care expenditures compared with synthetic grafts or central venous catheters. Early failure of fistulas due to thrombosis or inadequate maturation is a barrier to increasing the prevalence of fistulas among patients treated with hemodialysis. Small, inconclusive trials have suggested that antiplatelet agents may reduce thrombosis of new fistulas.

Objective.—To determine whether clopidogrel reduces early failure of hemodialysis fistulas.

Design, Setting, and Participants.—Randomized, double-blind, placebo-controlled trial conducted at 9 US centers composed of academic and community nephrology practices in 2003-2007. Eight hundred seventy-seven participants with end-stage renal disease or advanced chronic kidney disease were followed up until 150 to 180 days after fistula creation or 30 days after initiation of dialysis, whichever occurred later.

Intervention.—Participants were randomly assigned to receive clopidogrel (300-mg loading dose followed by daily dose of 75 mg; n=441) or placebo (n=436) for 6 weeks starting within 1 day after fistula creation.

Main Outcome Measures.—The primary outcome was fistula thrombosis, determined by physical examination at 6 weeks. The secondary outcome was failure of the fistula to become suitable for dialysis. Suitability was defined as use of the fistula at a dialysis machine blood pump rate of 300 mL/min or more during 8 of 12 dialysis sessions.

Results.—Enrollment was stopped after 877 participants were randomized based on a stopping rule for intervention efficacy. Fistula thrombosis occurred in 53 (12.2%) participants assigned to clopidogrel compared with 84 (19.5%) participants assigned to placebo (relative risk, 0.63; 95% confidence interval, 0.46-0.97; $P=.018$). Failure to attain suitability for dialysis did not differ between the clopidogrel and placebo groups (61.8% vs 59.5%, respectively; relative risk, 1.05; 95% confidence interval, 0.94-1.17; $P=.40$).

Conclusion.—Clopidogrel reduces the frequency of early thrombosis of new arteriovenous fistulas but does not increase the proportion of fistulas that become suitable for dialysis.

Trial Registration.—clinicaltrials.gov Identifier: NCT00067119.

▶ Obviously early patency is necessary for fistula maturation. However, there are clearly other aspects of fistula maturation other than early patency that are required for the fistula to ultimately be useful for dialysis. Distal stenoses in the draining vein, poor arterial inflow, and various patient factors such as the presence of diabetes and advanced age also can limit successful fistula maturation despite the use of an antiplatelet agent to prevent early thrombosis. Another key to fistula maturation may be surgical judgment. An adverse factor may be the zeal of many surgeons to try to construct an autogenous conduit, even when one is very unlikely to be successful. This study will be limited in its impact by the high percentage of fistulas, about 60%, that could never be used for dialysis. Perhaps the most important message here is the need to identify other mechanisms of failure of fistula maturation other than initial thrombosis. We also need realistic and improved criteria for selecting candidates for fistula creation in the first place. I am reasonably convinced a well-placed PTFE graft still has a role in dialysis access.

G. L. Moneta, MD

Fistula Elevation Procedure: Experience with 295 Consecutive Cases During a 7-Year Period

Bronder CM, Cull DL, Kuper SG, et al (Greenville Hosp System Univ Med Ctr, SC)
J Am Coll Surg 206:1069-1075, 2008

Background.—Up to 50% of AV fistulas fail to mature, primarily because of problems with fistula cannulation. Fistula elevation procedure (FEP) is a simple superficialization procedure where the fistula is surgically exposed, mobilized, and elevated into a more superficial position for the purpose of facilitating AV fistula cannulation. The purpose of this study is to review use of FEP as an adjunct to fistula maturation.

Study Design.—Two hundred ninety-five FEPs were performed between February 1999 and December 2005. FEP was performed if the fistula was considered too deep to cannulate or if nurses were unable to cannulate the fistula. Kaplan-Meier life-table analysis was used to determine patency and for a subanalysis by location of FEP performed (172 brachial-cephalic, 70 brachial-basilic, 46 radial-cephalic, 7 superficial femoral vein). Survival curves were compared using log-rank test.

Results.—Functional primary patency rates for patients undergoing an adjunctive FEP were 73% at 6 months, 60% at 1 year, and 46% at 2 years. Secondary functional patency rates were 81% at 6 months, 71% at 1 year, and 59% at 2 years. There was no statistical significance in any outcomes based on anatomic site of elevation.

Conclusions.—AV fistulas that might otherwise have been abandoned because of excessive depth or tortuosity can be successfully salvaged by an adjunctive FEP and achieve satisfactory longterm functional patency. FEP is a valuable adjunct to AV fistula creation, which will enhance fistula maturation rates.

▶ Many fistulas are patent and of reasonable caliber, but for various reasons the dialysis nurses and technicians cannot reliably access them. With increasing rates of obesity and diabetes, there are, and will be, many more obese patients with severe chronic kidney disease whose fistula is covered by a thick layer of adipose tissue that makes access difficult. The fistula elevation procedure, described in this report, consists of longitudinal incision covering the entire length of the fistula, mobilization of the vein, and then subcutaneous tissue closure beneath the fistula with a subcuticular skin closure over the vein itself. The patency rates described are in accordance with what one would expect for a nonmobilized fistula. The data indicate that no autogenous fistula should be abandoned simply because it is felt to be too deep or too tortuous for access.

G. L. Moneta, MD

Plication as Primary Treatment of Steal Syndrome in Arteriovenous Fistulas
Yaghoubian A, de Virgilio C (Harbor-UCLA Med Ctr, Los Angeles, CA)
Ann Vasc Surg 23:103-107, 2009

Steal syndrome is an uncommon complication following hemodialysis access. Options for management include fistula ligation, banding, and distal revascularization with interval ligation (DRIL). Plication is another technique that is simple yet infrequently reported. We have adopted plication as the procedure of choice for steal syndrome following autologous arteriovenous fistula (AVF) creation. We report seven cases managed by plication. All had immediate resolution of symptoms (Table 1). At follow-up, all AVFs were patent and continued to be used for hemodialysis. However, one patient experienced recurrence of symptoms and required re-plication. In conclusion, plication of the autologous AVF represents a simple alternative to the management of steal syndrome (Fig 1).

▶ There is always some steal in patients following creation of an arteriovenous fistula for hemodialysis. Blood is preferentially shunted to some degree or another to the low-resistance venous circulation. Pathologic steal, while uncommon, can produce devastating complications and has an overall incidence of between 1% to 9%. In many practices, the distal revascularization with interval ligation (DRIL) procedure has become the preferred method of treatment of steal syndrome. However, this operation requires a new bypass and results in ligation or division of the brachial artery distal to the fistula. While plication of an arteriovenous fistula is a known technique for dealing with steal syndrome, it is rarely reported. In this article, the authors describe their technique, in a small number of patients, for plication of arteriovenous fistulas associated with clinically significant steal. Plication was performed using a Satinsky clamp as a guide for the degree of plication with the vein narrowed by running horizontal mattress suture of 6-0 polypropylene (Fig 1). The length of vein plicated was approximately 1 cm, and the extent of plication determined by either return of a palpable pulse at the wrist or a change from monophasic to a biphasic distal Doppler signal. If the Doppler signal did not improve, the Satinsky clamp was reapplied and the plication repeated, further narrowing the plicated length of the fistula. The technique was effective and success was associated with preoperative restoration of the radial pulse with fistula compression.

Many patients with steal syndrome can be managed by observation. The inflow vessel dilates and symptoms may resolve within a few days to weeks. A basic principle of surgical therapy is to perform simple procedures that are effective in preference to more complex procedures. DRIL procedures are effective for steal with an 83% to 100% success rate; however, they are major operations and the brachial artery is ligated. This study serves as a reminder that simple plication may be an effective treatment for steal syndrome and should

TABLE 1.—Seven Cases of Steal Syndrome Treated with Plication of the Native Vein

	Type of Fistula	Time From Initial Access Surgery to Plication (Months)	Clinical Presentation	Preoperative Examination	Operative Procedure	Postoperative Examination
Patient 1	Left cephalic vein to brachial artery AVF	2	Numbness, coolness, and pain	Vascular exam: nonpalpable distal pulses, delayed capillary refill. Doppler: no ulnar signal, biphasic radial artery signals	Plication of AVF	Vascular exam: palpable radial pulse, brisk capillary refill. Doppler: biphasic ulnar and radial signals
Patient 2	Right basilic vein to brachial artery AVF	24	Pain with tingling and numbness	Vascular exam: +1 radial pulse, delayed capillary refill. Doppler: monophasic ulnar and biphasic radial artery signals	Superficialization and plication of AVF	Vascular exam: palpable ulnar and radial pulses, brisk capillary refill. Doppler: Biphasic radial and ulnar signals
Patient 3	Left cephalic vein to brachial artery AVF	6	Coolness with pain	Vascular exam: nonpalpable radial pulse, delayed capillary refill. Doppler: monophasic radial and ulnar signals	Superficialization and plication of AVF	Vascular exam: Nonpalpable radial pulse, brisk capillary refill. Doppler: Biphasic radial and ulnar signals
Patient 4	Left basilic vein to brachial artery AVF	36	Coolness and numbness	Vascular exam: nonpalpable radial pulse. Doppler: monophasic radial and ulnar signals	Superficialization and plication of AVF	Vascular exam: palpable radial pulse. Doppler: Biphasic radial and ulnar signals
Patient 5	Right cephalic vein to brachial artery AVF	3	Pain with tingling and numbness	Vascular exam: nonpalpable distal pulses. Doppler: monophasic radial and ulnar signals	Plication of AVF	Vascular exam: palpable radial and ulnar pulses, brisk capillary refill. Doppler: Biphasic radial and triphasic ulnar signals
Patient 6	Left cephalic vein to brachial artery AVF	24	Coolness, numbness and tingling	Vascular exam: +1 radial pulse. Doppler:	Plication of AVF and resection of aneurysmal portion of former anastomosis	Vascular exam: palpable radial pulse
Patient 7	Left cephalic vein to brachial artery AVF	96	Numbness and coolness	Vascular exam: Nonpalpable distal pulses, delayed capillary refill. Doppler:	Plication of AVF	Vascular exam: palpable radial pulse, brisk capillary refill

(Reprinted from Yaghoubian A, de Virgilio C. Plication as primary treatment of steal syndrome in arteriovenous fistulas. Ann Vasc Surg. 2009;23:103-107.)

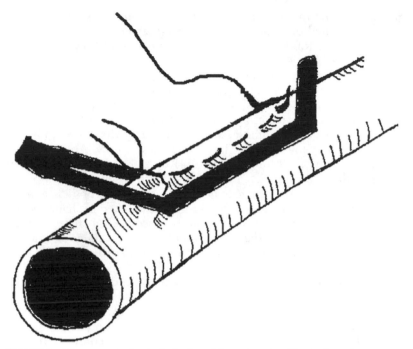

FIGURE 1.—Diagrammatic sketch of plication of the native vein with a horizontal mattress suture using a Satinsky clamp as a guide for degree of plication. (Reprinted from Yaghoubian A, de Virgilio C. Plication as primary treatment of steal syndrome in arteriovenous fistulas. *Ann Vasc Surg.* 2009;23:103-107.)

be considered as an alternative treatment for steal before performance of a DRIL procedure.

G. L. Moneta, MD

Risk of Hemodialysis Graft Thrombosis: Analysis of Monthly Flow Surveillance
Ram SJ, Nassar R, Work J, et al (Louisiana State Univ Health Sciences Ctr, Shreveport; Louisiana Tech Univ, Ruston; Emory Univ School of Medicine, Atlanta, GA; et al)
Am J Kid Dis 52:930-938, 2008

Background.—During clinical application of flow surveillance of hemodialysis grafts, the risk of thrombosis is assessed month after month, rather than after one or several measurements, as has been done in published studies. Adequate assessment of risk should consider the many measurements obtained over time.

Study Design.—Prospective cohort diagnostic test study.

Setting & Participants.—176 patients with hemodialysis grafts from 2 university-affiliated dialysis units during a 6-year period.

Index Tests.—Monthly measurement of graft blood flow or change in flow.

Outcome.—Graft thrombosis.

Results.—We used logistic regression analysis to compute the risk of thrombosis and used receiver operating characteristic (ROC) curves to assess the accuracy in predicting thrombosis within 1 month. Newer grafts were most likely to thrombose, whereas older grafts were unlikely to thrombose even at low flows or large decreases in flow. Areas under the ROC curves were 0.698 for flow and 0.713 for change in flow measured over 2 months. Flow predicted thrombosis with a sensitivity of 53% at a specificity of 79%, and change in flow had a sensitivity of 58% at a specificity of 75%. More than half the thromboses lacked a change in flow measurement, usually because thrombosis occurred before a change could be measured. Thus, the effective predictive accuracy of change in flow was much less than the ROC curves indicated because the curves do not consider missing measurements.

Limitations.—Performance characteristics of index tests may vary across patient populations.

Conclusion.—Flow and change in flow are inaccurate predictors of thrombosis. Many thromboses are not predicted, and intervention based on surveillance likely yields many unnecessary procedures. Thus, this study does not support routine application of surveillance to prevent thrombosis.

▶ Guidelines of the National Kidney Foundation Kidney Disease Outcomes Quality Initiative (NKF KDOQI) were updated in 2006 to indicate that surveillance of dialysis access grafts may, rather than does, improve patency and reduce thrombosis of dialysis access grafts.[1] Previous studies assessing risk of dialysis graft thrombosis associated with flow or change in flow assessed risk within an interval of only 1 or several measurements. Estimates of risk were therefore based on a relatively small number of measurements, whereas in actual practice risk is assessed repeatedly month after month. The authors, therefore, felt that accurate measurement of risk should involve many measurements observed over time. Indeed, low flow and change in flow were the predictors of graft thrombosis. However, despite this, more than half of thromboses lacked a change in flow measurement, likely because thrombosis occurred before the change could be measured. Unfortunately, sensitivity for both flow and change in flow to predict a thrombosis was only slightly more than 50%. Therefore, the data indicate that many thromboses of PTFE grafts will not be predicted by monthly surveillance, and intervention based on surveillance will likely yield many unnecessary procedures. The authors also postulate that because angioplasty may stimulate neointimal hyperplasia, acceleration of stenosis by unnecessary angioplasty may in fact promote graft failure and serve as an explanation for why surveillance with intervention has not prolonged graft life in randomized trials.

G. L. Moneta, MD

Reference

1. National Kidney Foundation: KDOQI Clinical Practice Guidelines and Clinical Practice Recommendations for Vascular Access 2006. *Am J Kidney Dis.* 2006;48 (Suppl 1):S176-S322.

Secondary Patency of Thrombosed Prosthetic Vascular Access Grafts with Aggressive Surveillance, Monitoring and Endovascular Management

Kakkos SK, Haddad GK, Haddad JA, et al (Henry Ford Hosp, Detroit, MI)
Eur J Vasc Endovasc Surg 36:356-365, 2008

Background.—To study the long-term patency of thrombosed prosthetic vascular access grafts treated with percutaneous mechanical thrombectomy (PMT) followed by aggressive surveillance and monitoring and repeated endovascular interventions.

Study design.—Two hundred seven vascular access grafts presented with first-time thrombosis were treated with PMT using the AngioJet device ($n = 185$) or the Arrow-Trerotola percutaneous thrombolytic device ($n = 22$) followed by angioplasty ($\pm$ stenting) of the anatomical lesion responsible for the thrombotic event. Clinical success was considered at least one successful subsequent hemodialysis session. Graft surveillance/monitoring included clinical and hemodialysis parameters to detect a failing or thrombosed graft.

Results.—PMT was technically successful in 202 cases (97.6%) and clinically successful in 193 cases (93.2%). During follow-up, 149 got thrombosed and either abandoned ($n = 33$) or underwent at least once repeat thrombectomy ($n = 116$); finally 100 grafts were abandoned ($n = 90$), ligated ($n = 5$) or removed ($n = 5$). Endovascular management (0.54 procedures per 100 graft-days, thrombectomy, $n = 307$ sessions and angioplasty, $n = 162$ sessions) increased significantly functional assisted-primary patency rates from 29% and 14% at 1 and 2 years to a secondary patency of 62% and 47%, respectively. Secondary patency was worse in loop grafts ($P = .02$) and intermediate graft thrombosis (occurred between 31–182 days after graft placement, $P < .001$) and better when renal failure was due to hypertension or diabetes (compared to other or cryptogenic causes, $P = .048$) or isolated angioplasty for graft dysfunction during follow-up had been performed ($P < .001$). Multivariate analysis identified intermediate graft thrombosis and isolated angioplasty as independent predictors of secondary patency ($P < .001$, relative risk 2.77 and $P < .001$, relative risk 0.28, respectively).

Conclusions.—PMT is a highly successful procedure with acceptable long-term secondary patency results, provided that aggressive endovascular management of subsequent thrombotic or dysfunction episode is performed. Further research to identify the causes of intermediate graft thrombosis is justified.

▶ Based on recommendations from updated Kidney Disease Outcomes Quality Initiative (KDOQI) guidelines, in restoring patency of thrombosed hemodialysis prosthetic grafts using endovascular techniques, clinical success rate should be > 85%, and primary patency should be > 40% at 3 months.[1] With the excellent results reported in this study, use of catheter-directed pharmacomechanical thrombectomy for thrombosed prosthetic vascular access grafts, aggressive surveillance and monitoring, and repeat endovascular interventions for underlying lesions seems to be an appropriate strategy to meet these guidelines. However, with the noted frequency of required endovascular procedures in this study, the cost-effectiveness of this approach may be a limiting factor.

M. A. Passman, MD

Reference

1. Foundation NK. KDOQI clinical practice recommendations for 2006 updates: hemodialysis adequacy, peritoneal dialysis adequacy and vascular access. *Am J Kidney Dis*. 2006;48:S1-322.

Brachial artery ligation with total graft excision is a safe and effective approach to prosthetic arteriovenous graft infections
Schanzer A, Ciaranello AL, Schanzer H, et al (Univ of Massachusetts Med School, Worcester; Massachusetts Gen Hosp, Boston; Mount Sinai Med School, NY)
J Vasc Surg 48:655-658, 2008

Objective.—While autogenous arteriovenous access is preferred, prosthetic arteriovenous grafts (AVG) are still required in a large number of patients. Infection of AVGs occurs frequently and may cause life-threatening bleeding or sepsis. Multiple treatment strategies have been advocated (ranging from graft preservation to excision with complex concomitant reconstructions), indicating a lack of consensus on appropriate management of infected AVGs. We undertook this study to evaluate if, in the setting of anastomotic involvement, brachial artery ligation distal to the origin of the deep brachial artery accompanied by total graft excision (BAL) is safe and effective.

Methods.—All prosthetic arteriovenous graft infections managed by a single surgeon between 1995 and 2006 were reviewed retrospectively. Patients were identified from a computerized vascular registry, and data were obtained via patient charts and the electronic medical record.

Results.—We identified 45 AVG infections in 43 patients. Twenty-one patients (49%) demonstrated arterial anastomotic involvement and were treated with BAL; these form the cohort for this analysis. Mean patient age was 53.2 (SD 9.5) years. The primary etiologies for end stage renal disease (ESRD) were hypertension (29%), HIV (24%), and diabetes (19%). An upper arm AVG was present in 95% of patients; one (5%) had a forearm AVG. The majority of grafts were polytetrafluoroethylene (PTFE) (90%). Follow-up was 100% at 1 month, 86% at 3 months, and 67% at 6 months. No ischemic or septic complications occurred in the 21 patients who underwent BAL.

Conclusion.—BAL is an effective and expeditious method to deal with an infected arm AVG in frequently critically ill patients with densely scarred wounds. In the short term, BAL appears to be well tolerated without resulting ischemic complications. Further study with longer duration of follow-up is necessary to ascertain whether BAL results in definitive cure, or whether patients may ultimately manifest ischemic changes and require additional intervention.

▶ Ligation of the brachial artery has been traditionally used in situations where reconstruction after injury or for infection is not possible or where graft failure or patch repair is predicted secondary to very high risk of infection. It has also been used for similar reasons in patients with infected dialysis prosthetic grafts. Here, however, the authors promote brachial artery ligation as first-line therapy for patients with infected loop prosthetic dialysis access grafts. In this study, no evidence of ischemia in the short term was seen in 21 patients treated with primary brachial artery ligation. All patients were cured of their infections and none required additional interventions. This article falls into the category of "what you can get away with." I see no reason to sacrifice a major artery if reconstruction is reasonably possible and would not advocate this approach for routine treatment of an infected access graft. The primary value of the article is to point out that ligation of the brachial artery can be well tolerated and should be an option under very selected circumstances. It is not that much trouble to close the brachial artery with a vein patch.

G. L. Moneta, MD

13 Carotid and Cerebrovascular Disease

The fate of patients with retinal artery occlusion and Hollenhorst plaque
Dunlap AB, Kosmorsky GS, Kashyap VS (The Cleveland Clinic, OH)
J Vasc Surg 46:1125-1129, 2007

Objective.—Ocular symptoms and signs often herald hemispheric neurological events associated with extracranial cerebrovascular disease. However, the presence of a Hollenhorst plaque (HP) or retinal artery occlusion (RAO) and the risk of stroke is unclear. The purpose of this study was to review the outcomes of all patients who presented with a HP or RAO at a single institution.

Methods.—Between 2000 and 2005, the management and outcome of 130 consecutive patients with a diagnosis of HP, central RAO, or branch RAO (ICD-9 codes 362.30 to 362.33) were reviewed. Patients with transient monocular visual loss (amaurosis fugax), retinal venous occlusion, and other ocular pathologies were excluded. Electronic and hardcopy medical records were reviewed for demographic data, clinical variables, radiological, and noninvasive vascular lab testing. Duplex and magnetic resonance angiography (MRA) of the carotid arteries were reviewed to confirm the presence of a lesion and quantify the degree of stenosis.

Results.—During the study interval, 70 males and 60 females, with a mean age of 68 ± 16 (±SD) years underwent ophthalmologic evaluation. Symptoms were present in 61% of patients and included eye pain, blurred vision, or atypical visual symptoms, while 39% were asymptomatic. Atherosclerotic risk factors in this population included the presence of hypertension (73%), diabetes (33%), hyperlipidemia (75%), and tobacco use (38%). A majority of patients underwent carotid interrogation via Duplex imaging (68%). Carotid bifurcation stenoses ipsilateral to the ocular findings were <30% in 68% of the patients, between 30 and 60% in 22% and >60% in only 8% of patients. Six patients with lesions greater than 60% went on to have either a carotid endarterectomy or carotid stenting. Follow-up data on this group ranged from 1 to 49 months (median, 22 months), with no stroke or transient ischemic attack identified. There were five deaths during follow-up; none related to stroke.

Serial carotid Duplex examinations failed to identify progression of carotid stenoses in this group of patients. Overall survival was 94% at 36 months for this cohort.

Conclusion.—The presence of a HP or RAO is associated with a low prevalence of extracranial cerebrovascular disease that requires intervention. Furthermore, in contradistinction to amaurosis fugax, these ocular findings are not associated with a high risk for hemispheric neurological events.

▶ Although this study shows a weak association between the presence of isolated Hollenhorst plaque or retinal artery occlusion, and a low prevalence of extracranial cerebrovascular disease, this conclusion should be tempered by a retrospective design, small sample size, and carotid Duplex ultrasound limited to only 68% of the study population. While the presence of significant extracranial cerebrovascular disease may be low (8% with > 60% stenosis) and no neurologic events were observed, with an association higher than the general population, isolated Hollenhorst plaque or retinal artery occlusion should still be considered a marker for potential cerebrovascular disease, especially in the presence of other atherosclerotic risk factors. Further cerebrovascular evaluation is still warranted.

M. A. Passman, MD

Aortic Atherosclerosis, Hypercoagulability, and Stroke. The APRIS (Aortic Plaque and Risk of Ischemic Stroke) Study
Di Tullio MR, Homma S, Jin Z, et al (Columbia Univ Med Ctr, NY)
J Am Coll Cardiol 52:855-861, 2008

Objectives.—Our goal was to assess the effect of hypercoagulability on the risk of stroke in patients with aortic plaques.

Background.—Atherosclerotic plaques in the aortic arch are a risk factor for ischemic stroke. Their relationship with blood hypercoagulability, which might enhance their embolic potential and affect treatment and prevention, is not known.

Methods.—We performed transesophageal echocardiography in 255 patients with first acute ischemic stroke and in 209 control subjects matched by age, gender, and race/ethnicity. The association between arch plaques and hypercoagulability, and its effect on the stroke risk, was assessed with a case-control design. Stroke patients were then followed prospectively to assess recurrent stroke and death.

Results.—Large (≥ 4 mm) arch plaques were associated with increased stroke risk (adjusted odds ratio [OR]: 2.4, 95% confidence interval [CI]: 1.3 to 4.6), especially when ulcerations or superimposed thrombus were present (adjusted OR: 3.3, 95% CI: 1.4 to 8.2). Prothrombin fragment F 1.2, an indicator of thrombin generation, was associated with large plaques in stroke patients (p = 0.02), but not in control subjects. Over a mean follow-up of 55.1 ± 37.2 months, stroke patients with large plaques and F 1.2 over the median value had a significantly higher risk of recurrent stroke and death than those with large plaques but lower F 1.2 levels (230 events per 1,000 person-years vs. 85 events per 1,000 person-years; $p = 0.05$).

Conclusions.—In patients presenting with acute ischemic stroke, large aortic plaques are associated with blood hypercoagulability, suggesting a role for coagulation activation in the stroke mechanism. Coexistence of large aortic plaques and blood hypercoagulability is associated with an increased risk of recurrent stroke and death (Figs 1 and 2).

▶ Large plaques in the proximal portion of the aorta are associated with an increased risk of ischemic stroke (Fig 1). Plaque thickness is related to stroke risk and a 4-mm thick plaque is considered clinically relevant for risk stratification. Ulcerations and mobile components of these plaques also contribute to embolic risk. It is suggested that superimposed thrombotic material on the aortic plaque may contribute to its thickness and enhanced stroke potential of the plaque. This study draws an association between activation of coagulation parameters and risk of stroke in patients with aortic arch plaques. Prothrombin fragment F 1.2 is a byproduct of the conversion of prothrombin to thrombin, and is an excellent indicator of thrombin generation. The results of the study suggest an overall association between hypercoagulability, aortic plaque thickness, and ischemic stroke. The best treatment for emboli likely originating from an aortic plaque is unknown. Anticoagulation agents are usually prescribed for

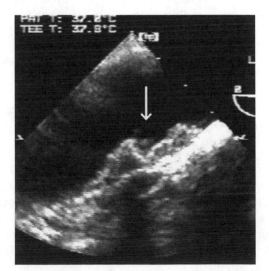

FIGURE 1.—Example of large, complex plaque in the aortic arch. An ulceration and 2 faintly echogenic superimposed thrombi are visualized (**arrow**). (Reprinted from Di Tullio MR, Homma S, Jin Z, et al. Aortic atherosclerosis, hypercoagulability, and stroke. The APRIS (Aortic Plaque and Risk of Ischemic Stroke) study. *J Am Coll Cardiol.* 2008;52:855-861, with permission from the American College of Cardiology Foundation.)

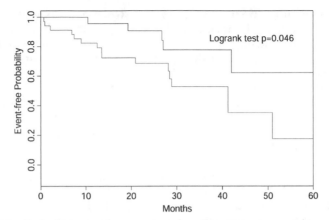

FIGURE 2.—Kaplan-Meier event-free curves in stroke patients. Data are presented according to arch plaque thickness and prothrombin fragment F 1.2 levels. **Blue lines** = large plaque and F 1.2 < median (n = 24, event = 5); **red lines** = large plaque and F 1.2 ≥ median (n = 34, event = 15). Editor's note: For interpretation of the references to color in this figure legend, the reader is referred to the web version of this article. (Reprinted from Di Tullio MR, Homma S, Jin Z, et al. Aortic atherosclerosis, hypercoagulability, and stroke. The APRIS (Aortic Plaque and Risk of Ischemic Stroke) study. *J Am Coll Cardiol* 2008;52:855-861, 2008 with permission from the American College of Cardiology Foundation.)

most thrombi, whereas anti-platelet agents are often used for plaques greater than 4 mm in but not without superimposed mobile thrombus. The results here suggest that patients with large nonmobile aortic plaques and ischemic strokes should have prothrombin fragment F 1.2 levels assessed at least for prognostic reasons (Fig 2). Future trials will be necessary to evaluate whether systemic anticoagulation may reduce the risk of subsequent stroke in patients with elevated fragment F 1.2 levels and large proximal aortic plaques.

G. L. Moneta, MD

The relationship between serum levels of vascular calcification inhibitors and carotid plaque vulnerability

Kadoglou NPE, Gerasimidis T, Golemati S, et al (Univ of Athens, Med School; Aristotle Univ of Thessaloniki; et al)
J Vasc Surg 47:55-62, 2008

Objective.—Osteopontin (OPN) and osteoprotegerin (OPG) are well-known vascular calcification inhibitors, which have been recently demonstrated to correlate with inflammation and cardiovascular events incidence. The aim of this cross-sectional study is to survey whether OPN and OPG are involved in carotid plaque vulnerability. For this reason, we assessed serum OPN and OPG levels in patients with carotid stenosis, and we explored their relationship with carotid plaque echogenicity and subsequent cerebrovascular ischemic events.

Methods.—A total of 164 Whites were selected from a large cohort of 297 subjects to participate. In particular, 114 patients (61 men, 53 women), aged 55 to 80, had recently-diagnosed ICA stenosis higher than 50%. A group of 50 age-, sex-, and body mass index (BMI)-matched healthy individuals served as healthy controls. Patients with renal failure, hypothyroidism, osteoporosis, and lipid-lowering therapy were excluded. Images of both carotids were obtained from all participants using a high-resolution color duplex ultrasound and the gray-scale median (GSM) score was calculated. Brain computed tomography (CT), and magnetic resonance imaging (MRI) scans when CT was questionable, were performed on all patients with carotid stenosis. Clinical parameters, lipid and glycemic indexes, hsCRP, fibrinogen, white blood cells (WBC) count, OPN, and OPG were measured. Independent t test, one-way ANOVA, Pearson correlation, and multiple regression analysis were used for statistical analysis.

Results.—Among patients with carotid stenosis, 60 had history of ipsilateral stroke or TIA and positive CT or MRI findings (group A), while 54 had no neurological symptoms and negative CT and MRI scan (group B). Overall, patients with carotid stenosis showed worse lipid profile and increased waist circumference, blood pressure, hsCRP, fibrinogen, WBC count, OPN, and OPG levels compared with healthy subjects (group C) ($P < .05$). Statistical analysis revealed that group A had significantly lower levels of GSM than group B (57.4 ± 38.19 vs 76.32 ± 36.72; $P = .008$) and higher levels of hsCRP, OPN, and OPG than groups B and C ($P < .05$). Concerning the latter, biochemical markers group B showed only elevated OPG levels compared with group C ($P = 038$). Notably, GSM was considerably associated with serum OPN and OPG and waist circumference in patients with carotid atherosclerosis in univariate ($r = -0.333$; $P = .032$, $r = -0.575$; $P < .001$, $r = -0.590$; $P = .006$, respectively) and multiple regression analysis ($R^2 = 0.445$; $P = .006$).

Conclusions.—The present study demonstrated elevated serum OPN and OPG levels in patients with carotid stenosis and documented an independent association between these biochemical markers, GSM and carotid-induced symptomatology. Therefore bone-matrix proteins combined with GSM could be potential markers for vulnerable carotid plaques.

▶ Osteopontin and osteoprotegerin are molecules that are thought to mediate tissue response to injury and inflammation. What remains unclear is whether these proteins have any relevance to vascular disease in humans. It is amazing that there appeared to be a measurable difference in serum levels between symptomatic versus asymptomatic and healthy individuals in the setting of such a small number of patients. The authors excluded patients with severe coronary artery disease, osteoporosis, or hypothyroidism. This may limit the applicability of these findings to women. Furthermore, patients who were on lipid-lowering therapy, angiotensin II receptor blockers, estrogen therapy, or warfarin were also excluded from this analysis. Further analysis of the correlation between the levels of these calcium inhibitors in patients with carotid and peripheral vascular disease is warranted.

M. T. Watkins, MD

Aspirin and Extended-Release Dipyridamole versus Clopidogrel for Recurrent Stroke

Sacco RL, Diener H-C, Yusuf S, et al (Univ of Miami, FL)
N Engl J Med 359:1238-1251, 2008

Background.—Recurrent stroke is a frequent, disabling event after ischemic stroke. This study compared the efficacy and safety of two antiplatelet regimens—aspirin plus extended-release dipyridamole (ASA–ERDP) versus clopidogrel.

Methods.—In this double-blind, 2-by-2 factorial trial, we randomly assigned patients to receive 25 mg of aspirin plus 200 mg of extended-release dipyridamole twice daily or to receive 75 mg of clopidogrel daily. The primary outcome was first recurrence of stroke. The secondary outcome was a composite of stroke, myocardial infarction, or death from vascular causes. Sequential statistical testing of noninferiority (margin of 1.075), followed by superiority testing, was planned.

Results.—A total of 20,332 patients were followed for a mean of 2.5 years. Recurrent stroke occurred in 916 patients (9.0%) receiving ASA–ERDP and in 898 patients (8.8%) receiving clopidogrel (hazard ratio, 1.01; 95% confidence interval [CI], 0.92 to 1.11). The secondary outcome occurred in 1333 patients (13.1%) in each group (hazard ratio for ASA–ERDP, 0.99; 95% CI, 0.92 to 1.07). There were more major hemorrhagic events among ASA–ERDP recipients (419 [4.1%]) than among clopidogrel recipients (365 [3.6%]) (hazard ratio, 1.15; 95% CI, 1.00 to 1.32), including intracranial hemorrhage (hazard ratio, 1.42; 95% CI, 1.11 to 1.83). The net risk of recurrent stroke or major hemorrhagic event was similar in the two groups (1194 ASA–ERDP recipients [11.7%], vs. 1156 clopidogrel recipients [11.4%]; hazard ratio, 1.03; 95% CI, 0.95 to 1.11).

Conclusions.—The trial did not meet the predefined criteria for noninferiority but showed similar rates of recurrent stroke with ASA–ERDP and with clopidogrel. There is no evidence that either of the two treatments was superior to the other in the prevention of recurrent stroke. (ClinicalTrials.gov number, NCT00153062.) (Fig 1).

▶ Surviving patients with ischemic stroke are at risk for recurrent stroke. Multiple trials have proven the efficacy of antiplatelet agents in prevention of recurrent stroke following noncardioembolic stroke. Which particular antiplatelet therapy may work best in the prevention of recurrent stroke is unknown and patients are essentially treated with differing antiplatelet medications based on physician preference. Here the authors investigated 2 widely used strategies of antiplatelet medications to prevent recurrent stroke. The study indicates no

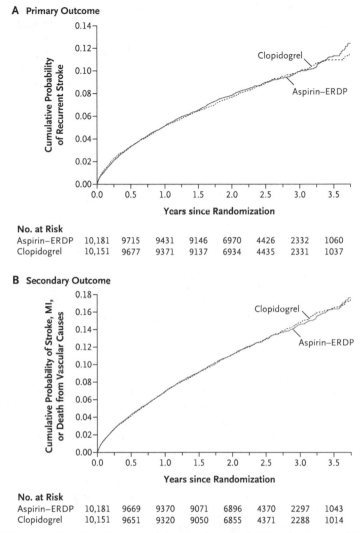

A Primary Outcome

No. at Risk

Aspirin–ERDP	10,181	9715	9431	9146	6970	4426	2332	1060
Clopidogrel	10,151	9677	9371	9137	6934	4435	2331	1037

B Secondary Outcome

No. at Risk

Aspirin–ERDP	10,181	9669	9370	9071	6896	4370	2297	1043
Clopidogrel	10,151	9651	9320	9050	6855	4371	2288	1014

FIGURE 1.—Kaplan–Meier Estimates of the Cumulative Probability of Primary and Secondary Outcomes, According to Treatment Group. The primary outcome of first recurrence of stroke (Panel A) occurred in 916 of 10,181 patients (9.0%) treated with aspirin plus extended-release dipyridamole (ERDP) and in 898 of 10,151 patients (8.8%) treated with clopidogrel (hazard ratio for aspirin–ERDP, 1.01; 95% confidence interval [CI], 0.92 to 1.11). The main secondary outcome of stroke, myocardial infarction (MI), or death from vascular causes (Panel B) occurred in 1333 patients (13.1%) in each of the two groups (hazard ratio for aspirin–ERDP, 0.99; 95% CI, 0.92 to 1.07). The estimated hazard ratios are based on a Cox model with covariates of baseline values of age, use or nonuse of angiotensin-converting–enzyme inhibitors, diabetes status, and score on the modified Rankin scale. (Reprinted from Sacco RL, Diener H-C, Yusuf S, et al. Aspirin and extended-release dipyridamole versus clopidogrel for recurrent stroke. *N Engl J Med.* 2008;359:1238-1251, with permission from Massachusetts Medical Society.)

significant difference between the use of aspirin/extended-release dipyridamole (ERDP) versus clopidogrel in preventing recurrent stroke. This was a huge study with large patient numbers and international representation from 35 countries or regions. The results of the study, therefore, should be generalizable worldwide. Although the study failed to identify a superior treatment to prevent recurrent stroke, we now know the expected risk of recurrent stroke in patients treated according to the study protocol. The study has also provided us safety and efficacy data for physicians concerning individual treatment decisions for their patients with ischemic stroke.

G. L. Moneta, MD

Markers of instability in high-risk carotid plaques are reduced by statins
Kunte H, Amberger N, Busch MA, et al (Charité-Universitätsmedizin Berlin, Germany)
J Vasc Surg 47:513-522, 2008

Background.—Macrophage infiltration and expression of matrix metalloproteinase-9 (MMP-9) are markers of high-risk atherosclerotic carotid plaques and strong indicators of plaque instability. Use of statins is associated with a decreased risk of stroke and reportedly improves stability of atherosclerotic plaques, but available data addressing the mechanism of this effect are conflicting.

Methods.—We retrospectively analyzed data from 94 consecutive patients with internal carotid artery stenosis who underwent carotid endarterectomy. Excised plaques underwent systematic quantitative immunohistochemical analysis to determine the percentage of macrophage area and the percentage of MMP-9 area. Associations between percentage of macrophage area and percentage of MMP-9 area and use of statins and cerebrovascular disease were examined by univariate and multivariate analysis.

Results.—We found significantly higher values of percentage of macrophage area and of MMP-9 area in recently symptomatic (n = 26) compared with asymptomatic (n = 68) internal carotid artery stenoses: median (IQR) percentage of macrophage area was 2.29 (1.53-4.129) vs 0.53 (0.27-0.96) and percentage of MMP-9 area was 0.61 (0.36-0.89) vs 0.08 (0.02-0.27; both $P < .0005$). Patients treated with statins (n = 49) showed lower percentage values of macrophage area and MMP-9 area than untreated patients: the percentage of macrophage area was 0.54 (0.31-1.18) vs 1.03 (0.57-2.08; $P = .01$) and percentage of MMP-9 area was 0.06 (0.02-0.22) vs 0.36 (0.16-0.62; $P < .0005$). These associations between statin treatment and percentages of macrophage area and MMP-9 area did not change after controlling for symptomatic cerebrovascular disease and the effects of other potential confounders in multivariable analysis.

Conclusions.—Our results confirm the value of percentage of macrophage area and percentage of MMP-9 area as markers of plaque instability and provide further evidence to support the hypothesis that statins reduce inflammatory responses and thereby stabilize carotid atherosclerotic plaques (Fig 3).

▶ Carotid plaques with a thin fibrous cap or a large lipid component may be unstable and prone to produce neurologic symptoms (Fig 3). Statins may have a "stabilizing effect" on atherosclerotic plaques, and the evidence is overwhelming that the pleiotropic effects of statins are independent of their lipid-lowering effects and are extremely important in reducing cardiovascular risk. Recently, investigations have begun targeting the anti-inflammatory effects of statins as a potential mediator of these pleiotropic effects. It is thought that a reduction of isoprenoids underlines the anti-inflammatory pleiotropic effects of statins. Isoprenoids participate in regulation of monocyte-adhesion molecules. Reduction in isoprenoids could result in reduced infiltration of macrophage into an atherosclerotic plaque, thereby enhancing plaque stability. Because macrophage infiltration may promote inflammatory signaling and contribute to matrix metalloproteinase-9 (MMP-9)–induced plaque instability,

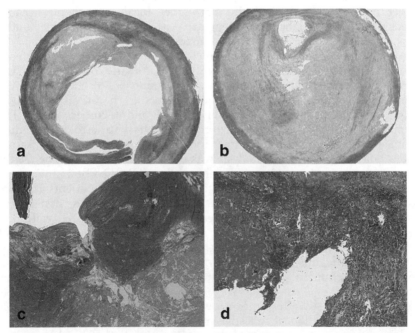

FIGURE 3.—Characteristic morphologic features of indirect plaque instability. **Panel a,** Representative cross section showing plaque with thin fibrotic cap and a fixed thrombus in the lumen of the vessel (staining with elastin van Gieson, ×15 original magnification). **Panel b,** Plaque cross-section with a very large lipid core (staining with elastin van Gieson, ×15 original magnification). **Panel c,** Plaque cross-section shows a plaque rupture with plaque content erupting from the lipid core (staining with elastin van Gieson, ×50 original magnification). **Panel d,** Plaque cross-section shows an intraplaque hemorrhage (staining with hematoxylin and eosin, ×50 original magnification). (Reprinted from Kunte H, Amberger N, Busch MA, et al. Markers of instability in high-risk carotid plaques are reduced by statins. *J Vasc Surg.* 2008;47:513-522, with permission from The Society for Vascular Surgery.)

the authors' observations that statins result in reduced plaque macrophage infiltration of the plaque and reduced MMP-9 production are consistent with an "isoprenoid" mechanism of statin benefit. The observation that the inflammatory markers linked to macrophage infiltration and MMP-9 production were reduced by statins independent of cholesterol levels should lead to even more investigations probing an anti-inflammatory mechanism, at least on the beneficial effects of statins.

G. L. Moneta, MD

General anaesthesia versus local anaesthesia for carotid surgery (GALA): a multicentre, randomised controlled trial
GALA Trial Collaborative Group (Western General Hosp, Edinburgh, UK)
Lancet 372:2132-2142, 2008

Background.—The effect of carotid endarterectomy in lowering the risk of stroke ipsilateral to severe atherosclerotic carotid-artery stenosis is offset by complications during or soon after surgery. We compared surgery under general anaesthesia with that under local anaesthesia because prediction and avoidance of perioperative strokes might be easier under local anaesthesia than under general anaesthesia.

Methods.—We undertook a parallel group, multicentre, randomised controlled trial of 3526 patients with symptomatic or asymptomatic carotid stenosis from 95 centres in 24 countries. Participants were randomly assigned to surgery under general (n = 1753) or local (n = 1773) anaesthesia between June, 1999 and October, 2007. The primary outcome was the proportion of patients with stroke (including retinal infarction), myocardial infarction, or death between randomisation and 30 days after surgery. Analysis was by intention to treat. The trial is registered with Current Control Trials number ISRCTN00525237.

Findings.—A primary outcome occurred in 84 (4·8%) patients assigned to surgery under general anaesthesia and 80 (4·5%) of those assigned to surgery under local anaesthesia; three events per 1000 treated were prevented with local anaesthesia (95% CI −11 to 17; risk ratio [RR] 0·94 [95% CI 0·70 to 1·27]). The two groups did not significantly differ for quality of life, length of hospital stay, or the primary outcome in the prespecified subgroups of age, contralateral carotid occlusion, and baseline surgical risk.

Interpretation.—We have not shown a definite difference in outcomes between general and local anaesthesia for carotid surgery. The anaesthetist and surgeon, in consultation with the patient, should decide which anaesthetic technique to use on an individual basis.

Funding.—The Health Foundation (UK) and European Society of Vascular Surgery (Fig 2).

▶ Stroke is the most feared complication of carotid surgery. There is considerable debate as to whether carotid endarterectomy under local or general

Subgroup		GA n/N	(%)	LA n/N	(%)		Odds ratio (95% CI)	p value
Prespecified								
Contralateral carotid	Yes	15/150	(10·0)	8/160	(5·0)		0·47 (0·20-1·15)	0·098
occlusion	No	69/1602	(4·3)	72/1611	(4·5)		1·04 (0·74-1·46)	
Age (years)	>75	26/489	(5·3)	21/453	(4·6)		0·87 (0·48-1·56)	0·741
	≤75	58/1263	(4·6)	59/1318	(4·5)		0·97 (0·67-1·41)	
Baseline surgical risk 1								
	High	6/146	(4·1)	7/152	(4·6)		1·13 (0·37-3·44)	0·933
	Medium	37/728	(5·1)	35/720	(4·9)		0·95 (0·59-1·53)	
	Low	41/878	(4·7)	38/899	(4·2)		0·90 (0·57-1·42)	
Post hoc								
Baseline surgical risk 2								
	High	17/243	(7·0)	14/236	(5·9)		0·84 (0·40-1·74)	0·261
	Medium	26/482	(5·4)	23/470	(4·9)		0·90 (0·51-1·60)	
	Low	36/695	(5·2)	31/734	(4·2)		0·81 (0·49-1·32)	
	Very low	5/332	(1·5)	12/331	(3·6)		2·46 (0·86-7·06)	
Trainee surgeon								
	Yes	7/242	(2·9)	7/210	(3·3)		1·16 (0·40-3·36)	0·702
	No	74/1476	(5·0)	71/1515	(4·7)		0·93 (0·67-1·30)	
Trainee anaesthetist								
	Yes	8/246	(3·2)	11/213	(5·2)		1·62 (0·63-4·10)	0·285
	No	60/1325	(4·5)	58/1356	(4·3)		0·94 (0·65-1·36)	
Asymptomatic stenosis								
	Yes	20/685	(2·9)	23/676	(3·4)		1·17 (0·64-2·15)	0·395
	No	64/1067	(6·0)	57/1095	(5·2)		0·86 (0·60-1·24)	
Country								
	UK	47/806	(5·8)	42/820	(5·1)		0·87 (0·57-1·34)	0·620
	Non-UK	37/946	(3·9)	38/951	(4·0)		1·02 (0·64-1·62)	

0·1   1   10

Odds ratio and 99% CI

Favours LA   Favours GA

FIGURE 2.—Subgroup analyses on primary outcome of stroke (including retinal infarction), myocardial infarction, or death between randomisation and 30 days after anaesthesia (or after randomisation for those patients who did not receive any anaesthetic). GA=general anaesthesia. LA=local anaesthesia. Big squares represent studies with small 95% CI (ie, with more information); the horizontal lines represent the 95% CIs. (Reprinted from GALA Trial Collaborative Group. General anaesthesia versus local anaesthesia for carotid surgery (GALA): a multicentre, randomised controlled trial. *Lancet.* 2008;372:2132-2142, with permission from Elsevier.)

anesthesia results in a more favorable outcome. It is postulated that carotid endarterectomy under local/regional anesthesia may be safer than under general anesthesia in that it allows awake testing of brain function during carotid clamping. A decrease in the neurologic status is used as an indication to place a shunt with, as a result, fewer shunts used. While shunts should protect the brain from stroke resulting from low cerebral blood flow during carotid clamping, they are also associated with complications of luminal damage and potentially transmitting emboli through the shunt itself. The general anaesthesia versus local anaesthesia for carotid surgery (GALA) trial sought to address the efficacy of local versus general anesthesia in the prevention of complications of carotid surgery. The trial failed to show a convincing difference between general and local anesthesia with respect to outcomes following carotid surgery. There were no significant differences with regard to perioperative stroke, myocardial infarction, or death overall or in any of the subgroups analyzed (Fig 2). The results are consistent with other clinical trials evaluating major surgical procedures, which have also failed to show a convincing benefit for local or regional anesthesia. The bottom line is that the surgeon and the anesthesiologist as a team should use whatever technique they are most comfortable with in performing carotid surgery.

G. L. Moneta, MD

Factors associated with stroke or death after carotid endarterectomy in Northern New England

Goodney PP, for the Vascular Study Group of Northern New England (Section of Vascular Surgery Dartmouth-Hitchcock Med Ctr, Lebanon, NH)
J Vasc Surg 48:1139-1145, 2008

Objective.—This study investigated risk factors for stroke or death after carotid endarterectomy (CEA) among hospitals of varying type and size participating in a regional quality improvement effort.

Methods.—We reviewed 2714 patients undergoing 3092 primary CEAs (excluding combined procedures or redo CEA) at 11 hospitals in Northern New England from January 2003 through December 2007. Hospitals varied in size (25 to 615 beds) and comprised community and teaching hospitals. Fifty surgeons reported results to the database. Trained research personnel prospectively collected >70 demographic and clinical variables for each patient. Multivariate logistic regression models were used to generate odds ratios (ORs) and prediction models for the 30-day postoperative stroke or death rate.

Results.—Across 3092 CEAs, there were 38 minor strokes, 14 major strokes, and eight deaths (5 stroke-related) ≤30 days of the index procedure (30-day stroke or death rate, 1.8%). In multivariate analyses, emergency CEA (OR, 7.0; 95% confidence interval [CI], 1.8-26.9; $P = .004$), contralateral internal carotid artery occlusion (OR, 2.8; 95% CI, 1.3-6.2; $P = .009$), preoperative ipsilateral cortical stroke (OR, 2.4; 95% CI, 1.1-5.1; $P = .02$), congestive heart failure (OR, 1.6; 95% CI, 1.1-2.4, $P = .03$), and age >70 (OR, 1.3; 95% CI, 0.8-2.3; $P = .315$) were associated with postoperative stroke or death. Preoperative antiplatelet therapy was protective (OR, 0.4; 95% CI, 0.2-0.9; $P = .02$). Risk of stroke or death varied from <1% in patients with no risk factors to nearly 5% with patients with ≥3 risk factors. Our risk prediction model had excellent correlation with observed results ($r = 0.96$) and reasonable discriminative ability (area under receiver operating characteristic curve, 0.71). Risks varied from <1% in asymptomatic patients with no risk factors to nearly 4% in patients with contralateral internal carotid artery occlusion (OR, 3.2; 95% CI, 1.3-8.1; $P = .01$) and age >70 (OR, 2.9; 95% CI, 1.0-4.9, $P = .05$). Two hospitals performed significantly better than expected. These differences were not attributable to surgeon or hospital volume.

Conclusion.—Surgeons can "risk-stratify" preoperative patients by considering the variables (emergency procedure, contralateral internal carotid artery occlusion, preoperative ipsilateral cortical stroke, congestive heart failure, and age), reducing risk with antiplatelet agents, and informing patients more precisely about their risk of stroke or death after CEA. Risk prediction models can also be used to compare risk-adjusted

TABLE 4.—Multivariate Analysis of Factors Associated with 30-day Stroke or Death After Carotid Endarterectomy[a]

Variable	OR	95% CI	P
Age >70 years	1.3	0.8-2.3	0.315
Contralateral ICA occlusion	2.8	1.3-6.2	0.009
Antiplatelet agent use	0.4	0.2-0.9	0.02
Congestive heart failure	1.6	1.1-2.4	0.03
Emergency procedure[b]	7.0	1.8-26.9	0.004
Pre-op ipsilateral cortical symptoms	2.4	1.1-5.1	0.02

CI, Confidence interval; *ICA*, internal carotid artery; *OR*, odds ratio.
[a]Area under receiver operating characteristic curve, 0.71.
[b]A procedure ≤6 hours of admission.
(Reprinted from Goodney PP, for the Vascular Study Group of Northern New England. Factors associated with stroke or death after carotid endarterectomy in Northern New England. *J Vasc Surg.* 2008;48:1139-1145, with permission from The Society for Vascular Surgery.)

outcomes between centers, identify best practices, and hopefully, improve overall results (Table 4).

▶ There is not a lot of new information here. The variables associated with stroke or death following carotid endarterectomy delineated in Table 4 are expected. Also, as shown in Fig 1 in the original article, as the number of risk factors increase, outcomes worsen; again, not unexpected. High-volume centers (Fig 3A in the original article), not necessarily high-volume surgeons (Fig 3B in the original article), seem to have better outcomes. These observations regarding surgeon and hospital volume stand in contrast to previous publications on this topic.[1,2] This may reflect heightened expertise in carotid surgery in the Northern New England area, or may represent simply a type 2 error from a limited sample size.

The authors point out that patients undergoing repair of an asymptomatic carotid stenosis who were more than 70 years of age and also had a contralateral internal carotid artery (ICA) occlusion, had a predicted stroke risk of > 4% with endarterectomy for asymptomatic ICA stenosis. A stroke and death rate of 4% exceeds acceptable levels for stroke and death for asymptomatic carotid surgery. They suggest that older patients with contralateral ICA occlusion may not be appropriate for intervention for asymptomatic carotid stenosis. Conversely, however, it can be argued that the natural history of this particular subgroup of patients may be sufficiently poor to justify a higher perioperative risk. It is probably inappropriate to extrapolate guidelines generated from randomized trials with strict entry criteria to specific subgroups of patients not represented with sufficient numbers in the trials to generate meaningful statistical data.

Overall, the surgeons in Northern New England are to be congratulated for their participation in this database. The information should be useful to the Northern New England surgeons and their patients. I doubt, given the relatively homogenous population of Northern New England, that the information can be applied to other regions of the United States with more ethnic diversity.

G. L. Moneta, MD

References

1. Birkmeyer JD, Stukel TA, Siewers AE, Goodney PP, Wennberg DE, Lucas FL. Surgeon volume and operative mortality in the United States. *N Engl J Med.* 2003;349:2117-2127.
2. Cowan JA Jr, Dimick JB, Thompson BG, Stanley JC, Upchurch GR Jr. Surgeon volume as an indicator of outcomes after carotid endarterectomy: an effect independent of specialty practice and hospital volume. *J Am Coll Surg.* 2002;195: 814-821.

Statistical modeling of the volume-outcome effect for carotid endarterectomy for 10 years of a statewide database
Nazarian SM, Yenokyan G, Thompson RE, et al (Johns Hopkins Univ, Baltimore, MD)
J Vasc Surg 48:343-350, 2008

Objective.—We aimed to achieve accurate statistical modeling of a putative relationship between carotid endarterectomy (CEA) annual surgeon and hospital volume and in-hospital mortality.

Design of Study.—We performed a secondary data analysis of 10 years (1994-2003) of the Maryland hospital discharge database. Annual volume was defined as the total number of procedures performed for the time in the dataset divided by the total years in the dataset. Non-linear relationships between death and average volumes were explored with logit-transformed lowess smoothing functions, followed by random effect models and inspection of data likelihood under each combination of spline knots. A marginal model with generalized estimating equations was used to represent population-average response as a function of covariates and to account for clustering in the data. Patient comorbidity was assessed using the Deyo modification of the Charlson Index.

Setting.—The Maryland hospital discharge database is a 100% sample of all hospitals in the state.

Subjects.—CEA was identified through ICD-9 and diagnosis codes, using a previously reported algorithm.

Main Outcome Measure.—Estimated odds ratios predicting in-hospital death, α set at 0.05.

Results.—During the study period, 22,772 patients with surgeon identifiers underwent CEA in Maryland, resulting in 123 in-hospital deaths (0.54%). The crude odds ratio of death for the entire surgeon dataset was 0.9838, meaning that the odds of death decreased by an average of 0.0162 for each additional annual procedure. Surgeon volume of four to 15 CEAs per year was highly significant: for an increase in annual surgeon volume by one procedure per year, the estimated odds of death decreased by 0.065 when controlling for hospital volume, age, and comorbidity ($P =.351$). Surgeons in other volume categories also demonstrated lower odds of death with increased annual volume, but these odds ratios did not attain statistical significance. Surgeons performing ≤3 CEA per year had an odds ratio of death of 0.802 per additional annual procedure ($P =.351$), whereas those performing >15 CEAs per year had an odds ratio of 0.997 ($P =.485$). Hospitals that saw >130 CEAs per year had an odds ratio of death of 0.945 per additional procedure, or 0.055 decrease in the odds of death ($P = 0.013$), whereas hospitals performing ≤130 CEAs per year had an odds ratio of 0.998 ($P = 0.563$).

Conclusion.—We have demonstrated a technique for rigorous statistical analysis of volume-outcome data and have found a volume effect for death after CEA in this 10-year Maryland dataset. Higher volume surgeons had lower estimated odds of death, particularly those performing four to 15 CEAs per year. These data suggest that a patient undergoing CEA by a surgeon performing an average of 16 CEAs annually has a statistically equivalent risk of death compared with one undergoing CEA by a surgeon performing any number higher than this, when controlling for hospital volume, patient comorbidity, and patient age. Hospital volume was not seen to be as significant a predictor of postoperative death in this study, with only high volume hospitals (≥130 CEAs per year) showing a statistically significant decrease in the odds ratio of death. As studies on volume-outcome relationships can have important implications for health policy and surgical training, such studies should consider non-linear effects in their modeling of procedural volume (Fig 1).

▶ The concept that experience with the procedure is associated with better results is pretty well accepted by almost everyone. However, one may argue

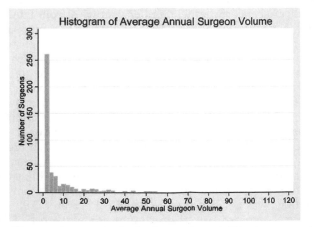

FIGURE 1.—Histogram demonstrating the distribution of annual CEA volume among the surgeons in the dataset. (Reprinted from Nazarian SM, Yenokyan G, Thompson RE, et al. Statistical modeling of the volume-outcome effect for carotid endarterectomy for 10 years of a statewide database. *J Vasc Surg.* 2008;48:343-350, with permission from The Society for Vascular Surgery.)

that volume is not necessarily an appropriate surrogate for experience and skill. It is reasonable that some level of ongoing experience with a procedure is desirable and likely to aid in producing good results. In that regard, an interesting finding of this article is that of the 442 individuals credited with performing endarterectomy in Maryland during the time of this study, 214 appear to perform 1 or less than 1 procedure per year (Fig 1). If this is true, that is a remarkable figure and indicates a problem with hospital credentialing committees in the state of Maryland. Finally, like all studies based on administrative databases, this one, despite its attempt to control for comorbidity, is severely limited by the fact that it is virtually impossible to stratify patients by indication and to truly stratify them by comorbidities with administrative databases. It is appropriate to be very skeptical about far-reaching conclusions derived from administrative database studies.

G. L. Moneta, MD

Association between minor and major surgical complications after carotid endarterectomy: Results of the New York Carotid Artery Surgery study
Greenstein AJ, Chassin MR, Wang J, et al (Mount Sinai School of Medicine and the Department of Neurology, Mount Sinai School of Medicine, NY)
J Vasc Surg 46:1138-1146, 2007

Objective.—Most studies on outcomes of carotid endarterectomy (CEA) have focused on the major complications of death and stroke. Less is known about minor, but more common, surgical complications such as hematoma, cranial nerve palsy, and wound infection. This study used data from a large, population-based cohort study to describe the incidence of minor surgical complications after CEA and examine associations between minor and major complications.

Methods.—The New York Carotid Artery Surgery (NYCAS) study examined all Medicare beneficiaries who underwent CEA from January 1998 to June 1999 in NY State. Detailed clinical information on preoperative characteristics and complications ≤ 30 days of surgery was abstracted from hospital charts. Associations between minor (cranial nerve palsies, hematoma, and wound infection) and major complications (death/stroke) were examined with χ^2 tests and multivariate logistic regression.

Results.—The NYCAS study had data on 9308 CEAs performed by 482 surgeons in 167 hospitals. Overall, 10% of patients had a minor surgical complication (cranial nerve (CN) palsy, 5.5%; hematoma, 5.0%; and wound infection, 0.2%). Cardiac complications occurred in 3.9% (myocardial 1.1%, unstable angina 0.9%, pulmonary edema 2.1%, and ventricular tachycardia 0.8%). In both unadjusted and adjusted analyses, the occurrence of any minor surgical complication, CN palsy alone, or hematoma alone was associated with 3 to 4-fold greater odds of perioperative stroke or combined risk of death and nonfatal stroke ($P < 0.0001$). Patients with cardiac complications had 4 to 5-fold increased odds of stroke or combined risk of death and stroke.

Conclusion.—Minor surgical complications are common after CEA and are associated with much higher risk of death and stroke. Patient factors, process factors, and direct causality are involved in this relationship, but future work will be needed to better understand their relative contributions.

▶ Analyses of large databases have become very popular. The results are often interesting, but because the data are analyzed retrospectively without predetermined end points, the results can seldom be considered definitive. This is such a study. The number of minor complications reported is probably an underestimate of the true numbers, and therefore, the idea that carotid endarterectomy (CEA) is associated with a surprising number of minor complications is probably correct. However, I doubt the database used here was designed to investigate the authors' hypothesis that these "minor" compilations after CEA convey a higher risk of stroke and death. Nevertheless, it makes sense that minor complications may indicate a more difficult procedure or a less-skilled surgeon, and therefore, a greater risk of a major complication, such as stroke or death. I would not, based on this study alone, be willing to suggest that minor complications after carotid surgery be monitored by hospital credentialing committees.

G. L. Moneta, MD

Carotid endarterectomy was performed with lower stroke and death rates than carotid artery stenting in the United States in 2003 and 2004
McPhee JT, Hill JS, Ciocca RG, et al (Univ of Massachusetts Med School, Worcester, MA)
J Vasc Surg 46:1112-1118, 2007

Objective.—Although carotid endarterectomy (CEA) is the gold standard for the treatment of carotid artery stenosis, the recent United States Food and Drug Administration approval of carotid artery stenting (CAS) may have led to its widespread use outside of clinical trials and registries. This study compared in-hospital postoperative stroke and mortality rates after CAS and CEA at the national level.

Methods.—The Nationwide Inpatient Sample (NIS) was queried to identify all patient-discharges that occurred for revascularization of carotid artery stenosis. The *International Classification of Diseases, 9th Revision, Clinical Modification* procedure codes for CEA (38.12), CAS (00.63), and insertion of noncoronary stents (39.50, 39.90) were used in conjunction with the diagnostic codes for carotid artery stenosis, with (433.11) and without (433.10) stroke. Primary outcome measures included in-hospital postoperative stroke and death rates. Multivariate logistic regressions were performed to evaluate independent predictors of postoperative stroke and mortality. Adjustment was made for age, sex, medical comorbidities, admission diagnosis, procedure type, year, and hospital type.

Results.—During the calendar years of 2003 and 2004, an estimated 259,080 carotid revascularization procedures were performed in the United States. CAS had a higher rate of in-hospital postoperative stroke (2.1% vs 0.88%, *P* < .0001) and higher postoperative mortality (1.3% vs 0.39%) than CEA. For asymptomatic patients (92%), the postoperative stroke rate was significantly higher for CAS than CEA (1.8% vs 0.86%, *P* < .0001), but the mortality rate was similar (0.44% vs 0.36%, *P* = .36). For symptomatic patients (8%), the rates for postoperative stroke (4.2% vs 1.1%, *P* < .0001) and mortality (7.5% vs 1.0%, *P* < .0001) were significantly higher after CAS. By multivariate regression, CAS was independently predictive of postoperative stroke (odds ratio [OR], 2.49; 95% confidence interval [CI], 1.91 to 3.25). CAS was also associated with in-hospital, postoperative mortality for asymptomatic (OR, 2.37; 95% CI, 1.46 to 3.84) and symptomatic (OR, 2.64; 95% CI, 1.89 to 3.69) patients.

Conclusions.—As determined from a large representative national sample including the years of 2003 and 2004, the in-hospital stroke rate after CAS for asymptomatic patients was twofold higher than after CEA. For symptomatic patients, the respective in-hospital stroke and mortality rates were fourfold and sevenfold higher. These unexpected results indicate that further randomized controlled trials with homogenous symptomatic and asymptomatic patient groups should be performed.

▶ This is another bit of evidence that carotid artery stenting (CAS) probably still has a way to go to catch up with carotid endarterectomy (CEA) with great differences in relative stroke rates favoring CEA over CAS (Fig 2 in the original article). There are, obviously, significant limitations to retrospective analysis of very large national databases, and therefore, these data are unlikely to change anyone's mind about the relative roles of CEA and CAS. It is, however, becoming clear that CEA is probably a much safer operation than it was 20 years ago. No matter how much CAS improves, I think it is actually going to be difficult for CAS to beat CEA in good- to moderate-risk patients when CEA is performed by experienced, well-trained surgeons. We still await the results of proper randomized controlled trials.

G. L. Moneta, MD

Significance of postoperative crossed cerebellar hypoperfusion in patients with cerebral hyperperfusion following carotid endarterectomy: SPECT study
Ogasawara K, Kobayashi M, Suga Y, et al (Iwate Med Univ, Uchimaru, Morioka, Japan)
Eur J Nucl Med Mol 35:146-152, 2008

Purpose.—Cerebral hyperperfusion after carotid endarterectomy (CEA) results in cerebral hyperperfusion syndrome and cognitive impairment. The goal of the present study was to clarify the clinical significance of postoperative crossed cerebellar hypoperfusion (CCH) in patients with cerebral hyperperfusion after CEA by assessing brain perfusion with single-photon emission computed tomography (SPECT).

Methods.—Brain perfusion was quantitatively measured using SPECT and the [^{123}I]N-isopropyl-p-iodoamphetamine-autoradiography method before and immediately after CEA and on the third postoperative day in 80 patients with ipsilateral internal carotid artery stenosis ($\geq$70%). Postoperative CCH was determined by differences between asymmetry of perfusion in bilateral cerebellar hemispheres before and after CEA. Neuropsychological testing was also performed preoperatively and at the first postoperative month.

Results.—Eleven patients developed cerebral hyperperfusion (cerebral blood flow increase of $\geq$100% compared with preoperative values) on SPECT imaging performed immediately after CEA. In seven of these patients, CCH was observed on the third postoperative day. All three patients with hyperperfusion syndrome exhibited cerebral hyperperfusion and CCH on the third postoperative day and developed postoperative cognitive impairment. Of the eight patients with asymptomatic hyperperfusion, four exhibited CCH despite resolution of cerebral hyperperfusion on the third postoperative day, and three of these patients experienced postoperative cognitive impairment. In contrast, four patients without postoperative CCH did not experience postoperative cognitive impairment.

Conclusions.—The presence of postoperative CCH with concomitant cerebral hyperperfusion reflects the development of hyperperfusion syndrome. Further, the presence of postoperative CCH in patients with cerebral hyperperfusion, following CEA, suggests development of postoperative cognitive impairment, even when asymptomatic.

▶ The article points out several not generally appreciated facets of cerebral hyperperfusion, and the cerebral hyperperfusion syndrome that can occur after carotid endarterectomy (CEA) for high-grade carotid stenosis. First of all, at least using the definition of a 100% increase in cerebral perfusion as measured by single-photon emission computed tomography scanning, cerebral hyperperfusion is more common than is clinically evident or generally acknowledged, and different patterns of cerebral hyperperfusion exist. (The authors do not detail the degree of carotid stenosis in the opposite internal carotid artery, but it seems unlikely all the patients had high-grade carotid stenosis bilaterally, further implying that the problem is more widespread than it is generally appreciated.) Another issue is that clinically evident hyperperfusion syndrome only develops in patients who have persistent cerebral hyperperfusion extending to the third postoperative day. Finally, and perhaps most disturbing, cognitive impairment occurs in patients with cerebral hyperperfusion after CEA, even in the absence of the clinically evident hyperperfusion syndrome (Fig 3 in the original article). Such patients may be able to be identified by the presence of cerebellar hypoperfusion after CEA.

G. L. Moneta, MD

Long-Term Results of Carotid Stenting versus Endarterectomy in High-Risk Patients

Gurm HS, Yadav JS, Fayad P, et al (Univ of Michigan School of Medicine, Ann Arbor; Piedmont Cardiovascular Inst, Atlanta; Univ of Nebraska Med Ctr, Omaha; et al)

N Engl J Med 358:1572-1579, 2008

Background.—We previously reported that, in a randomized trial, carotid stenting, with the use of an emboli-protection device, is not inferior to carotid endarterectomy for the treatment of carotid artery disease at 30 days and at 1 year. We now report the 3-year results.

Methods.—The trial evaluated carotid artery stenting with the use of an emboli-protection device as compared with endarterectomy in 334 patients at increased risk for complications from endarterectomy who had either a symptomatic carotid artery stenosis of at least 50% of the luminal diameter, or an asymptomatic stenosis of at least 80%. The prespecified major secondary end point at 3 years was a composite of death, stroke, or myocardial infarction within 30 days after the procedure or death or ipsilateral stroke between 31 days and 1080 days (3 years).

Results.—At 3 years, data were available for 260 patients (77.8%), including 85.6% of patients in the stenting group and 70.1% of those in the endarterectomy group. The prespecified major secondary end point occurred in 41 patients in the stenting group (cumulative incidence, 24.6%; Kaplan–Meier estimate, 26.2%) and 45 patients in the endarterectomy group (cumulative incidence, 26.9%; Kaplan–Meier estimate, 30.3%) (absolute difference in cumulative incidence for the stenting group, −2.3%; 95% confidence interval, −11.8 to 7.0). There were 15 strokes in each of the two groups, of which 11 in the stenting group and 9 in the endarterectomy group were ipsilateral.

Conclusions.—In our trial of patients with severe carotid artery stenosis and increased surgical risk, no significant difference could be shown in long-term outcomes between patients who underwent carotid artery stenting with an emboli-protection device and those who underwent endarterectomy.

▶ There are a number of significant limitations to this trial, all of which, to the authors' credit, are indicated on the last page of the article before the references. These include the absence of a medical therapy group, the fact that many of these patients in many practices would not be treated with any intervention, the small size of the randomized cohort that prevents meaningful subgroup analysis, incomplete follow-up at 3 years, the use of only 1 type of embolic protection device, and the lack of inclusion of moderate- or low-risk patients for carotid endarterectomy. Finally, 10 of the 12 named authors are financially linked to Cordis, the sponsor of the trial, or had patents linked to the cerebral protection device used in the trial.

G. L. Moneta, MD

Alert for increased long-term follow-up after carotid artery stenting: Results of a prospective, randomized, single-center trial of carotid artery stenting vs carotid endarterectomy

Steinbauer MGM, Pfister K, Greindl M, et al (Univ of Regensburg, Germany)

J Vasc Surg 48:93-98, 2008

Background.—Carotid endarterectomy (CEA) has been shown to be effective in stroke prevention for patients with symptomatic or asymptomatic carotid artery stenosis. Although several prospective randomized trials indicate that carotid artery stenting (CAS) is an alternative but not superior treatment modality, there is still a significant lack of long-term data comparing CAS with CEA. This study presents long-term results of a prospective, randomized, single-center trial.

Methods.—Between August 1999 and April 2002, 87 patients with a symptomatic high-grade internal carotid artery stenosis (>70%) were randomized to CAS or CEA. After a median observation time of 66 ± 14.2 months (CAS) and 64 ± 12.1 months (CEA), 42 patients in each group were re-evaluated retrospectively by clinical examination and documentation of neurologic events. Duplex ultrasound imaging was performed in 61 patients (32 CAS, 29 CEA), and patients with restenosis >70% were re-evaluated by angiography.

Results.—During the observation period, 23 patients (25.2%) died (10 CAS, 13 CEA), and three were lost to follow up. The incidence of strokes was higher after CAS, with four strokes in 42 CAS patients vs none in 42 CEA patients. One transient ischemic attack occurred in each group. A significantly higher rate of restenosis >70% (6 of 32 vs 0 of 29) occurred after CAS compared with CEA. Five of 32 CAS patients (15.6%) presented with high-grade (>70%) restenosis as an indication for secondary intervention or surgical stent removal, and three presented with neurologic symptoms. No CEA patients required reintervention (*P* < .05 vs CAS). A medium-grade (<70%) restenosis was detected in eight of 32 CAS patients (25%) and in one of 29 CEA patients (3.4%). In five of 32 CAS (15.6%) and three of 29 CEA patients (10.3%), a high-grade stenosis of the contralateral carotid artery was observed and treated during the observation period.

Conclusion.—The long-term results of this prospective, randomized, single-center study revealed a high incidence of relevant restenosis and neurologic symptoms after CAS. CEA seems to be superior to CAS concerning the development of restenosis and significant prevention of stroke. However, the long-term results of the ongoing multicenter trials have to be awaited for a final conclusion.

▶ This is a small study and it is not likely to change anyone's opinion regarding the relative efficacy of carotid artery stenting (CAS) versus carotid endarterectomy (CEA). In fact, the study is so small it probably should not change anyone's opinion about CAS and CEA. Nevertheless, the strengths of the study are that it was prospective and randomized and seems to have been well conducted. The relatively high rate of late neurologic events in the stented patients is at odds with data from other series of carotid stents where restenosis after stenting is associated with minimal neurologic morbidity. The idea is that restenotic stented arteries result from intimal hyperplasia, producing a relatively smooth lumen surface that is not prone to accumulation of platelet aggregates or thrombosis and the plaque itself is not subject to plaque rupture. The results of this study and the SPACE trial and the EVA-3S trials, which were also European randomized trials that failed to demonstrate noninferiority of CSA to CEA, are similar. One is left to wonder a bit why the US commerical trials with industry backing seem a bit more optimistic in their conclusions than those trials without industry funding.

G. L. Moneta, MD

Carotid Artery Stenting in High-Risk Patients: Midterm Mortality Analysis
Bianchi C, Ou HW, Bishop V, et al (Loma Linda Univ Med Ctr, CA)
Ann Vasc Surg 22:185-189, 2008

Carotid artery interventions are predicated on early and late survival to prevent ischemic strokes. The technical feasibility of carotid artery stenting (CAS) has been established. Short-term results have been conflicting. Despite this, many practices have adopted CAS as an alterative to carotid endarterectomy in high-risk patients. Long-term protective benefits, however, are less established in high-risk patients. Midterm results following CAS in our high-risk protocol were analyzed to determine specific and all-cause mortality rates (beyond 30 days). We retrospectively evaluated a prospective carotid artery stent registry from October 2003 to February 2006. Demographics, high-risk indication, presence of carotid symptoms, prior history of cancer, periprocedural success, complications, as well as follow-up including readmission rate, as well as specific etiology of death were recorded. Fifty patients with critical carotid stenosis (mean stenosis 90%) underwent CAS. This cohort met high-risk criteria due to physiologic reasons in 26 patients and anatomic factors in 22 cases. Two patients met both criteria. Indications were symptomatic disease in 14 (30%) and asymptomatic in 36 cases. The overall 30-day stroke, myocardial infarction, and death rate was 2%. No minor or major strokes were recorded within 30 days postprocedure. Overall average follow-up was 11-28 months. Stroke-free survival was 94% for all patients. Overall 1-year survival was 75% for all patients, significantly higher for the asymptomatic group (88%) ($p < 0.01$). Late mortality after 30 days was 11 cases (22%) at an average of 9 months post-CAS, ranging 3-13 months. No late mortality was due to ischemic stroke. Specific etiologies of mortality included end-stage cardiac disease ($n = 1$), recurrent or metastatic cancer ($n = 2$), acute cardiac event ($n = 1$), infectious complications ($n = 3$), and other ($n = 3$). Only symptomatic indication was predictive of late mortality. Clinicians may continue to cautiously offer CAS to asymptomatic high-risk patients given their anticipated longevity. Symptomatic patients, despite poor midterm survival, do achieve freedom from neurologic death following CAS.

▶ These authors, despite good intentions, need to be reined in a bit. Most high-risk patients in this study were asymptomatic, all were VA patients, and apparently none were stented, in the context of a clinical trial. Reimbursement for stenting of asymptomatic patients, outside the context of a clinical trial, is generally not available in the private sector, perhaps explaining why only VA patients were included in this study. Given the natural history of asymptomatic carotid stenosis and the limited numbers of patients available at a single institution, it is very unlikely, and entirely predictable, that the authors can ever show, in a single institution experience, a benefit of carotid stenting over medical treatment alone in high-risk patients with asymptomatic carotid stenosis. Inclusion of the patients in the SVS database is not a substitute for a proper multicenter trial. A cynic might hint that the patients were stented because they were in the VA system, and someone wanted to perform the procedure. Although intentions may be good, all the authors have shown is that they did not hurt their patients all that much. We do not know, and the authors will never know, if they actually benefited the patients.

G. L. Moneta, MD

Carotid artery stenting: Identification of risk factors for poor outcomes

Jackson BM, English SJ, Fairman RM, et al (Hosp of the Univ of Pennsylvania, Philadelphia, PA)
J Vasc Surg 48:74-79, 2008

Objectives.—Age greater than 80 has been identified as a risk factor for complications, including stroke and death, in patients undergoing carotid artery angioplasty and stenting (CAS). This study evaluates other potential predictors of perioperative complications in patients undergoing CAS.

Methods.—All cerebrovascular endovascular procedures performed by the vascular surgery division at our university hospital between July 2003 and December 2005 were retrospectively examined. During the course of 212 admissions, 198 patients underwent 215 procedures. Patient age, comorbidities, and admission status were analyzed as independent (predictor) variables. Complication rate, discharge disposition, and length of hospital stay were considered dependent (outcome) variables. Logistic regression and Fisher exact test or Student t test were performed, as appropriate.

Results.—Complications included major and minor stroke, myocardial infarction, femoral artery pseudoaneurysm, and death. The rates of perioperative major and minor stroke were 0.5% and 2.8%, respectively. Chronic renal insufficiency was a predictor of perioperative complications, including stroke: patients with serum creatinine greater than 1.3 mg/dL had a 37% complication rate and a 11.1% stroke rate, while those with normal renal function had a 13% complication rate ($P = .003$) and a 0.6% stroke rate ($P = .001$). Similar association was seen between creatinine clearance and both stroke and complications. Obesity was a risk factor for complications, but not stroke: obese patients had a complication rate of 28%, while others had a 16% complication rate ($P = .024$). Emergency admission predicted both extended hospital stay ($P < .001$) and requirement for further inpatient care in a rehabilitation or nursing facility ($P = .007$). There was no significant difference in complication rate or stroke rate between octogenarians and others.

Conclusion.—This experience demonstrates that chronic renal insufficiency, obesity, and emergent clinical setting are risk factors for patients undergoing CAS.

▶ There are a number of physiologic and anatomic variables that have been associated in some studies, but not all, with an increased risk of a poor outcome following carotid artery stenting. These include advanced age, very high-grade lesions, highly calcified lesions, echolucent plaques, tandem lesions, an occluded external carotid artery, a type 3 aortic arch, and the presence of aortic iliac occlusive disease. This reasonably large series adds additional risk factors to that list and includes an elevated creatinine, which was found to increase the risk of stroke substantially; obesity, which increased the risk of local access complications; and finally, an emergent admission, which predicted both the extended hospital stay and requirement for further inpatient care in a rehabilitation or nursing facility. That the authors found no increased risk with elderly patients highlights the fact that none of the risk factors for carotid artery angioplasty and stenting—with perhaps the exception of a type 3 aortic arch—are universally regarded as increasing the risk of carotid artery stenting. Like any other invasive procedure, ultimately who to stent and when to stent, comes down to a matter of individual physician judgment based on their relative skill and the individual patient.

G. L. Moneta, MD

A randomized trial of carotid artery stenting with and without cerebral protection
Barbato JE, Dillavou E, Horowitz MB, et al (Univ of Pittsburgh Med Ctr, PA)
J Vasc Surg 47:760-765, 2008

Background.—The use of a distal filter cerebral protection device with carotid artery stenting is commonplace. There is little evidence, however, that filters are effective in preventing embolic lesions. This study examined the incidence of embolic phenomenon during carotid artery stenting with and without filter use.

Methods.—This was a prospective, randomized, single-center study of carotid artery stenting with or without a distal cerebral protection filter. A 1:1 scheme was used to randomize 36 carotid artery stenting procedures in 35 patients. Diffusion-weighted magnetic resonance imaging (DW MRI) 24 hours after stenting was used to assess the occurrence of new embolic lesions. Blinded observers calculated lesion number and volume.

Results.—The mean age was 78.6 ± 7.0 in the cerebral protection group compared with 74.1 ± 8.7 in the no cerebral protection group (*P* = .92). Despite similar average age, the percentage of octogenarians was higher in the cerebral protection group (61.1% vs 22.2%; *P* = .04). Two procedures in the cerebral protection group were not successful. One was completed without protection because of inability to track the filter, and the second was aborted because of severe tortuosity with a later carotid endarterectomy. New MRI lesions were noted in 72% of the cerebral protection group compared with 44% in the no cerebral protection group (*P* = .09). The average number of lesions in these patients was 6.1 and 6.2, respectively, with mean DW MRI lesion size of 16.63 mm^3 vs 15.61 mm^3 (*P* = .79 and .49, respectively). Four strokes occurred (11%), two in each group, in patients aged 75, 80, 82, and 84 years. The only major stroke occurred in the no cerebral protection group.

Conclusions.—The use of filters during carotid artery stenting provided no demonstrable reduction of microemboli, as expected. Routine use of cerebral protection filters should undergo a more critical assessment before mandatory universal adoption.

▶ There is now a large industry that has grown around cerebral protection devices in conjunction with carotid stenting. The results of this study will, therefore, be heavily criticized by the pro-cerebral protection device mafia. What will the pro-cerebral protection people say? They will point out the small size of the study and indicate that an 11% stroke rate seems high, but that number is not really out of line with some other reported experiences with carotid angioplasty and stenting, and a 72% incidence of diffusion-weighted magnetic resonance imaging (DW MRI) lesions in the cerebral protection patients is excessive. Of course, this number is also consistent with other studies. The proper approach to this study is not immediate rejection but to think a bit about what seems obvious is always true.

G. L. Moneta, MD

Effects of Age and Symptom Status on Silent Ischemic Lesions after Carotid Stenting with and without the Use of Distal Filter Devices

Kastrup A, Gröschel K, Nägele T, et al (Univ of Göttingen, Germany; Univ of Tübingen, Germany; et al)
Am J Neuroradiol 29:608-612, 2008

Background and Purpose.—The routine use of distal filter devices during carotid angioplasty and stent placement (CAS) is controversial. The aim of this study was to analyze their effects on the incidence of new diffusion-weighted imaging (DWI) lesions as surrogate markers for stroke in important subgroups.

Materials and Methods.—DWI was performed immediately before and after CAS in 68 patients with and 175 without protection, and patients were further subdivided according to their age or symptom status.

Results.—The proportion of patients with new ipsilateral DWI lesion(s) was significantly lower after protected versus unprotected CAS (52% versus 68%), as well as in symptomatic patients (56% versus 74%) or those at or younger than 75 years of age (46% versus 67%; all $P < .05$). Similarly, the total number of lesions was significantly lower after protected versus unprotected CAS (median, 1; interquartile range [IQR], 0–2; versus median, 1; IQR 0–4.75) and in symptomatic patients (median, 1; IQR, 0–3; versus median, 2; IQR, 0–6) or those at or younger than 75 years of age (median, 0; IQR, 0–2; versus median, 1; IQR, 0–4; all $P < .05$). In contrast, for asymptomatic patients (48% versus 52%; $P = .8$; median, 0; IQR, 0–2; versus median, 1; IQR, 0–2.5; $P = .6$) or those older than 75 years of age (73% versus 69%; $P = .7$; median, 1; IQR, 0–4; versus median, 1.5; IQR, 0–5.75; $P = .6$), the proportion of patients with new lesion(s) and the total number of these lesions were not significantly different between protected and unprotected CAS.

Conclusions.—The use of distal filter devices generally reduces the incidence of new DWI lesions; however, this beneficial effect might not necessarily pertain to older and asymptomatic patients.

▶ Routine use of distal filter devices during carotid angioplasty and stenting (CAS) remains controversial. The authors sought to determine if certain subgroups of patients may benefit over others with the use of filter devices. They used new diffusion-weighted imaging (DWI) lesions as surrogate markers for stroke. DWI lesions at this time have uncertain long-term clinical significance. Nevertheless, no one considers such lesions as desirable, and their use as a surrogate marker to assess the results of carotid stenting is becoming more common. This was a retrospective and nonrandomized study. The nature of the study design does not truly permit conclusions with regard to the use of neuroprotective devices in symptomatic versus asymptomatic and younger versus older patients. The high prevalence of new DWI lesions in patients treated with and without neuroprotective devices and the lack of dramatic effects of neuroprotective devices on neurologic events associated with CAS makes one wonder about the efficacy of neuroprotective devices and/or the mechanism of new DWI lesions following CAS.

G. L. Moneta, MD

A risk score to predict ischemic lesions after protected carotid artery stenting

Gröschel K, Ernemann U, Schnaudigel S, et al (Univ of Göttingen, Germany; Univ of Tübingen, Germany)
J Neurol Sci 273:112-115, 2008

Background and Purpose.—While carotid artery stenting can be performed safely in many patients, some have a higher risk for periprocedural complications. The detection of embolic lesions after CAS with DWI could become a useful means to identify these patients. The aim of this study was to determine risk factors for new DWI lesions after CAS.

Methods.—One hundred seventy-six patients who had undergone protected CAS with pre- and postprocedural DWI between November 2000 and December 2006 were included in this retrospective investigation. The association of potential angiographic and clinical risk factors with the incidence of any new ipsilateral DWI lesion after CAS was analyzed with logistic regression analysis. Subsequently, a simple risk score was developed using area under the curve (ROC) statistics.

Results.—The proportion of patients with any new ipsilateral DWI lesion was 51%. Advanced age (odds ratio (OR) 1.06; 95% confidence interval (CI) 1.01–1.11, $p = 0.008$), the presence of an ulcerated stenosis (OR 2.28: 95% CI 1.10–4.75; $p = 0.027$) or a lesion length > 1 cm (OR 2.65; 95% CI 1.33–5.28, $p = 0.006$) were independent risk factors for new ipsilateral DWI lesions. A 4 point score ranging from 0 to 4 (age ≥ 70 years = 1 point, age ≥ 80 years = 2 points, lesion length > 1 cm = 1 point, and presence of an ulcerated stenosis = 1 point) reliably predicted the incidence of this outcome parameter (ROC = 0.70, $p < 0.001$).

Conclusions.—A simple risk score can be used to identify patients at a high risk for new DWI lesions as a possible surrogate of embolic complications after CAS (Fig 2).

▶ The appearance of new diffusion-weighted imaging (DWI) lesions following carotid artery stenting is now a common topic of investigation. They may not be bad, but they are surely not good. In reality, we really don't know all that much about them or what they mean in the long term. We do, however, know a few things. DWI lesions are very frequent following both protected and unprotected carotid artery stenting. The 51% incidence of new ipsilateral DWI lesions following protected carotid artery stenting in this series is consistent with previous reports. (Such lesions may be even more frequent with unprotected stenting.) The authors have tried to tell us which patients and which lesions are at most risk for new DWI lesions following carotid stents (Fig 2). Their proposed risk score is easy to use and remember. However, it is my guess that although everyone who performs carotid stenting would not personally want a DWI lesion in their brain, the occurrence of these lesions is not going to stop anyone from performing carotid stenting in their patients unless they can be shown to have short- or long-term clinical importance. Therefore, although this line of research is interesting, and a couple of years ago had

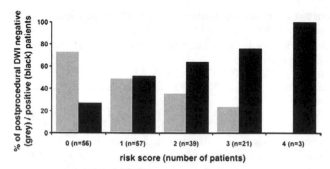

FIGURE 2.—Proportion of patients with any new ipsilateral DWI lesion according to their individual risk score. DWI positive patients are presented in black bars; DWI negative patients in grey bars, respectively. (Reprinted from Gröschel K, Ernemann U, Schnaudigel S, et al. A risk score to predict ischemic lesions after protected carotid artery stenting. *J Neurol Sci.* 2008;273:112-115, with permission from Elsevier.)

significant emotional impact, no one now is going to pay much attention to this sort of article that focuses only on the incidence of these lesions and finds no clinical impact. We need to know what, if anything, these lesions mean in the long term.

G. L. Moneta, MD

Endovascular treatment for carotid artery stenosis after neck irradiation

Favre J-P, Nourissat A, Duprey A, et al (Hôpital Nord, Saint-Etienne, Paris; Institut de Cancérologie de la Loire, Saint Priest en Jarez, Paris; et al)
J Vasc Surg 48:852-858, 2008

Background.—To lower the risk of complications, carotid angioplasty and stenting (CAS) has been proposed as an alternative to open surgery for carotid artery stenosis after neck irradiation. However, there are little postoperative data to support the benefits of this strategy. This study evaluated the outcome of CAS in patients who had undergone neck irradiation.

Methods.—This retrospective study was conducted at 15 vascular surgery or interventional radiology centers in France between January 1998 and July 2006. A total of 135 patients (115 men) with a mean age of 67 ± 8 years (range, 43-88) underwent CAS for 149 irradiation-induced lesions. The interval between irradiation and discovery of the lesions was 12 ± 8 years. Mean diameter reduction was 81% (range, 50%-95%), and stenosis was symptomatic in 34%. Contralateral carotid lesions were observed in 48% of patients, including thrombosis in 18 and stenosis >50% in 53.

Results.—Technical failure occurred during CAS in three cases. The overall technical success rate was 98%. A cerebral protection device was used in 59%. No death, one transient ischemic attack, and two strokes occurred during the first postoperative month. Mean follow-up was 30 months. Six patients were lost to follow-up. Survival rates were 93.9% at 1 year and 75.3% at 3 years. Complications after the first postoperative month included neurologic events in six, carotid thrombosis in nine, and restenosis in 18. The rates of freedom from neurologic and anatomic events were, respectively, 96.2% and 93.2% at 1 year and 93.1% and 85.9% at 3 years.

Conclusion.—The immediate outcome of CAS for irradiation-induced carotid artery stenosis was satisfactory. Medium-term neurologic outcome was acceptable, but the incidence of anatomic events such as thrombosis and restenosis was high. A randomized study is needed to confirm that the outcome of the endovascular and surgical therapy is comparable in this indication.

▶ This is an important study. Despite the limitations of being a retrospective study conducted across 15 centers between January 1998 and July 2006, this is a quite large study evaluating the outcome of carotid angioplasty and stenting (CAS) in patients with a previous history of neck irradiation for malignancy. One hundred sixty-seven lesions were treated in 149 carotid arteries in 135 patients. The interval between irradiation and treatment was 12 ± 8 years.

Complications were noteworthy in this study. The anatomic failure rate, defined as occlusion or restenosis, was significantly increased. There were 6 neurologic events, 9 carotid thromboses, and 18 restenoses within a mean of 18 months. The 30-day combined stroke and death rate was 1.5% in this high-risk population. Although this compares favorably with contemporary trials, one must consider that only 34% of the patients presented with symptoms.

One of the most interesting aspects of this article was that the authors found that the use of statins after CAS significantly decreased the incidence of anatomic events during follow up. This finding confirms the importance of medical treatment after interventions for radiation-induced stenosis of the carotid artery. The authors appropriately point out the value of a prospective-randomized trial for evaluating the utility of CAS versus an open approach for the management of postirradiation-induced carotid stenosis.

B. W. Starnes, MD

Results in a consecutive series of 83 surgical corrections of symptomatic stenotic kinking of the internal carotid artery
Illuminati G, Ricco J-B, Caliò FG, et al ("La Sapienza" Univ, Rome, Italy; Univ of Poitiers Med School, France)
Surgery 143:134-139, 2008

Background.—Although there is a growing body of evidence to document the safety and efficacy of operative treatment of carotid stenosis, surgical indications for elongation and kinking of the internal carotid

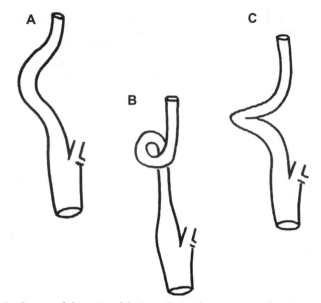

FIGURE 1.—Patterns of elongation of the internal carotid artery: type 1 elongation - tortuosity (A); type 2 elongation - coiling (B); type 3 elongation - kinking (C). (Reprinted from Illuminati G, Ricco J-B, Caliò FG, et al. Results in a consecutive series of 83 surgical corrections of symptomatic stenotic kinking of the internal carotid artery. *Surgery.* 2008;143:134-139, with permission from Elsevier.)

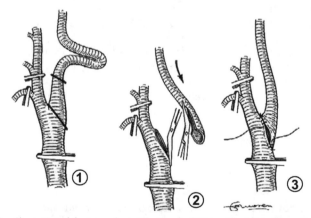

FIGURE 2.—Shortening of the internal carotid artery for kinking. The internal carotid artery is transected at the origin and shortened by reimplantation on the bulb. (Reprinted from Illuminati G, Ricco J-B, Caliò FG, et al. Results in a consecutive series of 83 surgical corrections of symptomatic stenotic kinking of the internal carotid artery. *Surgery.* 2008;143:134-139, with permission from Elsevier.)

artery remain controversial. The goal of this study was to evaluate the efficacy of surgical correction of internal carotid artery kinking in patients with persistent hemispheric symptoms, despite antiplatelet therapy.

Methods.—A consecutive series of 81 patients (mean age, 64 years) underwent 83 surgical procedures to correct kinking of the internal carotid

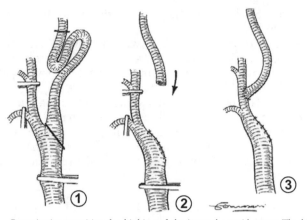

FIGURE 3.—Resection/transposition for kinking of the internal carotid artery. The kinked internal carotid artery is resected and the distal internal carotid artery is transposed onto the external carotid artery. (Reprinted from Illuminati G, Ricco J-B, Caliò FG, et al. Results in a consecutive series of 83 surgical corrections of symptomatic stenotic kinking of the internal carotid artery. *Surgery*. 2008;143:134-139, with permission from Elsevier.)

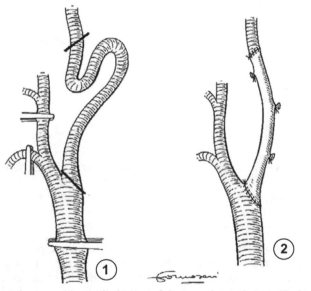

FIGURE 4.—Resection and bypass for kinking of the internal carotid artery. The kinked internal carotid artery is resected and a common-to-internal carotid saphenous graft is inserted. A PTFE graft may be used in place of the internal saphenous vein. (Reprinted from Illuminati G, Ricco J-B, Caliò FG, et al. Results in a consecutive series of 83 surgical corrections of symptomatic stenotic kinking of the internal carotid artery. *Surgery*. 2008;143:134-139, with permission from Elsevier.)

artery either by shortening and reimplanting the vessel on the common carotid artery, inserting a bypass graft, or transposing the vessel onto the external carotid artery. Mean follow-up was 56 months (range,

15-135 months). Study endpoints were 30-day mortality and any stroke occurring during follow-up.

Results.—No postoperative death was observed. The postoperative stroke rate was 1%. Primary patency, freedom from neurologic symptoms, and late survival at 5 years (x ± standard deviation) were 89 ± 4.1%, 92 ± 4%, and 71 ± 6%, respectively.

Conclusions.—The findings of this study indicate that surgical correction for symptomatic stenotic kinking of the internal carotid artery is safe and effective in relieving symptoms and preventing stroke. Operative correction should be considered as the standard treatment for patients with symptomatic carotid kinking that does not respond to antiplatelet therapy (Figs 1-4).

▶ This is a very interesting article. Often, a series of carotid operations for non-atherosclerotic indications comes along. It is important to recognize what the authors are operating on and what they are not operating on. These were kinked arteries with resulting high-grade stenotic lesions. Elongated, tortuous, or coiled arteries were not included (Fig 1). The article includes a good description of the technical aspects of the operations performed to correct stenotic kinks (Figs 2-4). Because this is a single-center case series, its overall level of evidence rating must be considered low. Also, one wonders how so many patients with relatively odd problems end up at a single center. Is carotid kinking a bit of a "regional disease," similar to celiac axis compression syndrome or neurogenic thoracic outlet syndrome? Nevertheless, this is a large series by experienced surgeons, and it should be read. Although I have never regarded carotid kinks as all that important, this article has made me re-examine that position.

G. L. Moneta, MD

Thrombolysis with Alteplase 3 to 4.5 Hours after Acute Ischemic Stroke
Hacke W, Kaste M, Bluhmki E, et al (Universität Heidelberg, Germany; Helsinki Univ Central Hosp, Finland; Boehringer Ingelheim, Biberach, Germany)
N Engl J Med 359:1317-1329, 2008

Background.—Intravenous thrombolysis with alteplase is the only approved treatment for acute ischemic stroke, but its efficacy and safety when administered more than 3 hours after the onset of symptoms have not been established. We tested the efficacy and safety of alteplase administered between 3 and 4.5 hours after the onset of a stroke.

Methods.—After exclusion of patients with a brain hemorrhage or major infarction, as detected on a computed tomographic scan, we randomly assigned patients with acute ischemic stroke in a 1:1 double-blind fashion to receive treatment with intravenous alteplase (0.9 mg per kilogram of body weight) or placebo. The primary end point was disability at 90 days, dichotomized as a favorable outcome (a score of 0 or 1 on the modified Rankin scale, which has a range of 0 to 6, with 0 indicating no symptoms at all and 6 indicating death) or an unfavorable outcome (a score of 2 to 6 on the modified Rankin scale). The secondary end point was a global outcome analysis of four neurologic and disability scores combined. Safety end points included death, symptomatic intracranial hemorrhage, and other serious adverse events.

Results.—We enrolled a total of 821 patients in the study and randomly assigned 418 to the alteplase group and 403 to the placebo group. The median time for the administration of alteplase was 3 hours 59 minutes. More patients had a favorable outcome with alteplase than with placebo (52.4% vs. 45.2%; odds ratio, 1.34; 95% confidence interval [CI], 1.02 to 1.76; P=0.04). In the global analysis, the outcome was also improved with alteplase as compared with placebo (odds ratio, 1.28; 95% CI, 1.00 to 1.65; P<0.05). The incidence of intracranial hemorrhage was higher with alteplase than with placebo (for any intracranial hemorrhage, 27.0% vs. 17.6%; P=0.001; for symptomatic intracranial hemorrhage, 2.4% vs. 0.2%; P=0.008). Mortality did not differ significantly between the alteplase and placebo groups (7.7% and 8.4%, respectively; P=0.68). There was no significant difference in the rate of other serious adverse events.

Conclusions.—As compared with placebo, intravenous alteplase administered between 3 and 4.5 hours after the onset of symptoms significantly improved clinical outcomes in patients with acute ischemic stroke; alteplase was more frequently associated with symptomatic intracranial hemorrhage. (ClinicalTrials.gov number, NCT00153036.)

▶ The only approved treatment for acute ischemic stroke is intravenous thrombolysis with alteplase. Approval is for administration < 3 hours after onset of symptoms. Efficacy has not been established for administration after 3 hours after onset of neurologic symptoms in patients with stroke. Early treatment of patients with ischemic stroke is, however, essential and there is a time-dependent effect of thrombolysis. This is now the second randomized trial to show treatment benefit with intravenous alteplase in patients with acute ischemic stroke. Surprisingly, although risk of symptomatic intracranial hemorrhage is increased with alteplase, mortality is not affected. The study should not be regarded as endorsing a larger time window for beginning thrombolysis in patients with acute ischemic stroke. Treatment with alteplase is nearly twice as effective when administered within < 1.5 hours compared with when administered between 1.5 to 3 hours after onset of symptoms. In this study the odds ratio for favorable treatment was 1.34 when the interval to treatment was between 181 and 270 minutes. Given the more favorable treatment effect with more rapid administration of alteplase, practitioners should still strive to administer the drug as early as possible. As the authors state: "Having more time does not mean we should be allowed to take more time."

G. L. Moneta, MD

14 Vascular Trauma

Blunt thoracic aortic injury: Open or stent graft repair?
Yamane BH, Tefera G, Hoch JR, et al (Univ of Wisconsin School of Medicine and Public Health, Madison)
Surgery 144:575-582, 2008

Background.—Despite a lack of level I evidence, endovascular stent grafting is frequently used for the treatment of blunt thoracic aortic injury. The purpose of this study is to compare the outcomes between open and endovascular repair of traumatic rupture of the thoracic aorta.

Methods.—This article is based on a single-institution review of all consecutive patients treated for blunt aortic injury at the University of Wisconsin Hospital and Clinics between October 1999 and May 2007. This study was reviewed and approved by the institutional review board. Patients were identified from our Level 1 trauma registry. Inclusion criteria for this study was based on computed tomographic or angiographic evidence of thoracic aortic injury distal to the left subclavian artery. Two groups were identified: patients who underwent open repair (OR) and, patients who underwent endovascular repair (ER). Patient demographics, mechanism of injury, Injury Severity Score, associated injuries, comorbid conditions, intraoperative findings, postoperative complications, and duration of hospital stay were analyzed. Data regarding these patients and their injuries were retrieved from our trauma registry as well as chart review and outpatient records. The outcomes from OR and ER were compared using the Fisher exact test. *P* values less than 0.05 were considered statistically significant.

Results.—During the 8-year period, 26 consecutive patients were treated for blunt aortic injury (OR = 12 and ER = 14). There were 20 men, and the mean age was 36 years. There were no differences between the groups in the mechanism of injury, Injury Severity Score, or number of associated injuries on initial presentation. On an intent-to-treat basis, the endovascular therapy was technically successful 100% of the time. There was no procedure-related mortality. There was 1 patient, however, in the OR group with presumed recurrent laryngeal nerve palsy. There was no incident of treatment-related paraplegia in either group. The 1-year survival for OR and ER patients was 93% and 92%, respectively. At 1 year, 25% of patients in the OR group and 18% of patients in the ER group required reinterventions. Mean operating room time was 309 minutes for the ERs and 383 minutes for the patients who underwent OR. Intraoperative blood product administration was

249

greater in the OR group $(P=.055)$; there was no difference between the groups, however, in the total blood products administered for a given hospital stay. The mean duration of hospital stay was 13 days for the OR group and 13.9 days for the ER group.

Conclusion.—There were no significant differences with respect to morbidity or mortality between these 2 groups. These data suggest that ER is at least as safe as OR for blunt aortic injury.

▶ Endovascular stent grafting has become near standard-of-care for treatment of blunt thoracic aortic injury. This is despite lack of any randomized data to support this paradigm change in the treatment of blunt aortic injury, but most case series on this subject have concluded endovascular repair of blunt thoracic injury has advantages over open repair. This article will not significantly detract from the trend for endovascular repair of blunt thoracic aortic injury. The number of patients treated here was relatively small, averaging only about 3 patients per year. In addition, the patients treated with open repair had a mean cross-club time of 27 minutes (these are quick surgeons), and half were able to be treated with primary repair (favorable injuries). Overall survival of the open repair group was higher than is usually seen in reports of open repair of thoracic aortic injury. This suggests a relatively favorable group of patients treated with open repair for blunt thoracic injury at the University of Wisconsin. More data are clearly needed, but despite this article, the trend for endovascular repair of blunt thoracic aortic injury will continue.

G. L. Moneta, MD

Endovascular Stenting for Traumatic Aortic Injury: An Emerging New Standard of Care

Moainie SL, Neschis DG, Gammie JS, et al (Univ of Maryland School of Med, Baltimore, MD)
Ann Thorac Surg 85:1625-1630, 2008

Background.—Thoracic aortic injury remains a leading cause of death after blunt trauma. Thoracic aortic stents have the potential to treat aortic tears using a less invasive approach. We have accumulated the largest series of patients treated with blunt thoracic aortic injury over a 2-year period.

Methods.—From July 2005 to present, 26 patients presenting with blunt aortic injury were treated with thoracic aortic endografting; these patients were retrospectively compared with the prior 26 patients presenting with similar aortic injury who were treated by open surgical repair. A Severity Characterization of Trauma score calculated for each patient predicts mortality based on severity of injury and degree of physiologic derangement on presentation.

Results.—Patients treated with endografting had a significantly shorter length of stay, less intraoperative blood loss, decreased 24-hour blood transfusion, and lower incidence of postoperative tracheostomy compared with patients undergoing open repair. Survival in both groups was similar despite a trend toward higher injury severity among patients treated with endografting.

Conclusions.—This early experience suggests that aortic endografting may provide a safe and efficient treatment of aortic tears that cardiac surgeons can be successful in employing.

▶ This is a large series of patients with blunt aortic trauma treated with thoracic endograft. Compared with historic controls, patients treated with endograft had shorter lengths of hospital stay, decreased blood loss, and similar survival despite a trend toward higher-injury severity scores. When used for treatment of thoracic-aortic trauma, endografts are being used in an off-label fashion. There are occasional dramatic complications of endograft collapse, but despite this, thoracic stent grafting has rapidly emerged as "standard-of-care" for patients with blunt thoracic aortic trauma. Unlike patients treated for degenerative aneurysms, patients with blunt thoracic aortic trauma are comparatively much younger. Their aortas will elongate and dilate as they age. The fate of these grafts over the very long term will therefore be very interesting to observe. Given the demographics of much of the trauma population, I wonder how many of these patients are actually returning for follow-up examination. Follow-up in this study was rather limited, to say the least. No data were presented beyond hospital discharge.

G. L. Moneta, MD

Endovascular repair of traumatic thoracic aortic disruptions with "stacked" abdominal endograft extension cuffs
Rosenthal D, Wellons ED, Burkett AB, et al (Atlanta Med Ctr, GA)
J Vasc Surg 48:841-844, 2008

Objective.—Endovascular stent graft repair of a traumatic thoracic aortic disruption (TTAD) is rapidly becoming an accepted alternative to open surgical repair. The use of currently approved thoracic stent grafts especially in younger patients with small, "steep," tapered aortas, remains a concern due to the acute thoracic endograft collapse and enfolding. The objective of this study, the largest report to date, was to evaluate the mid-term results of TTAD treated with abdominal aortic "stacked" extension cuffs, with follow-up extending to 41 months.

Methods.—Thirty-one patients with multi-system trauma (age range, 15 to 61; mean 31.4 years) were seen after motor vehicle accidents between January 1, 2003 and July 1, 2007. Chest x-ray findings warranted thoracic CT scans, which revealed disruptions of the thoracic aorta. Intra-operative arteriograms in all patients and intravascular ultrasound (IVUS) (n = 17) delineated the extent of the aortic injuries. The aortic length from the subclavian artery to the injury averaged 2.5 cm (range, 1.5 to 4.0 cm).

The repairs were performed with Gore (W.L. Gore & Associates, Flagstaff, Ariz) (n = 15), Aneuryx (Medtronic, Santa Rosa, Calif) (n = 15), and Zenith (Cook, Inc., Bloomington, Ind) (n = 1) Aortic Extension Cuffs. A femoral artery approach was used in 27 patients and a supra-inguinal retroperitoneal iliac approach in four. All patients underwent thoracic CT scans during follow-up.

Results.—In all patients, the stent-graft cuffs successfully excluded the TTAD: 21 patients had 2 cuffs, 9 had 3 cuffs, and 1 had 4 cuffs. The aorta adjacent to the injury mean diameter was 18.5 mm (range, 17-24 mm). No subclavian arteries were covered. Two patients required an additional cuff for exclusion of the Type I endoleaks at the distal attachment site within 6 weeks of initial endograft repair. There were no procedure-related deaths; 2 patients died of other injuries. At follow-up, extending to 41 months (range, 3 to 41 months), two pseudo-aneurysms occurred which required open operative repair: 1 due to infection (4 months) and a leaking pseudoaneurysm (14 months). A CT scan in all other survivors demonstrated no device-related complications, endoleaks, or cuff migrations.

Conclusion.—Stent-graft repair of TTAD is technically feasible. The technique of "stacked" aortic cuffs provides an acceptable option when urgent therapy is needed, when patients are deemed high-risk for open operative repair, or until thoracic endografts are designed which can safely treat focal, smaller aortic diameter injuries.

▶ This study is a single-center small series describing an endovascular approach to blunt aortic injury using commercially available "stacked cuffs." The authors describe their series retrospectively with follow-up extending to 41 months. As current thoracic endografts are approved only for the treatment of thoracic aneurysms and penetrating ulcers, the diameter of these grafts is often too large to treat young, healthy, injured aortas, which in this series was a mean diameter of 18.5 mm. Recently, the AAST 2 trial was published, which endorsed an endovascular approach for the overwhelming majority of these injuries and called for better device development specifically for the management of these injuries.[1]

Aside from the small size of this series, there are several obvious weaknesses of this descriptive report. The authors don't give crucial information on how many patients were admitted over the study period with injuries that were repaired using traditional open techniques or simply medical management alone. In addition, there are no data provided on patients who were evaluated and denied endovascular repair. Without this information, the reader must assume that there is potential for a huge selection bias, which would significantly impact the positive results described.

Notwithstanding, the authors' results are impressive and, while the definitive management of this disease is in evolution, provide a contemporary alternative using commercially available equipment.

B. W. Starnes, MD

Reference

1. Demetriades D, Velmahos GC, Scalea TM, et al. Operative repair or endovascular stent graft in blunt traumatic thoracic aortic injuries: results of an American Association for the Surgery of Trauma Multicenter Study. *J Trauma*. 2008;64: 561-570. discussion 570–571.

Blunt intraabdominal arterial injury in pediatric trauma patients: injury distribution and markers of outcome

Hamner CE, Groner JI, Caniano DA, et al (Columbus Children's Hosp, Ohio State Univ, USA; Schneider Children's Hosp, New Hyde Park, USA)
J Pediatr Surg 43:916-923, 2008

Background.—The epidemiology of pediatric blunt intraabdominal arterial injury is ill defined. We analyzed a multiinstitutional trauma database to better define injury patterns and predictors of outcome.

Methods.—The American College of Surgeons National Trauma Database was evaluated for all patients younger than 16 years with blunt intra- abdominal arterial injury from 2000 to 2004. Injury distribution, operative treatment, and variables associated with mortality were considered.

Results.—One hundred twelve intraabdominal arterial injuries were identified in 103 pediatric blunt trauma patients. Single arterial injury (92.2%) occurred most frequently: renal (36.9%), mesenteric (24.3%), and iliac (23.3%). Associated injuries were present in 96.1% of patients (abdominal visceral, 75.7%; major extraabdominal skeletal/visceral, 77.7%). Arterial control was obtained operatively (n = 46, 44.7%) or by endovascular means (n = 6, 5.8%) in 52 patients. Overall mortality was 15.5%. Increased mortality was associated with multiple arterial injuries ($P = .049$), intraabdominal venous injury ($P = .011$), head injury ($P = .05$), Glasgow Coma Score less than 8 ($P < .001$), cardiac arrest ($P < .001$), profound base deficit ($P = .007$), and poor performance on multiple injured outcomes scoring systems (Revised Trauma Score [$P < .001$], Injury Severity Score [$P = .001$], and TRISS [$P = .002$]).

Conclusion.—Blunt intraabdominal arterial injury in children usually affects a single vessel. Associated injuries appear to be nearly universal. The high mortality rate is influenced by serious associated injuries and is reflected by overall injury severity scores.

▶ Arterial injuries from blunt abdominal trauma in children are rare, with only 2.4% of 4265 blunt abdominal injuries in children, in a 5-year period, from the National Trauma database, complicated by an arterial injury. In most cases, only a single intra-abdominal artery is injured, and associated injuries are so common that they should be expected. Like a ruptured aneurysm or an adult arterial injury, how well the pediatric patient will do with an abdominal arterial injury from blunt trauma and who survives transport to the hospital, overall, are more determined by the severity of associated injuries than the arterial injury itself. A vascular surgeon is a useful member of the trauma team but should not be the dominant member of the trauma team, as the vascular injury, once repaired, will seldom prevent these patients from getting better.

G. L. Moneta, MD

Penetrating femoropopliteal injury during modern warfare: Experience of the Balad Vascular Registry
Woodward EB, Clouse WD, Eliason JL, et al (332nd EMDG/AFTH, Balad Air Base, Iraq; et al)
J Vasc Surg 47:1259-1265, 2008

Objective.—Wounding patterns, methods of repair, and outcomes from femoropopliteal injury have been documented in recent civilian literature. In Operation Iraqi Freedom, as in past conflicts, these injuries continue to be a therapeutic challenge. Therefore, the objective of the current study is to document the pattern of femoropopliteal injuries, methods of repair, and early outcomes during the current military campaign in Iraq.

Methods.—From September 1, 2004, to April 30, 2007, all vascular injuries arriving at the Air Force Theater Hospital (the central echelon III medical facility in Iraq; equivalent to a civilian level I trauma center), Balad Air Base, Iraq were prospectively entered into a registry. From this, injuries involving the lower extremities were reviewed.

Results.—During the 32-month study period, 9289 battle-related casualties were assessed. Of these, 488 (5.3%) were diagnosed with 513 vascular injuries, and 142 casualties sustained 145 injuries in the femoropopliteal domain. Femoral level injury was present in 100, and popliteal level injury occurred in 45. Injuries consisted of 59 isolated arterial, 11 isolated venous, and 75 combined. Fifty-eight casualties were evacuated from forward locations. Temporary arterial shunts were placed in 43, of which 40 (93%) were patent on arrival at our facility. Our group used shunts for early reperfusion before orthopedic fixation, during mass casualty care, or autogenous vein harvest in 11 cases. Arterial repair was accomplished with autogenous vein in 118 (88%), primary means in nine (7%), or ligation in seven (5%). Venous injury was repaired in 62 (72%). Associated fracture was present in 55 (38%), and nerve injury was noted in 19 (13%). Early limb loss due to femoropopliteal penetrating injury occurred in 10 (6.9%). Early mortality was 3.5% (n = 5).

Conclusions.—Femoropopliteal vascular injury remains a significant reality in modern warfare. Femoral injuries appear more prevalent than those in the popliteal region. Early results of in-theater repair are comparable with contemporary civilian reports and are improved from the Vietnam era. Rapid evacuation and damage control maneuvers such as

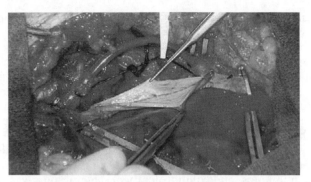

FIGURE 1.—Superficial femoral artery and femoral vein injuries. A temporary arterial shunt is in place while a panel graft repair of the femoral vein is undertaken. (Reprinted from Woodward EB, Clouse WD, Eliason JL, et al. Penetrating femoropopliteal injury during modern warfare: experience of the Balad Vascular Registry. *J Vasc Surg*. 2008;47:1259-1265. Copyright 2008, with permission from The Society for Vascular Surgery.)

temporary shunting and early fasciotomy assist timely definitive repair and appear effective (Fig 1).

▶ Regardless of how you feel about the war in Iraq, or the military in general, one thing no one can argue with is the desire of the military to take care of their people. The results presented here (7% amputation rate and a 3.5% mortality rate) for treatment of femoropopliteal penetrating injuries, many of which were associated with fractures or extensive soft tissue injury, are excellent and reflect the dedication of excellent surgeons, technicians, nursing staff, and a system that provides rapid evacuation of casualties and systematic usage of damage control measures, particularly temporary shunting (Fig 1) and early, very liberal, use of fasciotomy; that is, almost everyone received a fasciotomy. In particular, one should note how well the temporary arterial shunts worked, with 40 of 43 remaining functional during transport from a forward location. The take-home message is that shunts and fasciotomy can be valuable adjuncts in the treatment of lower extremity vascular trauma.

G. L. Moneta, MD

Post-Traumatic Ulnar Artery Thrombosis: Outcome of Arterial Reconstruction Using Reverse Interpositional Vein Grafting at 2 Years Minimum Follow-Up
Chloros GD, Lucas RM, Li Z, et al (Wake Forest Univ School of Med, Winston-Salem, NC)
J Hand Surg 33A:932-940, 2008

Purpose.—Treatment of posttraumatic symptomatic ulnar artery thrombosis (UAT) is controversial. This study reports the outcome at 2 years minimum follow-up of a uniform approach using reversed interpositional vein grafting to treat symptomatic patients with UAT.

Methods.—The records of all patients with vascular disease of the upper extremity who were revascularized at the authors' institution were retrospectively reviewed, and the following inclusion criteria were applied: (1) arteriographically proven UAT treated with excision of the involved segment and reversed interpositional vein grafting; (2) absence of collagen vascular disease, coagulopathy, or peripheral vascular disease, (3) minimum follow-up of 24 months. Twelve patients (13 hands) were identified and evaluated before surgery and at final follow-up using the following health-related quality of life outcome instruments: (1) McCabe cold sensitivity severity scale, (2) McGill visual analog pain scale, (3) Levine symptom and function scale, and (4) Wake Forest University symptom scale (pain, numbness, and cold intolerance). Digital microvascular perfusion testing (laser Doppler perfusion imaging and isolated cold stress testing) was also performed, and the final test was compared with 28 normal controls. All patients were evaluated for graft patency as determined by Allen's testing and/or Doppler ultrasound.

Results.—Ten of the 13 grafts were patent at final follow-up (77% patency rate). In all the patients with patent grafts, the Levine symptom

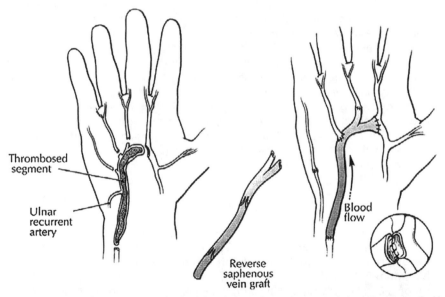

FIGURE 1.—In this case example, the thrombosed ulnar artery segment extends from the wrist crease to the origin of the common digital artery to the long-index finger. The thrombosed segment is excised, and a saphenous vein graft is harvested and subsequently reversed (RIVG). Distal anastomosis includes end-to-side anastomosis of the common digital to the ring finger–little finger into the vein graft, end-to-end repair of the vein branch to the common digital artery to the long finger–ring finger, and a complex end-to-end repair of the proximal vein to the junction of the common digital index finger–long finger and superficial radial artery. (Reproduced with permission from Koman LA, ed. Wake Forest University Orthopaedic Manual. Winston-Salem, NC: Wake Forest University Orthopaedic Press, 1997.) (Reprinted from Chloros GD, Lucas RM, Li Z, et al. Post-traumatic ulnar artery thrombosis: outcome of arterial reconstruction using reverse interpositional vein grafting at 2 years minimum follow-up. *J Hand Surg* 2008;33A:932-940, with permission from the American Society for Surgery of the Hand.)

scale, the McGill visual analog pain scale, the McCabe cold sensitivity severity scale, and the isolated cold stress testing responses of the patients were significantly improved at final follow-up. Isolated cold stress testing responses were not different from those of normal controls. The changes in the Levine function scale, Wake Forest University scale, and laser Doppler perfusion imaging were not significant. In the nonpatent grafts (3 of 13), 2 patients still complained of pain, numbness, and cold sensitivity, whereas 1 patient has minimal symptoms and continues to improve.

Conclusions.—Successful arterial reconstruction in symptomatic post-traumatic UAT decreases symptoms, improves function and microvascular physiology, and has a positive effect on the health-related quality of life.

Type of Study/Level of Evidence.—Therapeutic IV (Fig 1).

▶ Although the number of patients is small, this is actually a relatively large series with prolonged follow-up of an unusual condition infrequently treated by operation. Of particular interest is improvement in quality of life noted in these patients and the normalization of their physiologic response to cold testing. Interposition vein grafting of the distal ulnar artery is relatively straight-forward if the thrombosed segment does not involve the digital vessels. In such cases, the saphenous vein at the ankle is an appropriate conduit. The operation, of course, is considerably more technically demanding when digital arteries must be reimplanted into the saphenous vein graft. This may be done through individual anastomoses of the digital arteries to the saphenous vein graft or, more commonly in our experience, incorporation as a patch graft of the portion of the thrombosed ulnar artery from which the digital arteries originate onto a longitudinally oriented venotomy in the saphenous vein graft (Fig 1).

G. L. Moneta, MD

15 Nonatherosclerotic Conditions

Abdominal aortic coarctation: Surgical treatment of 53 patients with a thoracoabdominal bypass, patch aortoplasty, or interposition aortoaortic graft
Stanley JC, Criado E, Eliason JL, et al (Univ of Michigan Cardiovascular Ctr, Ann Arbor, MI)
J Vasc Surg 48:1073-1082, 2008

Objective.—Abdominal aortic coarctation is uncommon and often complicated with coexisting splanchnic and renal artery occlusive disease. This study was undertaken to define the clinical and anatomic characteristics of this entity, as well as the technical issues and outcomes of its operative treatment.

Methods.—Fifty-three patients, 34 males and 19 females, underwent surgical treatment of abdominal aortic coarctations from 1963-2008 at the University of Michigan. Patient ages in years ranged from 2-4 (n = 4), 5-8 (n = 17), 9-14 (n = 16), 15-20 (n = 11) and 25-49 (n = 5). The mean age was 11.9 years. Developmental disease (n = 48), inflammatory aortitis (n = 4), and iatrogenic trauma (n = 1) were suspected etiologies. Aortic coarctations were suprarenal (n = 37), intrarenal (n = 12), or infrarenal (n = 4). Patients often had coexisting occlusive disease of the splanchnic (n = 33) and renal (n = 46) arteries.

Results.—Major clinical manifestations included: aortic and renal artery-related secondary hypertension (n = 50), symptomatic lower extremity ischemia (n = 3), and intestinal angina (n = 3). Primary aortic reconstructive procedures included: thoracoabdominal bypass (n = 26), patch aortoplasty (n = 24), or an aortoaortic interposition graft (n = 3). Primary splanchnic (n = 19) or renal (n = 47) arterial reconstructions were performed as simultaneous (n = 45) or staged (n = 13) procedures in relation to the aortic surgery. Benefits existed regarding improved control of hypertension (n = 46), as well as elimination of extremity ischemia (n = 3) and mesenteric angina (n = 3). Secondary renal or splanchnic arterial reoperations (n = 8) were performed without mortality 5 days to 12 years postoperative for failed primary procedures. Secondary aortic procedures, 5 to 14 years postoperative, were performed for patch aortoplasties that became stenotic (n = 2) or aneurysmal (n = 1), and when thoracoabdominal bypasses developed an anastomotic narrowing (n = 1) or proved inadequate in size with patient growth (n = 1). No perioperative mortality accompanied either the primary or secondary aortic reconstructive procedures.

Conclusion.—Abdominal aortic coarctation represents a complex vascular disease. Individualized treatment changed little over the period of study, remaining dependent on the pattern of anatomic lesions, patient age, and anticipated growth potential. This experience documented salutary outcomes exceeding 90% following carefully performed operative therapy (Figs 1 and 4B).

▶ This article focuses on surgical treatment of abdominal coarctation: a fascinating problem that may be developmental in some cases or the end result of an inflammatory aortitis in others. Most vascular surgeons will never see this problem outside of the lecture hall, a textbook, or their oral certification examination. The authors do an outstanding job of describing the anatomic features and clinical characteristics of the so-called mid-aortic syndrome, and clearly

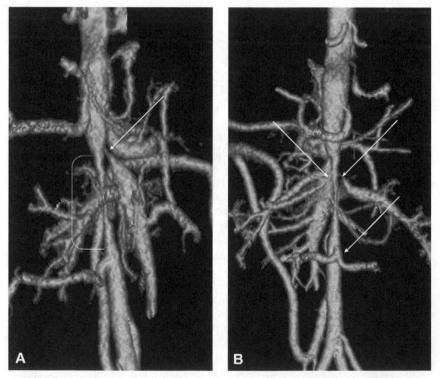

FIGURE 1.—A, *Suprarenal* abdominal aortic coarctation (*bracket*) with superior mesenteric artery stenosis (*arrow*) and (B) bilateral renal artery ostial stenoses (*arrows*). Note common trunk of lower lumbar artery (*arrow*). Preoperative computed tomographic angiography (CTA) (anterior and posterior projections, respectively). (Reprinted from Stanley JC, Criado E, Eliason JL, et al. Abdominal aortic coarctation: surgical treatment of 53 patients with a thoracoabdominal bypass, patch aortoplasty, or interposition aortoaortic graft. *J Vasc Surg*. 2008;48:1073-1082, with permission from the Society for Vascular Surgery.)

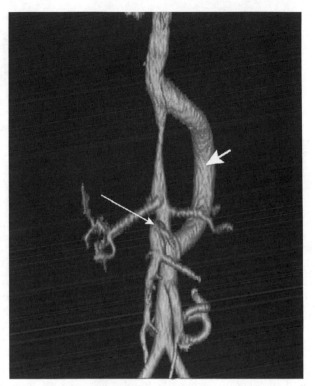

FIGURE 4.—B, Thoracoabdominal bypass (*broad arrow*) with aortic implantation of superior mesenteric artery (*arrow*). Postoperative computed tomographic angiography (CTA). (Reprinted from Stanley JC, Criado E, Eliason JL, et al. Abdominal aortic coarctation: surgical treatment of 53 patients with a thoracoabdominal bypass, patch aortoplasty, or interposition aortoaortic graft. *J Vasc Surg*. 2008;48:1073-1082, with permission from the Society for Vascular Surgery.)

detail technical options for reconstructive procedures in treating the broad range of problems associated with abdominal coarctation. Points to be emphasized are that hypertension is the clinical problem that drives treatment. Despite frequent involvement of the splanchnic vessels (Fig 1), mesenteric ischemia is uncommon in these patients. Lower extremity claudication is also uncommon, even in the setting of virtual obliteration of the upper abdominal or lower thoracic aorta. Untreated abdominal coarctation is associated with stroke, left ventricular hypertrophy, congestive heart failure, flash pulmonary edema, and, perhaps, renal failure.

There are a variety of reconstruction options for the aorta itself, including thoracoabdominal bypasses, patch aortoplasties, and interposition aortoaortic grafts with thoracoabdominal bypass (Fig 4B); patch aortoplasty is the most common. The latter is obviously reserved for those patients with an aorta of sufficient caliber that reconstruction of the native lumen is feasible. Visceral reconstruction is necessary in most patients and is usually performed at the time of the index procedure after completion of the aortoplasty or aortic bypass. Initial technical results are good, but not all patients are cured of their hypertension—only about 60% in this series. In addition, even in this extensive experience, follow-up is relatively limited, but failure of the aortic reconstruction over time appears extremely rare and no patient in this series appeared to require a secondary operation to reconstruct the aorta.

G. L. Moneta, MD

Complex vascular reconstruction of abdominal aorta and its branches in the pediatric population
Kaye AJ, Slemp AE, Chang B, et al (Hosp of the Univ of Pennsylvania, Philadelphia, PA; Children's Hosp of Philadelphia, PA)
J Pediatr Surg 43:1082-1088, 2008

Background.—Subdiaphragmatic aortic diseases in children are rare and form a heterogeneous group. The pediatric patient presents unique challenges because of their size, concerns about proper timing and conduit for repair, and anticipating expected growth.

Methods.—We performed a retrospective review of operations involving the abdominal aorta and called branches in children between January 2003 and April 2007, focusing on the details of preoperative evaluation, operative technique, and outcomes. The pertinent literature is reviewed.

Results.—Twenty-two children (age, 2 days to 17 years) were included. Mean follow-up was 28 months. Aneurysms were seen in 5 children; the remainder had stenotic disease. Aneurysms were typically asymptomatic and diagnosed incidentally, whereas stenotic lesions most commonly presented with hypertension (HTN). Fourteen complex vascular repairs were performed. All of the children with aneurysms underwent prompt surgery. The children with stenoses had operations for poorly controlled HTN, claudication, and/or mesenteric ischemia. Most patients with stenotic disease were treated medically for HTN and were followed closely while awaiting optimal size and availability of autogenous conduit for reconstruction. Cryopreserved allograft was used in 3 of the aneurysm operations. Dacron grafts were used to repair 5 aortic stenotic lesions. Renal and mesenteric revascularizations were performed with saphenous vein grafts. Pediatric, general, and transplant surgeons and nephrologic and cardiologic teams were integral to evaluation and management. No major operative complications occurred.

Conclusion.—Proper management of pediatric aortic vascular disease requires a multidisciplinary approach. It is best to use autologous grafts whenever possible. Children with stenotic disease should be treated medically for hypertension until they are large enough for an autologous graft reconstruction. Children with aneurysmal disease are at risk for embolism and thrombosis and therefore usually treated immediately using artificial graft material, if necessary.

▶ There is not a lot of science in this article, but it does provide an interesting overview of abdominal aortic problems in children. We don't need science all of the time; sometimes a "how I do it" article, such as this one, makes for a good reading. Some of the "principles" of treatment of pediatric vascular disease, championed in this article, are well known, such as use of end-to-side anastomoses, redundant grafts, and interrupted suture anastomotic techniques to plan for future growth of the child. The authors use prosthetic grafts, autogenous grafts, and cryoperserved allograft depending on age and size of the child and other individual circumstances. Perhaps, the main message is optimal medical management of the patients with mid-aortic syndrome, delaying operation as long as possible until the child reaches a size where there is optimum availability of autogenous conduit for reconstruction.

G. L. Moneta, MD

Quality of life of patients with Takayasu's arteritis
Abularrage CJ, Slidell MB, Sidawy AN, et al (Veterans Affairs Med Ctr, Washington, DC)
J Vasc Surg 47:131-137, 2008

Objective.—Takayasu's arteritis (TA) is a chronic immune vasculitis that causes inflammation of the aorta and its branches and is clinically characterized by exacerbations and remissions. This study examined the quality of life (QoL) of patients with TA using the Medical Outcomes Study Short Form 36 (SF-36) Health Survey, a validated health related QoL questionnaire.

Methods.—Questionnaires that included the SF-36 and demographic related variables were mailed to 392 patients enrolled in the Takayasu's Arteritis Research Association. Raw SF-36 scores, as well as Physical Health Summary (PHS) and Mental Health Summary (MHS) scores, were calculated according to standard protocols. Data were analyzed for predictors of superior QoL using univariate and stepwise logistic regression analysis. SF-36 scores were also compared with those of other chronic diseases associated with peripheral vascular disease (PVD) published in the literature. Results are reported as mean ± standard error of the mean.

Results.—A total of 158 patients (144 women, 14 men) with average age of 42.2 ± 1.1 years responded to the questionnaire. Mean onset of symptoms occurred at 30.5 ± 1.2 years, with a mean age at diagnosis of 34.7 ± 1.2, and a median of four doctors were seen before diagnosis. The group underwent 299 TA-related surgical procedures (1.9 ± 0.3), including coronary (38%), carotid (35%), upper extremity (30%), and lower extremity (26%) revascularization. PHS and MHS summary scores (39.2 ± 1.0 and 44.5 ± 1.0, respectively) were worse than mean scores for an age-matched healthy population as well as nationally reported scores for diabetes mellitus, hypertension, and coronary artery disease (all $P < .0001$). Multivariate predictors of better physical QoL were younger age ($P = .003$) and remission of the disease ($P = .0002$). The use of immunomodulating medications was associated with inferior physical QoL ($P = .02$). The sole predictor of better mental QoL was remission of disease ($P = .002$).

Conclusion.—TA is a rare disease with profound consequences on QoL. Scores for physical and mental health are worse compared with many other chronic diseases associated with PVD. Superior physical QoL is seen in younger patients, whereas inferior physical QoL is encountered in those who take immunomodulating medications. Because the only factor to influence positively both physical and mental QoL is disease remission, every effort should be directed to attenuate disease activity.

▶ This study is the largest published evaluation of quality of life in patients with Takayasu's arteritis. Not surprisingly, those responding to the questionnaire were within the typical age range and oftentimes required a vascular procedure (approximately 60%). However, what is new here is the observation that these patients are often left debilitated by Takayasu's primary and secondary effects, especially if disease occurred at a later age and was severe enough to require immunomodulating medications. While these findings are interesting, with only 158 respondents from the 392 questionnaires mailed to members enrolled in the Takayasu's Arteritis Research Association, there may be some selection bias. Also, the sampling was not time dependent, so whether these quality-of-life parameters will improve with time remains unclear.

M. A. Passman, MD

Intermittent claudication in diabetes mellitus due to chronic exertional compartment syndrome of the leg: An observational study of 17 patients

Edmundsson D, Svensson O, Toolanen G (Umeå Univ Hosp, Sweden)
Acta Orthop 79:534-539, 2008

Background and Purpose.—Intermittent claudication in diabetes mellitus is commonly associated with arterial disease but may occur without obvious signs of peripheral circulatory impairment. We investigated whether this could be due to chronic exertional compartment syndrome (CECS).

Patients and Methods.—We report on 17 patients (3 men), mean age 39 (18–72) years, with diabetes mellitus—12 of which were type 1—and leg pain during walking (which was relieved at rest), without clinical signs of peripheral arterial disease. The duration of diabetes was 22 (1–41) years and 12 patients had peripheral neuropathy, retinopathy, or nephropathy. The leg muscles were tender and firm on palpation. Radiography, scintigraphy, and intramuscular pressure measurements were done during exercises to reproduce their symptoms.

Results.—16 of the 17 patients were diagnosed as having CECS. The intramuscular pressures in leg compartments were statistically significantly higher in diabetics than in physically active non-diabetics with CECS ($p < 0.05$). 15 of the 16 diabetics with CECS were treated with fasciotomy. At surgery, the fascia was whitish, thickened, and had a rubber-like consistency. After 1 year, 9 patients rated themselves as excellent or good in 15 of the 18 treated compartments. The walking time until stop due to leg pain increased after surgery from less than 10 min to unlimited time in 8 of 9 patients who were followed up.

Interpretation.—Intermittent claudication in diabetics may be caused by CECS of the leg. The intramuscular pressures were considerably elevated in diabetics. One pathomechanism may be fascial thickening. The results after fasciotomy are good, and the increased pain-free walking time is especially beneficial for diabetics.

▶ Chronic exertional compartment syndrome (CECS) of the leg is primarily described in running athletes. It is characterized by increased muscle compartment pressure during exertion with resulting impaired tissue circulation, pain, and occasional neurologic deficits. Diagnosis is based on history of leg pain during exercise and increased intramuscular pressure. The anterior compartment of the leg is most frequently affected, but other compartments may be involved. The authors' small series suggests that CECS may be a cause of exercise-induced leg pain in patients with diabetes. These patients likely function at different levels than the traditional young athlete with CECS. Nevertheless, the apparent dramatic increase in pain-free walking in the diabetic patients treated in this series is gratifying. Patients with diabetes and walking impairment without evidence of peripheral vascular disease should be considered for a diagnosis of CECS. Fasciotomy in well-selected patients appears to be efficacious.

G. L. Moneta, MD

Predictors of Prosthetic Graft Infection after Infrainguinal Bypass

Brothers TE, Robison JG, Elliott BM (Med Univ of South Carolina, Charleston)
J Am Coll Surg 208:557–561, 2009

Background.—Some patients require major leg amputation after lower-extremity prosthetic bypass for graft occlusion or failure of wound healing, despite a patent graft. Amputation above or below the knee was hypothesized to increase susceptibility to prosthetic graft infection in the ipsilateral extremity.

Study Design.—All patients undergoing implantation of prosthetic infrainguinal arterial bypass grafts identified from a vascular surgical registry during a 12-year period were reviewed. Patient demographic data, comorbid conditions, and operative details were evaluated as risk factors, with graft infection among the primary outcomes of interest.

Results.—Prosthetic graft infection occurred in 25 of 141 (18%) infrainguinal grafts and occurred most frequently after major amputation (41% versus 6%; odds ratio [OR] = 12; 95% CI, 4.1 to 34) or early reoperation after initial grafting (70% versus 16%; OR = 11; 95% CI, 1.9 to 63). Risk was highest after amputation within 4 weeks of bypass (70% versus 32%; OR = 5.0; 95% CI, 1.1 to 23). Graft thrombosis (84% versus 39%;

OR = 8.3; 95% CI, 2.7 to 26) and presence of gangrene (52% versus 23%; OR = 3.6; 95% CI, 1.5 to 8.7) also increased infection risk. Independent predictors for development of graft infection were identified by stepwise regression analysis to be amputation (p < 0.001), early reoperation (p = 0.002), and absence of renal failure (p = 0.038) but not gangrene (p = 0.090). Amputations performed within 6 months of the initial bypass operation were more likely to be associated with prosthetic graft infection than those performed later than 6 months (52% versus 17%; OR = 5.3; 95% CI, 1.3 to 22).

Conclusions.—Amputation increases risk of prosthetic graft infection, especially when performed early or after failed revascularization. Consideration should be given to partial or complete removal of a prosthetic graft above the level of the amputation under these conditions (Fig 3).

▶ Prosthetic bypass is inferior to autogenous vein for infrainguinal arterial reconstructions. However, under certain circumstances, particularly lack of autogenous greater saphenous vein, prosthetic bypass can be used for femoral popliteal bypass. A significant disadvantage of infrainguinal prosthetic bypass is the increased infection rate compared with an autogenous bypass. It would seem intuitive that patients with poor wound healing, open wounds in the foot, or cellulitis would have higher rates of prosthetic bypass infection. Anecdotally, many surgeons have noticed late development of infection in prosthetic bypasses following ipsilateral above- or below-knee amputation. The authors hypothesized that major amputation of the lower limb would increase susceptibility of the prosthetic graft infection in the ipsilateral extremity.

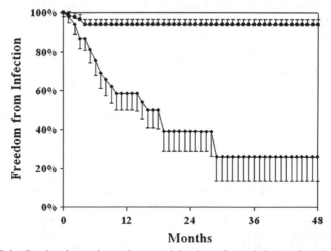

FIGURE 3.—Freedom from infection for expanded polytetrafluoroethylene grafts. Filled diamonds indicate patients who underwent major amputation at some time after initial revascularization. Filled squares indicate unamputated limbs. Standard error exceeds 10% at 28 months for amputated patients. (Reprinted from Brothers TE, Robison JG, Elliott BM. Predictors of prosthetic graft infection after infrainguinal bypass. *J Am Coll Surg.* 2009;208:557-561, with permission from the American College of Surgeons.)

The results presented are sobering. An overall incidence of 18% for infection of infrainguinal prosthetic grafts is astounding. It implies a high-risk patient population, and indeed very few of the grafts were placed for claudication alone. One might conclude the risk of prosthetic graft infection following amputation is sufficiently high that if the graft is occluded at the time of the amputation serious consideration should be given to concomitant graft removal. The other implication of the data is that if the patient has a significant likelihood of amputation with graft failure, the surgeon should consider other forms of revascularization rather than a prosthetic graft if possible. Such techniques might include the use of arm veins or even recanalization of an occluded superficial femoral artery. Of course, the best way to prevent an infrainguinal prosthetic graft infection is to never have placed an infrainguinal prosthetic graft in the first place.

G. L. Moneta, MD

16 Venous Thrombosis and Pulmonary Embolism

Incidence, clinical characteristics, and long-term prognosis of travel-associated pulmonary embolism

Lehmann R, Suess C, Leus M, et al (Johann Wolfgang Goethe-Univ Frankfurt, Germany; et al)

Eur Heart J 30:233-241, 2009

Aims.—Prolonged air travel is considered a risk factor for pulmonary embolism (PE). The clinical characteristics as well as the long-term prognosis of patients suffering from travel-associated PE ('economy-class syndrome', ECS) remain largely unknown. Owing to its proximity, our hospital is the primary referral centre for Frankfurt Airport, Europe's third-largest airport. The goal of our study was to follow-up all patients with ECS, who were admitted to our hospital between 1997 and 2006.

Methods and Results.—We systematically reviewed all medical charts from patients presenting with acute PE to our emergency room or intensive care unit (ICU) and performed a telephone follow-up on patients discharged alive. Together with the data provided from the statistics department of Fraport Inc., the operating company of the Frankfurt International Airport, we were also able to put the medical data in context with the corresponding number of passengers and flight distances. A total of 257 patients with acute PE were admitted to our emergency and ICU between 1997 and 2006. Out of these, 62 patients suffered from ECS (45 flight-associated PE and 17 from other travel-associated PE). ECS patients were prone to more haemodynamic relevant acute events, reflected by a higher rate of initial cardiopulmonary resuscitation (4.8% vs. 1.5%; $P = 0.153$) and higher percentage of massive PE (8% vs. 3%; $P = 0.064$). Nevertheless, intrahospital mortality was similar in both groups (ECS 4.8%, others 4.1%; $P = 0.730$). Interestingly, the long-term outcome of ECS patients was excellent (Kaplan–Meier analysis; P log-rank: 0.008 vs. other entities). In general, ECS was a rare event (one event/5 million passengers), where long-haul flights over 5000 km lead to a 17-fold risk increase compared with shorter flights.

TABLE 3.—Risk of Pulmonary Embolism in Dependence on Flight Duration

Flight Duration (h)	Flight Distance km	No. of Patients with PE	No. (Millions) of Passengers 1997–2006	Cases Per Million Passengers
Unknown	Unknown	2	–	–
0–6	0–5000	5	165.7	0.03
6–9	5000–7499	22	27.9	0.8
9–12	7500–9999	12	39.1	0.3
> 12	> 10 000	4	5.8	0.7
Total		45	238.7 million	0.2

(Reprinted from Lehmann R, Suess C, Leus M, et al. Incidence, clinical characteristics, and long-term prognosis of travel-associated pulmonary embolism. *Eur Heart J.* 2009;30:233-241, permission from The European Society of Cardiology.)

Conclusions.—Travel-associated PE was a common cause of PE in our hospital, with patients showing excellent long-term prognosis after discharge. The risk of ECS is rather low and strictly dependent on the flight distance (Table 3).

▶ Retrospective analyses of travelers arriving at Charles de Gaulle airport in Paris and the Madrid-Barajas airport have determined that distance traveled is a significant contributing risk for pulmonary embolism (PE)-associated air travel.[1,2] The incidence of PE among passengers traveling > 5000 km is 1.5 cases per million compared with 0.01 cases per million in those traveling < 5000 km. In this article, the authors sought to determine the proportion of travel-associated PE compared with other associated causes of PE, and the long-term prognosis of affected patients. Travel-associated PE was defined as that occurring within 2 months of travel. The study followed patients with travel-related PE who admitted to the University of Frankfurt Hospital between 1997 and 2006. This hospital serves as the primary referral center for Frankfurt airport, the largest airport in Germany and third largest in Europe. Approximately one-third of the passengers arriving at this airport have traveled > 5000 km. The main points of this study are that travel-related PE is exceedingly rare and is vanishingly rare in shorter haul flights (Table 3). Virtually all patients with travel-related PE have additional risk factors for venous thromboembolism. Overall, the patients do well with no difference in hospital mortality compared with other patients with PE, and the patients with travel-related PE have a better long-term prognosis.

G. L. Moneta, MD

References

1. Lapostolle F, Surget V, Borron SW, et al. Severe pulmonary embolism associated with air travel. *N Engl J Med.* 2001;345:779-783.
2. Perez-Rodriguez E, Jiminez D, Diaz G. Incidence of air travel-related pulmonary embolism at the Madrid-Barajas airport. *Arch Intern Med.* 2003;163:2766-2770.

Clinical Predictors for Fatal Pulmonary Embolism in 15520 Patients With Venous Thromboembolism: Findings From the Registro Informatizado de la Enfermedad TromboEmbolica venosa (RIETE) Registry

Laporte S, Mismetti P, Décousus H, et al (Univ Hosp, Saint-Etienne, France; et al)
Circulation 117:1711-1716, 2008

Background.—Clinical predictors for fatal pulmonary embolism (PE) in patients with venous thromboembolism have never been studied.

Methods and Results.—Using data from the international prospective Registro Informatizado de la Enfermedad TromboEmbolica venosa (RIETE) registry about patients with objectively confirmed, symptomatic acute venous thromboembolism, we determined independent predictive factors for fatal PE. Between March 2001 and July 2006, 15 520 consecutive patients (mean age ± SD, 66.3 ± 16.9 years; 49.7% men) with acute venous thromboembolism were included. Symptomatic, deep-vein thrombosis without symptomatic PE was observed in 58.0% (n=9008) of patients, symptomatic nonmassive PE in 40.4% (n=6264), and symptomatic massive PE in 1.6% (n=248). At 3 months, the cumulative rates of overall mortality and fatal PE were 8.65% and 1.68%, respectively. On multivariable analysis, patients with symptomatic nonmassive PE at presentation exhibited a 5.42-fold higher risk of fatal PE compared with patients with deep-vein thrombosis without symptomatic PE (*P*<0.001). The risk of fatal PE was multiplied by 17.5 in patients presenting with a symptomatic massive PE. Other clinical factors independently associated with an increased risk of fatal PE were immobilization for neurological disease, age >75 years, and cancer.

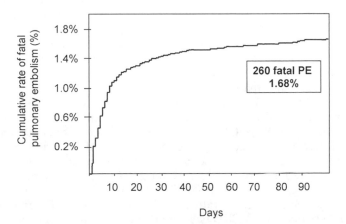

FIGURE 1.—Cumulative rate of fatal PE. (Reprinted from Laporte S, Mismetti P, Décousus H, et al. Clinical predictors for fatal pulmonary embolism in 15 520 patients with venous thromboembolism: findings from the Registro Informatizado de la Enfermedad TromboEmbolica venosa (RIETE) registry. *Circulation*. 2008;117:1711-1716, with permission from the American Heart Association, Inc.)

Conclusion.—PE remains a potentially fatal disease. The clinical predictors, identified in the present study, should be included in any clinical risk stratification scheme to optimally adapt the treatment of PE to the risk of the fatal outcome (Fig 1).

▶ There are a large number of articles being produced from the Registro Informatizado de la Enfermedad TromboEmbolica (RIETE) registry. Most, like this one, really have no particular or stunning new insights, but the data do provide some quantification of the variables analyzed. The rate of fatal pulmonary embolism (PE) at 6 months, in patients with venous tromboembolism, is interesting and is in line with previous reports. The data indicate that if you initially survive a massive PE, you are likely to survive longer term as 50% and 75% of the deaths directly attributed to PE occurred within 5 and 12 days, respectively, of the massive PE (Fig 1). I was a bit surprised that the study did not find cardiac or respiratory insufficiency to be predictive of death from pulmonary embolism. This may reflect insufficiency numbers or, more likely, it is a function of the type of data available in a registry where no specific testing was systemically performed, that were of cardiac and pulmonary functional status.

G. L. Moneta, MD

Chronic Kidney Disease Increases Risk for Venous Thromboembolism
Wattanakit K, Cushman M, Stehman-Breen C, et al (Univ of Minnesota, Minneapolis, MN; Univ of Washington, Seattle; et al)
J Am Soc Nephrol 19:135-140, 2008

Chronic kidney disease (CKD) is associated with increased risk for cardiovascular disease morbidity and mortality, but its association with incident venous thromboembolism (VTE) in non–dialysis-dependent patients has not been evaluated in a community-based population. With the use of data from the Longitudinal Investigation of Thromboembolism Etiology (LITE) study, 19,073 middle-aged and elderly adults were categorized on the basis of estimated GFR, and cystatin C (available in 4734 participants) was divided into quintiles. During a mean follow-up time of 11.8 yr, 413 participants developed VTE. Compared with participants with normal kidney function, relative risk for VTE was 1.28 (95% confidence interval [CI] 1.02 to 1.59) for those with mildly decreased kidney function and 2.09 (95% CI 1.47 to 2.96) for those with stage 3/4 CKD, when adjusted for age, gender, race, and center. After additional adjustment for cardiovascular disease risk factors, an increased risk for VTE was still observed in participants with stage 3/4 CKD, with a multivariable adjusted relative risk of 1.71 (95% CI 1.18 to 2.49). There was no significant association between cystatin C and VTE. In conclusion, middle-aged and elderly patients with CKD (stages 3 through 4) are at increased risk for incident VTE, suggesting that VTE prophylaxis may be particularly important in this population.

▶ It is known that chronic kidney disease (CKD) is associated with increased risk for morbidity and mortality of cardiovascular disease. This study sought to evaluate the risk of venous thromboembolism (VTE) in nondialysis-dependent patients with CKD in a community-based population. This is the first study demonstrating the association between mild to moderately decreased kidney function and VTE in the general population. It is important to remember that estimation of renal function in this study was based on a single measurement of serum creatinine that occurred on average 11.8 years before incident VTE events. It is unclear whether changes in kidney function during the almost 12-year interval could have resulted in systematic misclassification of CKD status at the time of the VTE event. Therefore, the data should be regarded as suggestive, but not definitive, that patients with mild to moderate CKD are at increased risk for VTE.

G. L. Moneta, MD

Activated Partial Thromboplastin Time and Risk of Future Venous Thromboembolism
Zakai NA, Ohira T, White R, et al (Brown Univ and Boston Univ, Providence, RI; Univ of Minnesota, MI; Univ of California Davis Med Ctr, Sacramento; et al)
Am J Med 121:231-238, 2008

Background.—Lower activated partial thromboplastin times are associated with higher levels of some coagulation factors and may represent a procoagulant tendency.

Methods.—In the Atherosclerosis Risk in Communities study, we studied the 13-year risk of venous thromboembolism in relation to baseline activated partial thromboplastin time in 13,880 individuals. We also studied 258 venous thromboembolism cases and 589 matched controls with measurements of additional coagulation factors.

Results.—After adjustment for demographics and procoagulant factors reflected in the activated partial thromboplastin time (fibrinogen, factors VIII, IX, and XI, and von Willebrand factor), participants in the lowest 2 quartiles of activated partial thromboplastin time compared with the fourth quartile had 2.4-fold (95% confidence interval [CI], 1.4-4.2) and 1.9-fold (95% CI, 1.1-3.2) higher risks of venous thromboembolism. The risk associated with activated partial thromboplastin times below the median was higher for idiopathic (odds ratio 5.5; 95% CI, 2.0-15.5) than secondary venous thromboembolism (odds ratio 1.74; 95% CI, 0.88-3.43). Subjects with both activated partial thromboplastin times below the median and factor V Leiden were 12.6-fold (95% CI, 5.7-28.0) more likely to develop venous thromboembolism compared with those with neither risk factor (*P* interaction <.01). A lower activated

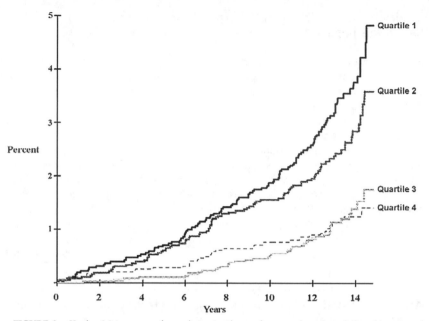

FIGURE 2.—Kaplan-Meier curve of cumulative incidence of venous thromboembolism by activated partial thromboplastin time quartile (full cohort): quartile 1: 21.1-27.0 seconds; quartile 2: 27.1-28.7 seconds; quartile 3: 28.8-30.6 seconds; quartile 4: 30.7-35.8 seconds. (Reprinted from Zakai NA, Ohira T, White R, et al. Activated partial thromboplastin time and risk of future venous thromboembolism. *Am J Med.* 2008;121:231-238, with permission from Elsevier.)

partial thromboplastin time also added to the thrombosis risk associated with obesity and elevated D-dimer.

Conclusion.—A single determination of the activated partial thromboplastin time below the median increased the risk of future venous thromboembolism. Findings were independent of coagulation factor levels, and a low activated partial thromboplastin time added to the risk associated with other risk factors (Fig 2).

▶ The coagulation cascade is obviously complicated. New abnormalities increasing the risk of venous thromboembolism (VTE) seem to appear in the literature on a regular basis. This article proves that you do not have to discover a new coagulation defect to contribute to the ability to stratify risk for VTE. Lower activated partial thromboplastin times (aPTTs) have long been suspected to be indicative of a relative hypercoagulable state—the question has been *how* hypercoagulable. This important study helps to quantify the risk of decreased aPPTs (Fig 2). The authors determined aPTTs below the median, which doubled the risk of VTE independent of other coagulation factors. aPTTs below the median were supra-additive with obesity, elevated D-dimer, and especially factor V Leiden in increasing the risk of VTE. This type of information should be immediately useful in evaluating patients with VTE and also for prophylaxis of VTE in at-risk patients. Perhaps patients with VTE and lowered aPTTs should be considered for a longer period of anticoagulation to treat their VTE event. In addition, further study of high-risk groups, such as those with situational or permanent risk factors for VTE, will be needed to see whether lower aPTTs are truly useful in stratifying risk for initial or recurrent VTE.

G. L. Moneta, MD

Etiology and VTE risk factor distribution in patients with inferior vena cava thrombosis
Linnemann B, Schmidt H, Schindewolf M, et al (Johann Wolfgang Goethe Univ Hosp, Frankfurt, Germany; Univ of Würzburg, Germany; et al)
Thromb Res 123:72-78, 2008

Introduction.—Inferior vena cava (IVC) thrombosis is a rare event and data detailing the underlying etiology are scarce.

Materials and Methods.—Therefore, we reviewed all available cases of IVC thrombosis consecutively registered in the MAISTHRO (MAin-ISar-THROmbosis) database and described the prevalence of VTE risk factors and other conditions contributing to IVC thrombosis development.

Results.—53 patients (35 F, 18 M) with IVC thrombosis aged 12 to 79 years were identified. 40 patients (75.5%) developed thrombosis under the age of 45. Local problems, such as IVC anomalies or external venous compression, contributed to the development of thrombosis in 12 cases (22.6%). Lupus anticoagulants (10.9 vs. 2.3%, $p = 0.013$) and malignoma (17.0 vs. 6.4%, $p = 0.023$) were more prevalent in IVC thrombosis patients compared to 265 age and sex matched controls with isolated lower extremity DVT. No difference was identified with regard to inherited thrombophilia or other known VTE risk factors. Symptomatic pulmonary embolism (PE) occurred in 32.1% of IVC thrombosis patients compared to 15.2% of controls ($p = 0.005$).

Conclusions.—Local problems such as IVC anomalies and external venous compression, malignancy and the presence of lupus anticoagulants contribute to the risk of IVC thrombosis. The risk of symptomatic pulmonary embolism in the acute setting is high.

▶ Inferior vena cava (IVC) thrombosis is relatively rare, and venous thromboembolism (VTE) risk factors that contribute to the development of IVC thrombosis are not well characterized. The authors have performed a valuable service in trying to use a large VTE registry to provide some insight into vena cava thrombosis. IVC thrombosis is a subset of deep vein thrombosis (DVT), but, based on data presented here, it appears to have slightly different predisposing factors compared with patients with DVT isolated to the lower extremity. In particular, the study identified local abnormalities of the vena cava, external compression of the vena cava from neighboring pathologic processes, malignancy, and the presence of antiphospolipid antibody syndrome as important predisposing factors to IVC thrombosis. Patients with IVC thrombosis should therefore be investigated for malignancy and the presence of antiphospholipid antibody syndrome. The risk of symptomatic pulmonary embolism (PE) appears quite high. It may be reasonable to consider the placement of a prophylactic vena cava filter.

G. L. Moneta, MD

Incidence of deep vein thrombosis related to peripherally inserted central catheters in children and adolescents

Dubois J, Rypens F, Garel L, et al (Ctr hospitalier universitaire Sainte-Justine, Montréal, Que)
Can Med Assoc J 177:1185-1190, 2007

Background.—Peripherally inserted central catheters (PICC) in children and adolescents are being used with increasing frequency. We sought to determine the incidence and characterize risk factors of deep vein thrombosis associated with peripherally inserted central catheters in a pediatric population.

Methods.—We conducted a prospective study involving consecutive patients referred to the radiology department of a tertiary care university-affiliated hospital for insertion of a peripherally inserted central catheter. We included patients, ages 18 years or less, who weighed more than 2.5 kg and had a peripherally inserted central catheter successfully inserted in his or her arm between June 2004 and November 2005. The primary outcome was the occurrence of partial or complete deep vein thrombosis evaluated by clinical examination, ultrasonography and venous angiography.

Results.—A total of 214 patients (101 girls, 113 boys) were included in the study. Partial or complete deep vein thrombosis occurred in 20 patients, for an incidence of 93.5 per 1000 patients and 3.85 per 1000 catheter-days. Only 1 of the cases was symptomatic. In the univariable analyses, the only variable significantly associated with deep vein thrombosis was the presence of factor II mutation G20210A (odds ratio 7.08, 95% confidence interval 1.11–45.15, $P = 0.04$), a genetic mutation that increases the risk of a blood clot and that was present in 5 (2.3%) of the 214 patients.

Interpretation.—The incidence of deep vein thrombosis, related to peripherally inserted central catheters in our study, was lower than the incidence related to centrally inserted venous catheters described in the pediatric literature (11%–50%).

▶ Despite the relatively high incidence of deep vein thrombosis (DVT) associated with peripherally inserted central catheters (PICCs), the incidence of DVT with PICC catheters appears lower than those reported with centrally inserted venous catheters. Because only one of the patients with DVT in this study was symptomatic, the study argues that objective diagnosis of DVT in patients with upper extremity catheters must be used to determine the true incidence of this complication. The authors do not address the incidence of superficial venous thrombosis involving the basilic or cephalic veins in patients with PICC because it is probably a more frequent complication of a PICC line than a DVT.

G. L. Moneta, MD

A 10-year analysis of venous thromboembolism on the surgical service: The effect of practice guidelines for prophylaxis
Shackford SR, Rogers FB, Terrien CM, et al (Univ of Vermont College of Medicine, Burlington)
Surgery 144:3-11, 2008

Background.—There is a national effort to decrease the incidence of venous thromboembolism (VTE) in surgical patients by encouraging compliance with established guidelines for prophylaxis. Reported compliance with these guidelines has been poor. The outcome of noncompliance in terms of morbidity and mortality in surgical patients is unknown. We sought to determine if there has been a decrease in the incidence of symptomatic VTE since implementation of the guidelines and whether there has been compliance with the guidelines in individual patients; we also analyzed the outcome of a cohort with VTE.

Methods.—We reviewed the records of all patients with symptomatic VTE on 3 surgery services over the 10-year period since initial publication of the guidelines. We determined, in each patient, whether there was compliance with the guidelines. We weighted the morbidity of each episode of VTE based on the likelihood of short-term mortality and long-term morbidity to determine the disease burden.

Results.—Of 37,615 patients, 172 developed a VTE (0.46%), and the incidence increased gradually over the years of the study. There was partial or complete compliance with the guidelines in 84% of the patients, but 37% of the VTEs were considered to be preventable. The disease burden was greatest in the higher-risk patients–there were 20 deaths (6%), 4 of which were caused by a pulmonary embolus.

Conclusions.—Despite one of the highest published rates of compliance with the guidelines for prophylaxis, the rate of symptomatic VTE is increasing.

▶ The authors report one of the highest rates of compliance with American College of Chest Physicians (ACCP)–suggested guidelines for prophylaxis of venous thromboembolism (VTE) in surgical patients. Despite this, their rate of symptomatic VTE has increased from 0.13% to 0.41% over the 10-year period included in the study. A number of things may play a role in this increased incidence of symptomatic VTE. They include more aggressive diagnostic approaches to pulmonary embolism with the availability of rapid multislice CT scanners, an increase in the comorbidity burden of patients undergoing surgical care, and the possibility that the prophylactic measures suggested by the ACCP guidelines are inadequate for higher-risk patients. Despite the efforts of the Joint Commission, the ACCP, Medicare and Medicaid, and just about everyone else, VTE, as a complication of surgical care, will continue to be a clinically important problem for the future.

G. L. Moneta, MD

Clinical probability assessment and D-dimer determination in patients with suspected deep vein thrombosis, a prospective multicenter management study
Elf JL, Strandberg K, Nilsson C, et al (Lund Univ, Sweden)
Thromb Res 123:612-616, 2009

Objectives.—To investigate the reliability of a combined strategy of clinical assessment score followed by a local D-dimer test to exclude deep vein thrombosis. For comparison D-dimer was analysed post hoc and batchwise at a coagulation laboratory.

Design.—Prospective multicenter management study.

Setting.—Seven hospitals in southern Sweden.

Subjects.—357 patients with a suspected first episode of deep vein thrombosis (DVT) were prospectively recruited and pre-test probability score (Wells score) was estimated by the emergency physician. If categorized as low pre-test probability, D-dimer was analysed and if negative, DVT was considered to be ruled out. The primary outcome was recurrent venous thromboembolism (VTE) during 3 months of follow up.

Results.—Prevalence of DVT was 23.5% (84/357). A low pre-test probability and a negative D-dimer result at inclusion was found in 31% (110/357) of the patients of whom one (0.9%, [95% CI 0.02–4.96]) had a VTE at follow up. Sensitivity, specificity, negative predictive value and negative likelihood ratio for our local D-dimer test in the low probability group were 85.7%, 74.5%, 98.2%, and 0,19 respectively compared to 85.6%, 67,6%, 97.9% and 0,23 using batchwise analysis at a coagulation laboratory.

Conclusion.—Pre-test probability score and D-dimer safely rule out DVT in about 30% of outpatients with a suspected first episode of DVT. One out of 110 patients was diagnosed with DVT during follow up. No significant difference in diagnostic performance was seen between local D-dimer test and the post hoc batch analysis with the same reagent in the low probability group.

▶ It is well known that there are far more patients in emergency departments with suspected deep vein thrombosis (DVT) than those that actually have DVT. Recent studies that indicate low clinical probability scores along with a negative D-dimer can exclude DVT in about 30% to 50% of outpatients with suspected DVT. This combination, therefore, likely safely obviates the need for further diagnostic testing in such patients.[1,2] The authors point out that previous studies have occurred in the setting of a low prevalence of

DVT, and that the probability that a patient has a disease following diagnostic testing is determined by the estimated probability before the test in combination with the accuracy of the test. This study involves Scandinavian patients where it appears there is a higher prevalence (30% to 50%) of confirmed DVT in outpatients suspected of DVT than that observed in other countries.[3,4] This should increase the pretest probability of the disease actually being present, and therefore potentially increase the risk of false-negative results. In addition, D-dimer assays are not standardized; therefore, there is a theoretic possibility of different results with different assays. Based on all this the authors sought to determine whether a combined strategy of using a clinical assessment score followed by D-dimer testing was safe for patients in a clinic setting where the prevalence of DVT in outpatients is high. The approach seemed to be effective. The "competition" is of course routine ultrasound testing in patients suspected of DVT. What we really need is an analysis of under what circumstances pretest probability scoring and D-dimer actually are useful fiscally and from physician and patient perspective. One can postulate that during the day, when an ultrasound test is readily available, patients and the emergency room are better served by a definitive quick ultrasound examination. On the other hand, at night when the availability of ultrasound technologists may be more limited, the approach of pretest probability scoring and D-dimer testing may be more attractive.

G. L. Moneta, MD

References

1. Kearon C, Ginsberg JS, Douketis J, et al. Management of suspected deep venous thrombosis in outpatients by using clinical assessment and D-dimer testing. *Ann Intern Med.* 2001;135:108-111.
2. Anderson DR, Kovacs MJ, Kovacs G, et al. Combined use of clinical assessment and d-dimer to improve the management of patients presenting to the emergency department with suspected deep vein thrombosis (the EDITED Study). *J Thromb Haemost.* 2003;1:645-651.
3. Lindahl TL, Lundahl TH, Ranby M, Fransson SG. Clinical evaluation of a diagnostic strategy for deep venous thrombosis with exclusion by low plasma levels of fibrin degradation product D-dimer. *Scand J Clin Lab Invest.* 1998;58:307-316.
4. Hansson PO, Eriksson H, Eriksson E, Jagenburg R, Lukes P, Risberg B. Can laboratory testing improve screening strategies for deep vein thrombosis at an emergency unit? *J Intern Med.* 1994;235:143-151.

Evaluation of Wells score and repeated D-dimer in diagnosing venous thromboembolism

Ljungqvist M, Söderberg M, Moritz P, et al (Karolinska Institutet, Stockholm, Sweden; et al)
Eur J Intern Med 19:285-288, 2008

Background.—Patients presenting with symptoms suggestive of venous thromboembolism (VTE), i.e., deep vein thrombosis (DVT) and pulmonary embolism (PE), are common at the emergency departments.

However, of those, only 15–25% actually have the disease. The aims of this study were to determine (1) if low pre-test probability (PTP) using the Wells score, together with a normal D-dimer, safely excludes VTE in outpatients and (2) if a follow-up D-dimer adds extra information.

Methods.—Patients ($n = 151$, 68% women) with suspected VTE, a PTP below 1.5, and a D-dimer test (TinaQuant®) below 0.5 mg/L were included in the study and underwent no further diagnostic investigations. Patients ($n = 177$, 54% women) with D-dimer levels of 0.5 mg/L or higher or a PTP of 1.5 or higher were excluded. A follow-up D-dimer test was conducted 3–7 days after the initial hospital visit and further diagnostic investigations were made if test results were abnormal. Patients were studied for 3 months.

Results.—A follow-up D-dimer test was conducted in 101/151 cases (67%), 13/101 of which revealed elevated D-dimer levels. None of these 13 patients had persistent symptoms or was diagnosed with VTE. All 151 patients were contacted after 3 months; none of them had clinical signs of VTE. Of the 177 patients excluded, 45 (25%) were diagnosed with VTE. Of the 176/328 (151 + 177) patients with normal D-dimer levels, only 1 had VTE (< 0.01%).

Conclusion.—A normal PTP using the Wells score and a normal D-dimer safely excludes VTE at the emergency department. A follow-up D-dimer test adds no further information.

▶ Every day, in emergency rooms throughout the world, many thousands of patients undergo evaluation for possible venous thromboembolism (VTE). Overall, less than one-fourth of the patients evaluated for VTE in an emergency room setting will actually have the disease. The data presented here support the use of a clinical algorithm that includes both the Wells criteria pretest probability score and D-dimer levels to reduce the number of ultrasound investigations in patients with low risk of VTE. There were no symptomatic VTEs within 3 months in 151 patients with low pretest probability scores and a normal D-dimer level. A follow-up D-dimer test did not add clinically important information. The overall concept of this study is therefore interesting and may serve to improve the efficiency of evaluation of patients in the emergency room for possible VTE. It must be remembered, however, that there are many assays for D-dimer. The data here apply only to that assay used in this study.

G. L. Moneta, MD

D-dimer and factor VIII are independent risk factors for recurrence after anticoagulation withdrawal for a first idiopathic deep vein thrombosis
Cosmi B, Legnani C, Cini M, et al (S. Orsola-Malpighi Univ Hosp, Bologna, Italy)
Thromb Res 122:610-617, 2008

Background and objectives.—To assess the predictive value of D-dimer (D-d) and Factor VIII (FVIII) in combination for recurrent venous thromboembolism (VTE) after vitamin K antagonist (VKA) therapy suspension.

Design and methods.—Consecutive outpatients with a first episode of idiopathic proximal deep vein thrombosis of the lower limbs were enrolled on the day of VKA suspension. After 30 ± 10 days, D-d (cut-off value: 500 ng/mL), chromogenic FVIII activity and inherited thrombophilia were determined. Follow-up was 2 years.

Results.—Overall recurrence rate was 16.4% (55/336; 95% CI:13–21%). The multivariate hazard ratio (HR) for recurrence was 2.45 (95% CI: 1.24–4.99) for abnormal D-d and 2.76 (95% CI:1.57–4.85) for FVIII above the 75th percentile (2.42 U/mL) after adjustment for age, sex, thrombophilia, VKA duration and residual venous obstruction. When compared with normal D-d and FVIII, the multivariate HR was 4.5 (95% CI: 1.7–12.2) for normal D-d with FVIII above 2.42 U/mL and 2.7 (95% CI: 1.2–6.6) and 7.1 (95% CI:2.8–17.6) for abnormal D-d with FVIII, respectively, below and above 2.42 U/mL.

Interpretation and conclusions.—D-d and FVIII at 30 ± 10 days after VKA withdrawal are independent risk factors for recurrent VTE (Fig 1 and 2).

▶ It is unknown what the appropriate length of treatment with vitamin K antagonist (VKA) therapy is for patients with idiopathic venous thromboembolism

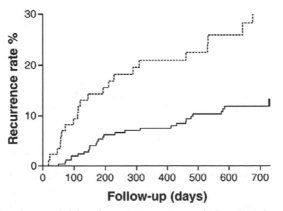

FIGURE 1.—Cumulative probability of recurrence in patients with idiopathic index event according to FVIII: 1 - FVIII <75th percentile (solid line); 2 - FVIII >75th percentile (dotted line). (Reprinted from Cosmi B, Legnani C, Cini M, et al. D-dimer and factor VIII are independent risk factors for recurrence after anticoagulation withdrawal for a first idiopathic deep vein thrombosis. *Thromb Res.* 2008:122:610-617.)

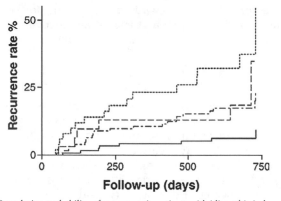

FIGURE 2.—Cumulative probability of recurrence in patients with idiopathic index event according to combination of D-d and FVIII at T2: 1 - normal D-d with FVIII <75th percentile (reference group: solid line); 2 - abnormal D-d with FVIII <75th percentile (semi-dotted line); 3 - normal D-d with FVIII >75th percentile (dashed line) and 4 - abnormal D-d with FVIII >75th percentile (dotted line). (Reprinted from Cosmi B, Legnani C, Cini M, et al. D-dimer and factor VIII are independent risk factors for recurrence after anticoagulation withdrawal for a first idiopasthic deep vein thrombosis. *Thromb Res.* 2008:122:610-617.)

(VTE). There is, therefore, intense interest in stratifying patients with idiopathic VTE with respect to risk factors that may increase rates of recurrence. The available data do suggest that the longer the treatment period with VKA, the less the recurrence rates of VTE. Of course, VKAs are associated with increased risk of bleeding and are inconvenient for the patient. There is, therefore, intense interest in stratifying risk among those patients with idiopathic VTE. This is another article that attempts to do just that. The percentage of patients in this study with both normal D-dimer (D-d) and Factor VIII less than the 75th percentile was 37%. This implies that at least a third of patients with idiopathic VTE have a low risk of VTE recurrence. Clearly, larger studies are warranted to determine if the combination of Factor VIII and D-d analysis can be used to tailor the duration of VKA therapy following idiopathic VTE.

G. L. Moneta, MD

Identifying unprovoked thromboembolism patients at low risk for recurrence who can discontinue anticoagulant therapy

Rodger MA, Kahn SR, Wells PS, et al (Univ of Ottawa, ON; McGill Univ, Montréal, Quebec, Canada)
Can Med Assoc J 179:417-426, 2008

Background.—Whether to continue oral anticoagulant therapy beyond 6 months after an "unprovoked" venous thromboembolism is controversial. We sought to determine clinical predictors to identify patients who are at low risk of recurrent venous thromboembolism who could safely discontinue oral anticoagulants.

Methods.—In a multicentre prospective cohort study, 646 participants with a first, unprovoked major venous thromboembolism were enrolled over a 4-year period. Of these, 600 participants completed a mean 18-month follow-up in September 2006. We collected data for 69 potential predictors of recurrent venous thromboembolism while patients were taking oral anticoagulation therapy (5–7 months after initiation). During follow-up after discontinuing oral anticoagulation therapy, all episodes of suspected recurrent venous thromboembolism were independently adjudicated. We performed a multivariable analysis of predictor variables ($p < 0.10$) with high interobserver reliability to derive a clinical decision rule.

Results.—We identified 91 confirmed episodes of recurrent venous thromboembolism during follow-up after discontinuing oral anticoagulation therapy (annual risk 9.3%, 95% CI 7.7%–11.3%). Men had a 13.7% (95% CI 10.8%–17.0%) annual risk. There was no combination of clinical predictors that satisfied our criteria for identifying a low-risk subgroup of men. Fifty-two percent of women had 0 or 1 of the following characteristics: hyperpigmentation, edema or redness of either leg; D-dimer ≥ 250 µg/L while taking warfarin; body mass index ≥ 30 kg/m²; or age ≥ 65 years. These women had an annual risk of 1.6% (95% CI 0.3%–4.6%). Women who had 2 or more of these findings had an annual risk of 14.1% (95% CI 10.9%–17.3%).

Interpretation.—Women with 0 or 1 risk factor may safely discontinue oral anticoagulant therapy after 6 months of therapy following a first unprovoked venous thromboembolism. This criterion does not apply to men. (http://Clinicaltrials.gov trial register number NCT00261014).

▶ This study is consistent with the previously determined adverse effect of male sex on recurrence of venous thromboembolism (VTE).[1] There are 3 major points that are discussed here. First, identification of risk factors after 5 to 7 months of oral anticoagulation therapy are strong predictors of recurrent VTE. Second, D-dimer levels after stopping oral anticoagulation may not be sufficient to identify patients at low risk of recurrence, whereas D-dimer levels while taking oral anticoagulation may be a strong predictor of recurrent VTE. The point is particularly interesting in that it allows more efficient care of patients. Stopping anticoagulation and testing D-dimer levels 1 month later and subsequently restarting anticoagulation therapy if necessary is impractical and exposes potentially high-risk patients to a period without anticoagulation. Finally, the authors identified a clinical decision rule that identifies women at low risk of VTE. Such rules with respect to venous thrombosis are interesting but unfortunately not all that widely used.

G. L. Moneta, MD

Reference

1. McRae S, Tran H, Schulman S, Ginsberg J, Kearon C. Effect of patient's sex on risk of recurrent venous thromboembolism: a meta-analysis. *Lancet.* 2006;368: 371-378.

Thromboembolic Consequences of Subtherapeutic Anticoagulation in Patients Stabilized on Warfarin Therapy: The Low INR Study
Clark NP, Witt DM, Delate T, et al (Kaiser Permanente Colorado, Lafayette; et al)
Pharmacotherapy 28:960-967, 2008

Study Objective.—To quantify the absolute risk of thromboembolism associated with a significant subtherapeutic international normalized ratio (INR) in patients with previously stable anticoagulation while receiving warfarin.

Design.—Retrospective, matched cohort analysis.

Setting.—Centralized anticoagulation service in an integrated health care delivery system.

Patients.—A total of 2597 adult patients receiving warfarin from January 1998–December 2005; 1080 patients were in the low INR cohort and were matched to 1517 patients in the therapeutic INR cohort based on index INR date, indication for warfarin, and age.

Measurements and Main Results.—Stable, therapeutic anticoagulation was defined as two INR values, measured at least 2 weeks apart, within or above the therapeutic range. The low INR cohort included patients with a third INR value of 0.5 or more units below their therapeutic range. The therapeutic INR cohort included patients with a third therapeutic INR value and no INR value 0.2 or more units below their target INR range in the ensuing 90 days. The primary outcome was anticoagulation-related thromboembolism during the 90 days after the index INR. Secondary outcomes were times to the first occurrence of anticoagulation-related complications (bleeding, thromboembolism, or death) in the 90 days after the index INR. Four thromboembolic events (0.4%) occurred in the low INR cohort and one event (0.1%) in the therapeutic INR cohort (p=0.214). The differences in the proportions of thromboembolism, bleeding, or death were not significant between the cohorts (p>0.05). No significant differences were noted in the hazard of thromboembolism, bleeding, or death between the cohorts (p>0.05).

Conclusion.—Patients with stable INRs while receiving warfarin who experience a significant subtherapeutic INR value have a low risk of thromboembolism in the ensuing 90 days. The risk was similar to that observed in a matched control population in whom therapeutic anticoagulation was maintained. These findings do not support the practice of anticoagulant bridge therapy for patients stabilized on warfarin therapy to reduce their risk for thromboembolism during isolated periods of subtherapeutic anticoagulation.

▶ Optimal use of warfarin is hampered by unpredictable pharmokinetics. In specialized anticoagulation clinics, about 40% of international normalized ratios (INRs) fall outside the target therapeutic range, with most of these abnormal INR values being below the target range.[1] The authors conducted a retrospective, longitudinal investigation to quantify the risk associated with isolated subtherapeutic anticoagulation.

The study has several strengths, including its large sample size, carefully defined patient population, and essentially complete follow-up in outcome assessment of the patients in this anticoagulation clinic. Although there were not many events, many patients did fall into the low INR cohort; approximately 40% of the patients managed in this anticoagulation clinic. Therefore, the data seem fairly strong and indicate that a single low INR value is of very little consequence in a patient with an otherwise stable anticoagulation profile. The findings do not support bridge therapy with heparins in patients previously stable on warfarin who have a period of subtherapeutic anticoagulation. Of course, this was a retrospective study and therefore there may have been incomplete capture of outcome events. Nevertheless, it does not appear that one needs to be too concerned when a patient, who is otherwise stable on warfarin anticoagulation, presents with a diminished INR.

G. L. Moneta, MD

Reference

1. Witt DM, Sadler MA, Mazzoli G, Tillman DJ. Effect of a centralized clinical pharmacy anticoagulation service on the outcomes of anticoagulation therapy. *Chest.* 2005;127:1515-1522.

Deep Vein Thrombosis of Lower Extremity: Direct Intraclot Injection of Alteplase Once Daily with Systemic Anticoagulation—Results of Pilot Study
Chang R, Chen CC, Kam A, et al (Natl Insts of Health, Bethesda, MD)
Radiology 246:619-629, 2008

Purpose.—To prospectively evaluate the outcome of patients with acute deep vein thrombosis (DVT) of the lower extremity treated with "lacing" of the thrombus with alteplase (recombinant tissue plasminogen activator, or rTPA).

Materials and Methods.—This HIPAA-compliant study was approved by the Institutional Review Board of the National Heart, Lung, and Blood Institute and was funded by the National Institutes of Health. After giving written consent, 20 patients with first-onset acute DVT were treated with direct intraclot lacing of the thrombus with alteplase (maximum daily dose, 50 mg per leg per day; maximum of four treatments) and full systemic anticoagulation. Alteplase was chosen because its high fibrin affinity obviates continuous infusion of this thrombolytic agent. Ventilation-perfusion (V/Q) scans were performed for evaluation of embolic risks, and clinical and imaging examinations were supplemented with pharmacokinetic studies to enable further assessment of treatment outcomes.

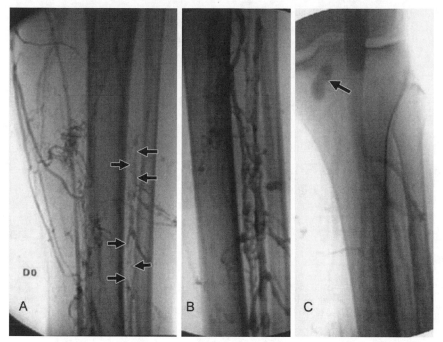

FIGURE 1.—Femoropopliteal DVT. Serial venograms (anteroposterior views) obtained with foot vein injection in 79-year-old man with left leg DVT. *A*, Before treatment, most of the injected contrast material diverts into superficial veins, despite use of tourniquets at ankle. Only a segment of a peroneal vein is visualized and shows filling defects (arrows) due to thrombosis. Above this level, deep popliteal and femoral veins in the thigh were also occluded (not shown). *B*, Venogram obtained 1 day after pulse-spray intraclot injection of alteplase shows preferential filling of calf veins. Although there is evidence of residual thrombus in calf veins, flow was reestablished in calf, popliteal, and femoral veins. The patient's calf discomfort had resolved, and no additional thrombolytic therapy was given. Anticoagulation was continued for 6 months. *C*, Foot venogram obtained 6 weeks after initial therapy shows restoration of flow in calf and popliteal veins. Mild incompetence of perforating veins allows visualization of small varicose vein segment (arrow) in superficial venous system. (Reprinted from Chang R, Chen CC, Kam A, et al. Deep vein thrombosis of lower extremity: direct intraclot injection of alteplase once daily with systemic anticoagulation—results of pilot study. *Radiology.* 2008;246:619-629, with permission from RSNA.)

Results.—The 20 patients included 13 men and seven women aged 18–79 years. Antegrade blood flow was restored through-out the deep venous system in 16 patients (80%) during thrombolytic therapy, with complete resolution of symptoms in 18 patients (90%) after 6 months of anticoagulation. Pharmacokinetic studies showed rapid clearance of circulating alteplase and recovery of plasminogen activator inhibitor-1 levels within 2 hours after termination of alteplase treatment. V/Q scans revealed a 40% incidence of pulmonary embolism before treatment and a 15% incidence of asymptomatic pulmonary embolism during thrombolytic therapy. There were no cases of clinically important pulmonary embolism or serious bleeding during thrombolytic therapy. During a mean follow-up period of 3.4 years, no patient developed a postthrombotic syndrome or recurrent thromboembolism.

Conclusion.—Intraclot injection or lacing of the thrombus with a fibrin-binding thrombolytic agent such as alteplase is an alternative to continuous-infusion thrombolytic regimens and minimizes the duration of systemic exposure to thrombolytic agents (Fig 1).

▶ The standard method for administering thrombolytic therapy for the treatment of deep vein thrombosis (DVT) is continuous infusion of the lytic agent directly into the thrombus through catheters embedded in the thrombus. However, continuous infusion of lytic agents is logistically difficult; in many hospitals it requires an ICU bed, and results in prolonged exposure of the systemic circulation to the thrombolytic agents. An alternative is to lace the thrombus with a thrombolytic agent that binds to fibrin in the clot and is rapidly cleared from the general circulation. This can allow the thrombolytic agent to work at the site where it is needed, but minimize the duration of systemic exposure to the thrombolytic agent.

The data indicate the approach presented here can be effective (Fig 1). There are also a number of potential advantages to this intermittent approach of thrombolytic therapy. The most obvious practical advantage is that patients do not require intensive monitoring of a continuous infusion of a thrombolytic agent. However, the administration of alteplase directly into the thrombus does require a substantial commitment of time in the imaging department. In this study, typical procedure times for first treatment of an uncomplicated iliofemoral DVT was 1½ hours. If there was extensive calf vein thrombus, initial procedure times could be doubled or almost tripled. Procedure times for subsequent treatments are shorter because catheters are left in place after the initial treatment and can be exchanged using standard guidewire techniques. Overall it appears that if one has the catheter skills and the time, intermittent administration of thrombolytic agent directly into the clot may be a viable alternative to more standard continuous infusion techniques.

G. L. Moneta, MD

17 Chronic Venous and Lymphatic Disease

Determinants and Time Course of the Postthrombotic Syndrome after Acute Deep Venous Thrombosis
Kahn SR, Shrier I, Julian JA, et al (McGill Univ Health Ctr and McGill Univ; et al)
Ann Intern Med 149:698-707, 2008

Background.—The reason some patients with deep venous thrombosis (DVT) develop the postthrombotic syndrome is not well understood.

Objective.—To determine the frequency, time course, and predictors of the postthrombotic syndrome after acute DVT.

Design.—Prospective, multicenter cohort study.

Setting.—8 Canadian hospital centers.

Patients.—387 outpatients and inpatients who received an objective diagnosis of acute symptomatic DVT were recruited from 2001 to 2004.

Measurements.—Standardized assessments for the postthrombotic syndrome using the Villalta scale at 1, 4, 8, 12, and 24 months after enrollment. Mean postthrombotic score and severity category at each interval was calculated. Predictors of postthrombotic score profiles over time since diagnosis of DVT were identified by using linear mixed modeling.

Results.—At all study intervals, about 30% of patients had mild (score, 5 to 9), 10% had moderate (score, 10 to 14), and 3% had severe (score >14 or ulcer) postthrombotic syndrome. Greater postthrombotic severity category at the 1-month visit strongly predicted higher mean postthrombotic scores throughout 24 months of follow-up (1.97, 5.03, and 7.00 increase in Villalta score for mild, moderate, and severe 1-month severity categories, respectively, vs. none; $P < 0.001$). Additional predictors of higher scores over time were venous thrombosis of the common femoral or iliac vein (2.23 increase in score vs. distal [calf] venous thrombosis; $P < 0.001$), higher body mass index (0.14 increase in score per kg/m^2; $P < 0.001$), previous ipsilateral venous thrombosis (1.78 increase in score; $P = 0.001$), older age (0.30 increase in score per 10-year age increase; $P = 0.011$), and female sex (0.79 increase in score; $P = 0.020$).

Limitations.—Decisions to prescribe compression stockings were left to treating physicians rather than by protocol. Because international normalized ratio data were unavailable, the relationship between anticoagulation quality and Villalta scores could not be assessed.

Conclusion.—The postthrombotic syndrome occurs frequently after DVT. Patients with extensive DVT and those with more severe postthrombotic manifestations 1 month after DVT have poorer long-term outcomes.

▶ The Villalta scale, used to quantify the severity of the post-thrombotic syndrome in this study, is a clinical measure of post-thrombotic syndrome that grades severity from 0-absent to 3-severe of 5 patient-related symptoms (pain, cramps, heaviness, pruritus, and paresthesia) and 6 clinician-related clinical signs (edema, redness, skin induration, hyperpigmentation, venous ectasia, and pain on calf compression). A score of 5 or more indicates the presence of post-thrombotic syndrome. The scale has been validated when measured against quality-of-life instruments as well as anatomic and physiologic markers of post-thrombotic syndrome. It appears to have good to excellent interobserver reproducibility and responds to clinical change. However, it seems a bit cumbersome to use, and the other factors identified by the authors as predicting post-thrombotic syndrome are already well appreciated. I don't see use of the Villalta score becoming a routine component of clinical practice.

G. L. Moneta, MD

A Randomized, Double-Blind Multicentre Clinical Trial Comparing the Efficacy of Calcium Dobesilate with Placebo in the Treatment of Chronic Venous Disease
Martínez-Zapata MJ, Moreno RM, Gich I, et al (Iberoamerican Cochrane Ctr, Spain; Hosp Clínico San Carlos, Madrid, Spain; et al)
Eur J Vasc Endovasc Surg 35:358-365, 2008

Objective.—To assess the efficacy of calcium dobesilate on the quality-of-life (QoL) of patients with chronic venous disease (CVD).

Design.—Randomized, parallel, double blind, placebo-controlled clinical trial.

Methods.—Patients were recruited from vascular surgery clinics and randomized to 500 mg capsules of calcium dobesilate twice a day for 3 months or placebo. The primary outcome measure was 'QoL after 3 months' treatment measured by the specific Chronic Insufficiency Venous International Questionnaire (CIVIQ). Secondary outcomes were QoL at 12 months and assessment of the CVD signs and symptoms. The principal analysis was undertaken on the intention-to-treat (ITT) data.

Results.—Five hundred and nine patients were recruited (246 to calcium dobesilate and 263 to placebo). The analysis of the 'QoL after 3 months' showed no significant differences between groups (p = 0.07). For secondary outcomes, oedema and symptoms of CVD, there were no significant differences between groups. In a multi-factorial analysis, the 'QoL at 12 months' was better in the calcium dobesilate group than in placebo group (p = 0.02).

Conclusions.—Treatment with calcium dobesilate was not found to be superior to placebo on the QoL of CVD patients. The sustained effect of calcium dobesilate observed after treatment should be confirmed in future studies.

▶ It is always difficult to publish negative results. Negative results are, to some, not very interesting; however, they can be very important, and I think the results here should be taken seriously. The trial was well-designed, contained a large number of patients, had a reasonably long follow-up, and was well analyzed. At the dosages of the drug used, the results using the quality of life instrument have to be considered valid. It is especially important to note the improvement in the placebo group. The placebo effect is well recognized and clearly played a role in the negative results of this trial. It should be noted that although this study focused on quality-of-life analysis, other studies assessing calcium dobesilate in the treatment of venous disease have found that calcium dobesilate can reduce edema in patients with chronic venous disease. If edema precedes many of the more serious manifestations of chronic venous disease, a possible overall conclusion is that calcium dobesilate does not improve patient-oriented, short-term outcomes, but may be effective in the long term in preventing late manifestation of venous insufficiency. Patient perception of improvement, therefore, may be different if follow-up was for many years rather than 1 year or less.

G. L. Moneta, MD

Comparisons of side effects using air and carbon dioxide foam for endovenous chemical ablation

Morrison N, Neuhardt DL, Rogers CR, et al (Morrison Vein Inst, Scottsdale, AZ; Compudiagnostics, Inc., Scottsdale, AZ)
J Vasc Surg 47:830-836, 2008

Objective.—This clinical study evaluated prospectively adverse events immediately following ultrasound-guided foam sclerotherapy (UGFS) for the treatment of lower extremity venous valvular insufficiency. Incidence of side effects associated with carbon dioxide (CO_2) foam was compared with a historical control using air-based foam. The literature on the subject was reviewed.

Methods.—Vital signs were monitored during and immediately after UGFS, and adverse events were recorded for 24 hours following the procedure. The air-based foam group had 49 patients: 44 women and 5 men. The CO_2-based foam group had 128 patients: 115 women and 13 men. CEAP class was C2EpAsPr, describing varicose veins, primary etiology, and saphenous reflux. UGFS followed thermal ablation of the great saphenous vein. Foam was prepared using the three-way tap technique to mix gas with 1% polidocanol in a 4:1 ratio. Segments of the great and small saphenous veins and their tributaries were treated with UGFS. Foam volumes injected were 27 ± 10 (SD) (6-46 range) and 25 ± 12 (6-57 range) mL for air- and CO_2-based foams respectively ($P = .39$). Incidence of adverse events was compared by χ^2 statistics. Vital signs were compared by paired t test.

Results.—During the procedure, the average heart rate decreased by less than 5 bpm for both groups ($P < .001$), and blood pressure decreased by less than 3 mm Hg in the CO_2 group ($P < .02$). Respiratory rate, electrocardiogram, and pulse oxymetry did not change significantly in both air- and CO_2-foam series ($P > .05$). Visual disturbances were experienced by 3.1% (4/128) and 8.2% (4/49) patients in the CO_2 and air groups respectively ($P = .15$). Respiratory difficulties or circumoral paresthesia each occurred in 0.8% (n = 1) of the CO_2 patients. Incidence of chest tightness (3.1% vs 18%), dry cough (1.6% vs 16%), or dizziness (3.1% vs 12%) were significantly lower in the CO_2 vs air groups ($P < .02$). Nausea occurred in 2% and 4% of the CO_2 and air-based foam groups ($P = .53$). Overall, the proportion of patients describing side effects decreased from 39% (19/49) to 11% (14/128) as CO_2 replaced air for foam preparation ($P < .001$). Similar findings were described in the literature of air-based foam but data on the use of physiological gas were rare.

Conclusions.—Side effects decreased significantly if CO_2 rather than air was employed to make the sclerosing foam for chemical ablation of superficial veins of the lower extremity.

▶ Foam sclerotherapy is clearly a hot item in the sclerotherapy world. But we really do not know much about the complications of foam sclerotherapy. Clearly, the impression is side effects, adverse reactions, and minor or major complications following foam sclerotherapy are limited. Different studies have different objectives and varying descriptions of complications. This all makes it difficult to analyze the information on complications presented in the literature. Although this study used historic controls, it does a nice job of quantifying the complications of foam sclerotherapy when foam is used to treat branches or segments of the greater and lesser saphenous veins (the information presented here does not apply to treatment of spider veins). The study also does a nice job of bringing, to the nonsclerotherapist, attention to some of the lesser known complications such as dry cough, metallic or medicinal taste, and chest tightness. From my reading of the article, it appears that with the exception of the most minor complications and despite the concluding sentence of the abstract, complications are not all that different with carbon dioxide versus air.

G. L. Moneta, MD

The importance of deep venous reflux velocity as a determinant of outcome in patients with combined superficial and deep venous reflux treated with endovenous saphenous ablation

Marston WA, Brabham VW, Mendes R, et al (Univ of North Carolina School of Med, Chapel Hill)

J Vasc Surg 48:400-406, 2008

Introduction.—Twenty to thirty percent of patients with symptomatic chronic venous insufficiency (CVI) are found to have combined superficial and deep venous reflux on duplex testing. It is currently unclear whether endovenous ablation (EVA) of the saphenous vein will result in correction of CVI without addressing the deep venous reflux. In this study, we examined deep venous reflux velocities to determine whether these would predict outcome after endovenous ablation.

Methods.—Patients with symptomatic CVI and both saphenous and deep venous reflux were identified using duplex ultrasonography. Reflux times and maximal reflux velocity (MRV) in each examined vein segment were determined. In each limb, the venous filling index (VFI) and the venous clinical severity score (VCSS) were obtained both before and after laser ablation of the great and/or small saphenous veins. Preoperative venous reflux velocities were correlated with improvement in VFI and VCSS after ablation.

Results.—75 limbs with both deep and superficial venous reflux were identified. Seventy-five percent of limbs were CEAP clinical class 3 or 4 and the other 25% were class 5 or 6. Forty limbs demonstrated deep venous reflux in the femoral and/or popliteal vein. After EVA, significant improvements in VFI and VCSS were seen, but this depended on MRV in the deep vein. When MRV in the popliteal or femoral vein was <10 cm/sec, limbs had significantly better outcomes than limbs with MRV >10 cm/sec as measured by both VFI ($P = .01$) and VCSS ($P = .03$). In 35 limbs, deep venous reflux was identified only in the CFV. In this group, the average pre-procedure VFI (6.54 ± 3.9 cc/sec) decreased significantly to 2.2 ± 1.9 cc/sec ($P < .001$) and the VCSS improved markedly from 7.0 ± 2.8 to 1.3 ± 1.4 ($P < .001$).

Conclusions.—EVA of the saphenous veins can be performed in patients with concomitant deep venous insufficiency with hemodynamic and clinical improvement in most cases. Patients with popliteal or femoral reflux velocities lower than 10 cm/sec usually experience marked improvement in both the VFI and the VCSS. Patients with femoral or popliteal reflux velocities greater than 10 cm/sec have a high incidence of persistent symptoms after EVA (Fig 1).

▶ It has been pointed out in a number of studies that correction of saphenous vein reflux can frequently result in correction of coexisting common femoral vein reflux. However, not all patients with common femoral vein reflux have resolution of the reflux after removal or ablation of a refluxing greater saphenous vein (GSV). Up until this point, there were no guidelines as to which

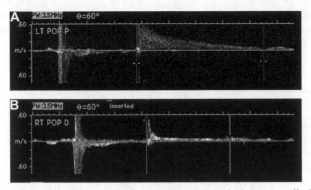

FIGURE 1.—Measurement of maximal reflux velocity (MRV). In both images, cuff release occurs at the first vertical line. The x-axis is time with the large hash marks indicating 1 second. At 0.5 seconds after cuff release, the velocity of reverse flow (in cm/sec) is identified and recorded as MRV. **A,** High velocity reflux in the popliteal vein of 38 cm/sec. **B,** Low velocity reflux in the popliteal vein of 8 cm/sec. (Reprinted from Marston WA, Brabham VW, Mendes R, et al. The importance of deep venous reflux velocity as a determinant of outcome in patients with combined superficial and deep venous reflux treated with endovenous saphenous ablation. *J Vasc Surg.* 2008;48:400-406, with permission from The Society for Vascular Surgery.)

patients with coexisting GSV and deep venous reflux were likely to benefit from treatment of the GSV reflux. The study is valuable in that it points out that patients with maximum reflux velocities (Fig 1) in their deep veins of < 10 cm/s will do quite well both in terms of hemodynamic improvement and symptom improvement with correction of GSV reflux. In addition, the study brings to our attention that popliteal reflux with a low maximum reflux velocity may not be a significant problem if there is GSV reflux that can be corrected. This article should be carefully read by anyone performing procedures for correction of saphenous vein reflux.

G. L. Moneta, MD

Endovenous laser ablation: Does standard above-knee great saphenous vein ablation provide optimum results in patients with both above- and below-knee reflux? A randomized controlled trial
Theivacumar NS, Dellagrammaticas D, Mavor AID, et al (Leeds Vascular Inst, UK)
J Vasc Surg 48:173-178, 2008

Background.—Following above-knee (AK) great saphenous vein (GSV) endovenous laser ablation (EVLA) 40% to 50% patients have residual varicosities. This randomized controlled trial (RCT) assesses whether more extensive GSV ablation enhances their resolution and influences symptom improvement.
Method.—Sixty-eight limbs (65 patients) with varicosities and above and below-knee GSV reflux were randomized to Group A: AK-EVLA (n = 23); Group B: EVLA mid-calf to groin (n = 23); and Group C:

AK-EVLA, concomitant below-knee GSV foam sclerotherapy (n = 22). Primary outcomes were residual varicosities requiring sclerotherapy (6 weeks), improvement in Aberdeen varicose vein severity scores (AVVSS, 12 weeks), patient satisfaction, and complication rates.

Results.—EVLA ablated the treated GSV in all limbs. Sclerotherapy requirements were Group A: 14/23 (61%); Group B: 4/23 (17%); and Group C: 8/22 (36%); $\chi^2 = 9.3$ (2 *df*) $P = .01$ with $P_{A-B} = 0.006$; $P_{B-C} = 0.19$; $P_{A-C} = 0.14$. AVVSS scores improved in all groups as follows: A: 14.8 (9.3-22.6) to 6.4 (3.2-9.1), (P < .001); B: 15.8 (10.2-24.5) to 2.5 (1.1-3.7), (P < .001); and C: 15.1 (9.0-23.1) to 4.1 (2.3-6.8), (P < .001) and $P_{A-B} = 0.011$, $P_{A-C} = 0.042$. Patient satisfaction was highest in Group B. BK-EVLA was not associated with saphenous nerve injury.

Conclusions.—Extended EVLA is safe, increases spontaneous resolution of varicosities, and has a greater impact on symptom reduction. Similar benefits occurred after concomitant BK-GSV foam sclerotherapy.

▶ It is basic dogma in the venous world that ablation or stripping of the greater saphenous vein should be confined to the above-knee segment of the vein. This stems from the fact that the saphenous nerve runs deep in the thigh and only accompanies the saphenous vein below the knee. By avoiding treatment of the greater saphenous vein distally, postoperative saphenous neuralgia is hopefully avoided. However, there are many patients with saphenous reflux both above and below the knee in the saphenous vein. Some authors have observed an increased need for retreatment in patients with below-knee saphenous reflux when only the above-knee saphenous vein has been treated. This is a relatively small study, but it does indicate, at least in this center's patients, that both above- and below-knee saphenous reflux treatment of the below-knee segment of the vein with either foam-square therapy or laser ablation results in better control of varicosities without saphenous nerve injury. Based on this study, it would seem reasonable to consider beginning the point of ablation of the greater saphenous vein with laser or radiofrequency ablation from the lowest observed site of reflux. Data here obviously do not apply to standard stripping of the saphenous vein and most, although clearly not all, surgeons would still advocate limiting stripping of the greater saphenous vein to the above-knee portion of the vein.

G. L. Moneta, MD

A Prospective Study of Incidence of Saphenous Nerve Injury after Total Great Saphenous Vein Stripping
Flu HC, Breslau PJ, Hamming JF, et al (HagaHospital, The Hague, The Netherlands; Leiden Univ Med Ctr, The Netherlands)
Dermatol Surg 34:1333-1339, 2008

Background and Objectives.—Total stripping of the great saphenous vein (GSV) is a validated surgical strategy of treating patients with primary varicose veins (PVV). An often cited, but not well documented and studied, complication of total stripping is postoperative damage of the saphenous nerve (SN).

Objective.—The objective was to evaluate the incidence of SN damage and to assess the therapeutic efficacy after total stripping of the GSV.

Materials and Methods.—Patients undergoing total stripping of the GSV because of PVV in the entire lower limb were enrolled. Pre- and postoperative neurologic examination was performed to identify potential sensory neurologic deficits.

Results.—Total stripping of the GSV in 69 limbs occurred because of pain (9%) or a tired feeling in the limbs (77%) or for cosmetic reasons (14%). The overall incidence of postoperative sensory neurologic deficits was 7 and 6%, respectively, after 6-week follow-up and both 3% after 3-month follow-up. In 99% of the patients, total stripping of the GSV resulted in reduction of the primary signs and symptoms.

Conclusion.—The incidence of SN damage after total stripping of the GSV is low. Thus, total stripping of the GSV resulted in improvement of the primary complaint in almost all patients. Total stripping of the GSV is an effective surgical strategy in treating PVV.

▶ In the era of endovenous ablation, partial stripping of the great saphenous vein (GSV) is still an option for treatment of some patients with primary varicose veins. Even with GSV reflux above and below the knee, clinicians generally perform a partial stripping of the GSV, leaving the below-knee segment in situ because of fear of saphenous nerve (SN) injury. There are, however, very little data on the incidence of SN injury after total GSV. The study suggests it is reasonable to treat the GSV below the knee when total saphenous reflux is present. These surgical results parallel a similar study using endovenous techniques to treat total GSV reflux. It appears that when there is GSV reflux both above and below the knee, a complete treatment of the vein, whether by endovascular or open surgical techniques, results in a very low incidence of SN injury. There should be a randomized trial to evaluate symptom reduction and SN injury in patients with total GSV reflux treated with total versus above-knee-only saphenous stripping or endovenous ablation.

G. L. Moneta, MD

The appropriate length of great saphenous vein stripping should be based on the extent of reflux and not on the intent to avoid saphenous nerve injury
Kostas TT, Ioannou CV, Veligrantakis M, et al (Univ Hosp of Heraklion, Greece; et al)
J Vasc Surg 46:1234-1241, 2007

Objective.—To investigate the effect of stripping the below knee great saphenous vein (GSV) segment on varicose vein recurrence as well as any disability induced after saphenous nerve injury (SNI) during a 5-year period.

Methods.—One hundred and six limbs (86 patients, 64 female, mean age 46 years), that underwent GSV stripping, to the knee or ankle level, were prospectively followed up at 1 month and 5 years postoperatively with clinical examination and color duplex imaging (CDI), in order to evaluate SNI and the development of recurrence. The extent of GSV stripping complied with preoperative CDI in 84 limbs (79%) that were subjected to GSV stripping to the ankle and full abolishment of duplex-confirmed reflux. Furthermore, 19 limbs (18%) underwent stripping restricted to the below knee level since the distal GSV was competent. On the contrary, in three limbs (3%), the extent of stripping did not comply with preoperative CDI due to the absence of varicosities in the tibia, and stripping was restricted to the knee level, although they had reflux along the whole GSV length.

Results.—Overall recurrence was found in 24 out of 106 operated limbs (23%) after 5 years. Recurrence was found to be 20% (17/84) in the limbs with total GSV stripping and 32% (7/22) in the limbs with restricted GSV stripping ($P > .05$). However, the recurrence rate in the tibial area was significantly lower in limbs subjected to GSV stripping, which was in compliance with the preoperative CDI (9/103, 9%) compared with those that had undergone GSV stripping that was not in agreement with the preoperative CDI (3/3, 100%; $P < .005$). Neurological examination at 1 month postoperatively, revealed SNI in 17 limbs (16%). However, at the 5-year neurological reassessment, we found that seven out of these limbs (40%) were alleviated from SNI adverse symptoms presenting only deficits in sensation. In addition, no significance was found concerning SNI between limbs subjected to total and restricted GSV stripping (16/84 vs 1/22; $P > .05$).

Conclusions.—Though SNI may occur after both restricted and total GSV stripping, this does not influence limb disability since any related symptoms seem to regress in almost half of the limbs 5 years postoperatively. Additionally, it seems that recurrence could be reduced in the tibial area if the level of GSV stripping complies with the extent of the ultrasonographically proven GSV reflux. Therefore, the extent of GSV stripping should not be guided by the intent of avoiding SNI.

▶ The authors performed a reasonable study with good long-term follow-up. In this article, the authors report that although saphenous nerve injury may occur after both restricted and total great saphenous vein (GSV) stripping, it did not influence limb disability postoperatively because symptoms regressed in almost half of the limbs 5 years postoperatively. In contrast to previous reports, they found that the extent of GSV stripping did not seem to reduce the incidence of saphenous nerve injury. They showed that the extent of GSV reflux had no impact on the overall likelihood of developing recurrence due to unavoidable causes of recurrence such as neovascularization and chronic venous disease progression. Lastly, the authors suggest that recurrence, following GSV varicose veins surgery, could be reduced if the level of GSV stripping was based on preoperative duplex-confirmed venous reflux mapping.

D. L. Gillespie, MD

A prospective evaluation of the outcome after small saphenous varicose vein surgery with one-year follow-up

O'Hare JL, Vandenbroeck CP, Whitman B, et al (Gloucestershire Royal Hosp, Gloucester, UK; et al)

J Vasc Surg 48:669-674, 2008

Objective.—The aim was to examine the effect of various surgical maneuvers during standard surgery for small saphenous varicose veins (SSV).

Methods.—This was a prospective cohort study of patients that underwent small saphenous varicose vein surgery. Two-hundred nineteen consecutive patients (234 legs) with isolated primary or recurrent small saphenous varicose veins undergoing surgery were enrolled in a multicenter study involving nine vascular centers in the United Kingdom. Operative technique was determined by individual surgeon preference; clinical and operative details, including the use of stripping, were recorded. Clinical examination (recurrence rates) and duplex imaging (superficial and deep incompetence) were evaluated at six weeks and one year after surgery.

Results.—A total of 204 legs were reviewed at one year; 67 had small saphenous varicose vein stripping, 116 had saphenopopliteal junction (SPJ) disconnection only, and the remainder had miscellaneous procedures. The incidence of visible recurrent varicosities at one year was lower after SSV stripping (12 of 67, 18%) than after disconnection only (28 of 116, 24%), although this did not reach statistical significance. There was no significant difference in the rate of numbness at one year between those who had SSV stripping (20 of 71, 28%) and those who had disconnection only (38 of 134, 28%). The rate of SPJ incompetence detected by duplex at one year was significantly lower in patients who underwent SSV stripping (9 of 67, 13%) than in those who did not (37 of 115, 32%) ($P < .01$).

Conclusion.—Stripping of the SSV significantly reduced the rate of SPJ incompetence after one year without increasing the rate of complications.

▶ The potential for damage to the sural nerve has discouraged most surgeons from stripping the small saphenous vein in patients being treated for lateral venous ulcer or varicosities in the small saphenous distribution. The preferred procedure has been ligation and disconnection of the saphenopopliteal junction (SPJ) rather than small saphenous stripping. However, in this study, patients undergoing stripping of the small saphenous vein had a reduced instance of recurrent varicositites and a reduced rate of SPJ incompetence when compared with those who underwent merely high ligation or disconnection of the SPJ. There was no difference in the rate of numbness in the sural nerve distribution at 1 year in those with stripping versus those who had disconnection only. However, what is surprising is the high rate of numbness seen in both the stripping and disconnection patients. This study was performed before endovenous methods for treating the short saphenous vein were in widespread use. One would hope, and results of case series suggest, endoluminal techniques provide better overall results than small saphenous stripping. It may be that the primary message from this article is to avoid any type of surgery in the popliteal fossa for venous disease whether it be for disconnection of the short saphenous vein or stripping of the short saphenous vein.

G. L. Moneta, MD

Iliac vein compression syndrome: Outcome of endovascular treatment with long-term follow-up

Oguzkurt L, Tercan F, Ozkan U, et al (Baskent Univ Faculty of Medicine, Ankara, Turkey)
Eur J Radiol 68:487-492, 2008

Objective.—To retrospectively evaluate technical success and long-term outcome of endovascular treatment in patients with iliofemoral deep vein thrombosis (DVT) due to iliac vein compression syndrome (IVCS).

Materials and Methods.—Between March 2003 and September 2006, 36 consecutive patients (26 women [72%], 10 men, mean age 50 ± 18 years) with acute or chronic iliofemoral deep vein thrombosis due to iliac vein compression syndrome were evaluated for outcome of endovascular treatment. Stent patency was estimated by using the Kaplan–Meier method.

Results.—Technical success was achieved in 34 of 36 patients (94%). Six patients with acute or subacute thrombosis had chronic occlusion of the left common iliac vein. Rethrombosis of the stents was observed in four patients. Primary and secondary patency rates were 85 and 94% at 1 year, and 80 and 82% at 4 years. Resolution of symptoms was achieved in 17 of 20 patients (85%) with acute and subacute DVT, and 4 of 16 patients (25%) with chronic DVT. Major complication was seen in one patient (3%).

Conclusion.—Intimal changes in the left common iliac vein are mostly chronic in nature even in patients with acute DVT secondary to IVCS. Endovascular treatment with stent placement has a high technical success rate and good long-term patency in the treatment of acute and chronic DVT due to IVCS. Symptomatic improvement seems to be better in patients with acute than chronic DVT due to IVCS.

▶ Iliac vein compression syndrome (IVCS) (so-called May-Thurner syndrome) can cause both lower extremity deep vein thrombosis (DVT) and venous hypertension without thrombosis. Prevalence of the condition is unknown, but it does seem common among patients with symptomatic left lower extremity DVT. In this study, the authors report their venographic findings and outcome of endovascular treatment with catheter-directed thrombolysis, manual aspiration thrombectomy, and stent placement in patients with iliofemoral DVT secondary to IVCS. This is a relatively small series compared with what is coming from some centers in the United States. Nevertheless, it does point out that catheter-based techniques can be useful in relieving symptoms of acute iliofemoral DVT. This is becoming more and more accepted. Efficacy in preventing long-term problems associated with postphlebitic syndrome following iliofemoral DVT and relief of chronic symptoms in patients with long-standing iliac vein obstruction is much less clear. Complications of treatment are infrequent and relatively minor.

G. L. Moneta, MD

Ovarian vein incompetence: a potential cause of chronic pelvic pain in women

Tropeano G, Di Stasi C, Amoroso S, et al (Università Cattolica del Sacro Cuore, Roma, Italy)

Eur J Obstet Gynecol Reprod Biol 139:215-221, 2008

Objective.—To evaluate whether ovarian vein incomplete may be a source of chronic pelvic pain (CPP) in women.

Study Design.—Twenty-two women, aged 19–50 years, with chronic pelvic pain, no laparoscopically detected pelvic pathology, and evidence of reflux in dilated pelvic veins on transvaginal color Doppler ultrasound underwent retrograde ovarian venography and sclerotherapy of the ovarian vein(s) if incompetent. The primary outcome was symptom change as assessed by a symptom questionnaire and visual analog pain scales (VAS) at 3, 6, and 12 months of follow-up. Changes in pelvic circulations after sclerotherapy procedure were also evaluated by serial ultrasound examinations. Differences between baseline and post-procedural VAS scores were analysed using the Wilcoxon signed-rank test.

Results.—Twenty (91%) of the 22 women had venographic evidence of incompetent ovarian vein(s) and received sclerotherapy. There were no immediate or late complications. Variable symptom relief was observed in 17 (85%) of the 20 treated women, with follow-up at 12 months showing marked-to-complete relief in 15 patients and mild-to-moderate relief in the remaining 2 patients. Three (15%) women had no improvement in symptoms. Median VAS scores at 3 (2.0), 6 (2.5), and 12 months (3.0) were significantly lower than at baseline (8.0) $(P < .001)$. Follow-up ultrasound examinations showed absence of pelvic venous reflux in all but 3 patients, in whom recurrence of reflux was seen at 3 months.

Conclusion(s).—Ovarian vein sclerotherapy provided symptomatic relief and improved pelvic circulation in most patients. These findings suggest that ovarian vein incompetence was the likely source of chronic pain in these women, and that sclerotherapy was a safe and effective treatment for this condition.

Condensation.—Ovarian vein incompetence leading to pelvic circulatory changes may be a cause of chronic pelvic pain in women.

▶ As in many things in medicine, when it comes to ovarian vein incompetence as a cause of chronic pelvic pain, you are either a believer or a nonbeliever. The authors' conclusion that "ovarian vein incompetence leading to pelvic circulatory changes may be a cause of chronic pelvic pain in women" is a safe conclusion given their data. Unfortunately, there are no really good data on this subject anywhere. The interesting point in this article is the association of the detection of pelvic varicosities with laparoscopy. All the women in this study underwent laparoscopy. Less than half had pelvic varicosities detected by their laparoscopy. This indicates the absence of pelvic varicosities at the time of laparoscopy does not rule out the diagnosis. The data suggest that if you believe in pelvic congestion syndrome, patients who have had a thorough history, clinical evaluation, and negative standard diagnostic tests, then ovarian venography should be considered if one is going to treat potentially underlying ovarian vein reflux.

G. L. Moneta, MD

18 Technical Notes

EVAR of Aortoiliac Aneurysms with Branched Stent-grafts
Dias NV, Resch TA, Sonesson B, et al (Malmö Univ Hosp, Sweden)
Eur J Vasc Endovasc Surg 35:677-684, 2008

Introduction.—Branched iliac stent-grafts (bSG) have recently been developed in order to preserve internal iliac artery (IIA) flow in patients with aneurysmal or short common iliac arteries. The aim of this study is to evaluate a single-center experience with bSG for the IIA.

Methods.—Twenty-two male patients (70 (IQR 65–79) years old) underwent EVAR with 23 bSG (1 bilateral repair) between September 2002 and August 2007. Median AAA diameter was 52 (37–60) mm while common iliac diameter on the side of the bSG was 34 (27–41) mm. Two in-house modified Zenith SG and subsequently 21 commercially available bSG (18 Zenith Iliac Side and 3 Helical Branches) were used. Follow-up (FU) included CT at one month and yearly thereafter. Data was prospectively entered in a database.

Results.—Primary technical success was 91% (21 bSG). Median FU duration was 20 (8–31) months. One patient (5 %) died after discharge from acute myocardial infarction on day 13. Another patient died 30 months after EVAR of an unrelated cause. The overall bSG patency was 74% due to 6 branch occlusions (2 intraoperative and 4 late). All patients with patent bSG were asymptomatic. Three occlusions were asymptomatic findings on CT, while the other three developed claudication (two patients with contralateral IIA occlusion and one with simultaneous occlusion of the external iliac). One patient (5%) developed an asymptomatic type III endoleak at 1 month and was successfully treated with a bridging SG. Overall, four patients (18%) required reinterventions (1 bilateral stenting of the external iliac arteries, 1 external and 1 internal SG extensions and 1 femoro-femoral cross-over bypass). Nine out of 16 patients (56%) with CT-FU ≥ 1 year had shrinking aneurysms. There were no postoperative aneurysm expansions.

Conclusions.—EVAR of aortoiliac aneurysms with IIA bSG is a good alternative to occlusion of the IIA in patients with challenging distal anatomy.

▶ This important article describes a small, early European experience with commercially available branched stent grafts for the treatment of short or aneurismal common iliac arteries to preserve blood flow into internal iliac arteries during endovascular aneurysm repair. The authors report an immediate technical success rate of 91% with a 74% patency rate during a mean follow-up of 20 months. Six internal iliac vessels occluded—2 intraoperatively and 4 postoperatively—with 50% of these patients having symptoms of buttock or leg claudication.

The authors point out that these procedures are quite demanding with a mean operative time of 279 minutes and a fluoroscopy time ranging from 67 to 108 minutes. What is unfortunately not well described is the quality of the revascularized internal iliac artery. One might assume that as endovascular branched-vessel technology and operator experience advances, target vessel occlusions will decrease in incidence. These techniques represent exciting new technologies for the management of more complex aortoiliac aneurismal disease.

B. W. Starnes, MD

Successful devascularization of carotid body tumors by covered stent placement in the external carotid artery
Scanlon JM, Lustgarten JJ, Karr SB, et al (Georgetown Univ and Washington Hosp Ctr; Kaiser Permanente (Mid-Atlantic))
J Vasc Surg 48:1322-1324, 2008

Management of highly vascular carotid body tumors can involve preoperative percutaneous embolization before definitive surgical resection.

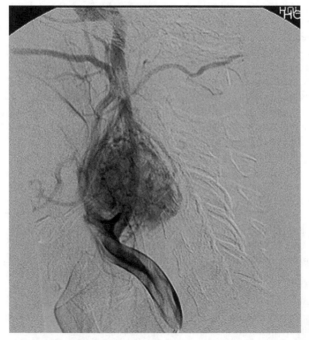

FIGURE 1.—Pre-stenting angiogram demonstrating a carotid body tumor in a 40-year-old man. (Reprinted from Scanlon JM, Lustgarten JJ, Karr SB, et al. Successful devascularization of carotid body tumors by covered stent placement in the external carotid artery. *J Vasc Surg.* 2008;48:1322-1324, with permission from The Society for Vascular Surgery.)

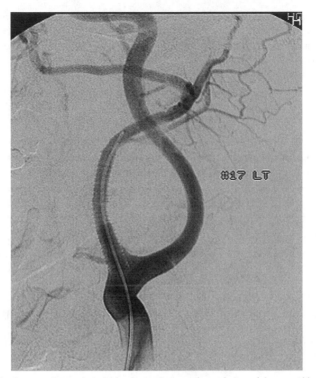

FIGURE 2.—Post-stenting angiogram demonstrating vascular exclusion of the carotid body tumor. At surgery the tumor was found to be enveloping the external carotid artery. (Reprinted from Scanlon JM, Lustgarten JJ, Karr SB, et al. Successful devascularization of carotid body tumors by covered stent placement in the external carotid artery. *J Vasc Surg.* 2008;48:1322-1324, with permission from The Society for Vascular Surgery.)

This step reduces tumor size, reduces operative blood loss, and makes for a less hazardous dissection with the goal of reducing morbidity and mortality. The effectiveness of a recently described technique of interrupting vascular supply via covered stent placement in the external carotid artery is further described in a series of three recent cases. This technique may be useful for large tumors with a primary blood supply from the external carotid since it avoids the intracranial embolic risk of coils used for this purpose (Figs 1 and 2).

▶ In my opinion, routine attempts of devascularization of carotid body tumors before their resection are not warranted. Small tumors can be resected without the added risk and inconvenience of devascularization before surgical treatment. However, when a larger tumor is encountered or when the tumor is suspected to circumferentially involve the external carotid artery (Shamblin 3), devascularization before resection is prudent. The authors' technique of using a covered stent in the external carotid artery to devascularize the tumor may be less challenging and time consuming than the painstaking process of embolization. In addition, obviously, the use of the authors' technique rather than embolization eliminates the risk of unwanted distal embolization of particulate matter. I am not sure this technique will be widely adopted by those who routinely perform carotid body surgery, but it does seem to be a reasonable technique to be aware of for the occasional carotid body tumor that truly requires devascularization before operation (Figs 1 and 2).

G. L. Moneta, MD

Repair of complex renal artery aneurysms by laparoscopic nephrectomy with ex vivo repair and autotransplantation

Gallagher KA, Phelan MW, Stern T, et al (Univ of Maryland Med Ctr, Baltimore)
J Vasc Surg 48:1408-1413, 2008

Objective.—Renal artery aneurysms are being discovered more frequently due to increased use of non-invasive imaging. Complex renal artery aneurysms involving multiple secondary or tertiary branches are not amenable to in vivo or endovascular treatment and often require ex vivo repair with autotransplantation. In order to minimize incisional morbidity and hasten recovery, we developed a technique of laparoscopic nephrectomy combined with backbench ex vivo repair, followed by autotransplantation through a small laparoscopic extraction incision. This

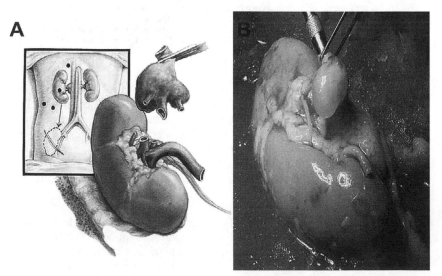

FIGURE 2.—**A,** Schematic drawing illustrating resection of the renal artery aneurysm. Inset in left upper corner demonstrates standard laparoscopic port placement and Gibson extraction incision for laparoscopic nephrectomy. **B,** Aneurysm resection following laparoscopic nephrectomy. (Reprinted from Gallagher KA, Phelan MW, Stern T, et al. Repair of complex renal artery aneurysms by laparoscopic nephrectomy with ex vivo repair and autotransplantation. *J Vasc Surg.* 2008;48:1408-1413, with permission from The Society for Vascular Surgery.)

study describes our initial experience with this combined technique in patients that were not candidates for endovascular techniques or in vivo arterial reconstruction.

Methods.—Seven patients with complex renal artery aneurysms underwent laparoscopic nephrectomy and ex vivo repair with multiple saphenous vein grafts and autotransplantation through the small laparoscopic extraction incision. The aneurysms ranged from 2.5 to 5.0 cm. In all cases, the aneurysm was resected ex vivo, leaving multiple branch arteries that were extended with saphenous vein grafts. Arterial inflow was then re-established with sequential saphenous vein anastomoses to the external iliac artery. Ureteral reconstruction was performed via standard Lich ureteroneocystostomy. Patients were followed postoperatively for two to eight years.

Results.—Laparoscopic nephrectomy with ex vivo repair of complex aneurysms was successfully employed in seven patients with renal aneurysms that were not amenable to endovascular or in vivo repair. There were no incisional morbidities and all patients had significant improvements in symptoms post-operatively. Renal function remained unchanged and there were no ureteral complications following surgery. All patients had postoperative ultrasound imaging done at two years which demonstrated patency of the anastomoses. The mean hospital stay was four days (range, two to seven days).

Conclusion.—Repair of complex renal artery aneurysms involving distal branch arteries remains a challenge. This new technique combines the

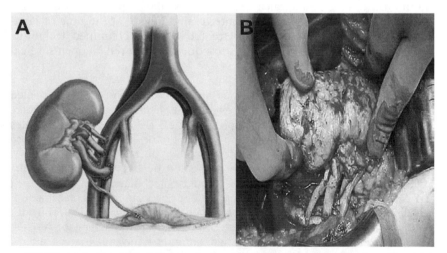

FIGURE 4.—A, Illustration depicting reimplantation of the kidney following successful arterial, venous and ureteral anastomoses. B, Successful ileo-renal bypass following nephrectomy and aneurysmectomy. (Reprinted from Gallagher KA, Phelan MW, Stern T, et al. Repair of complex renal artery aneurysms by laparoscopic nephrectomy with ex vivo repair and autotransplantation. *J Vasc Surg.* 2008;48:1408-1413, with permission from The Society for Vascular Surgery.)

advantages of minimally invasive surgery with the effectiveness of ex vivo aneurysm repair (Figs 2 and 4).

▶ The authors have taken 2 relatively standard techniques and combined them into a new approach to repair complex renal artery aneurysms. Certainly ex vivo repair of complex renal artery aneurysms is not new. Laparoscopic nephrectomy is also routinely used in cases of living-related renal transplantation. The principal advantage of the technique is basically the avoidance of an upper abdominal incision with hopefully decreased perioperative morbidity and chronic postoperative pain from the upper abdominal incision. The article is beautifully illustrated (Figs 2 and 4) and should be of interest to vascular surgeons who practice in an institution with individuals skilled at laparoscopic nephrectomy.

G. L. Moneta, MD

Intraoperative Retrograde Mesenteric Angioplasty for Acute Occlusive Mesenteric Ischaemia: A Case Series
Moyes LH, McCarter DHA, Vass DG, et al (Glasgow Royal Infirmary, UK)
Eur J Vasc Endovasc Surg 36:203-206, 2008

Acute mesenteric ischaemia secondary to atherosclerotic disease of the superior mesenteric artery is a surgical emergency associated with a poor prognosis, and requires prompt diagnosis and early revascularisation in order to improve outcome. The traditional management of surgical resection of necrotic bowel plus mesenteric revascularisation by surgical bypass is associated with significant morbidity and mortality. We describe the use of a combined surgical and endovascular approach, using intraoperative retrograde superior mesenteric angioplasty at the time of laparotomy. Four patients have been treated by this combined technique with three surviving, although one subsequently required an open surgical revascularisation procedure.

▶ The individual with acute mesenteric ischemia (AMI) who cannot be treated with thrombectomy and will otherwise require a prosthetic graft is a candidate for this procedure (Fig 1 in the original article). Other possible candidates include patients unstable at the time of exploratory laparotomy and those requiring a supraceliac aortic clamp for construction of the proximal anastomosis. Surgeons unfamiliar with the retrograde bypass technique from the iliac artery but who are familiar with angioplasty techniques would also want to consider this procedure. The authors do not advocate routine placement of stents following dilatation of the superior mesenteric artery (SMA). This may be because of concern of potential stent infection in the setting of AMI. In this technique, the SMA is approached retrograde through a small arterial branch dissected from the mesentery. A 0.35 glide wire is passed into the SMA and through the stenosis or occlusion at the SMA origin. The branch through which the glide wire was placed is dilated to accommodate a 6-French sheath. Angioplasty is performed with a 7-mm balloon. Following dilatation the access vessel is ligated. Second-look laparotomies were performed as needed. Three out of the 4 patients who underwent this procedure survived, although one did require a definitive surgical bypass later on during the same hospital admission. Intraoperative retrograde SMA angioplasty can be a useful technique in the management of selected patients with AMI. In my opinion, however, in a patient with an appropriate vein and who is hemodynamically stable, a vein bypass procedure is still preferable.

G. L. Moneta, MD

Midterm Patency following Atherectomy for Infrainguinal Occlusive Disease: A Word of Caution

Chung SW, Sharafuddin MJ, Chigurupati R, et al (Univ of Iowa Roy and Lucille Carver College of Medicine)
Ann Vasc Surg 22:358-365, 2008

There has been widespread initial enthusiasm for peripheral atherectomy using the SilverHawk device. We sought to evaluate our midterm patency following infrainguinal atherectomy. Nineteen consecutive patients underwent 23 separate atherectomy procedures on 20 limbs from March 2005 through June 2006 (11 males, age 66 ± 14 years). The primary lesions were atherosclerotic (n = 18) and vein graft stenoses (n = 2). Three additional procedures were redo atherectomies for restenotic lesions. The TASC classification of the primary lesions was A in 3, B in 9, and C in 8. The median number of treated lesions per limb was 2 (range 1-4). The location of the most distal native vessel stenosis was the superficial femoral artery in 12, popliteal artery in six, and crural artery in two. Atherectomy was successful in 18 primary procedures and all three repeat atherectomy procedures. Touch-up balloon dilatation was used in five procedures. Complications included one groin hematoma and two perforations, treated with stenting in one and bypass grafting in one. Preoperative ankle-brachial index and transmetatarsal pulse volume recording were 0.51 ± 0.16 and 3.3 ± 0.8, respectively, which at 1-month improved to 0.80 ± 0.16 and 2.4 ± 0.4 ($p < 0.001$). Only two vessels remained patent at 12 months. Recurrence developed in 16 of the successful primary procedures, including both vein graft lesions and all three repeat atherectomy procedures. The mode of recurrence was restenosis in 14 and occlusion/thrombosis in five. Secondary interventions included balloon angioplasty/thrombolysis in two, stenting in three, redo atherectomy in three, vein bypass grafting in five, and observation alone in one. Major limb amputation was required in five patients. Primary patency rates per treated limb at 3, 6, and 12 months were 38%, 10%, and 10%. The corresponding assisted patency rates were 50%, 23%, and 10%. Our experience suggests a very poor midterm patency of excisonal atherectomy using the SilverHawk device, although a 74% limb salvage rate was maintained through secondary interventions. Liberal use of this technology is associated with high cost and frequent requirement of reintervention.

▶ This is a study that documents 1-year poor patency rate of excisional atherectomy using the SilverHawk atherectomy device. A cynic might say that the evaluation of endoluminal devices for treatment of infrainguinal occlusive disease takes a frighteningly similar pattern independent of device. Initially there is great enthusiasm for a new device. Pundits espouse the virtue of the device. Physicians become consultants. Testimonials appear on the Internet and articles touting the virtues of the device appear in throwaway journals often accompanied by pictures of the authors. As time goes by, articles begin to appear in more reputable journals and enthusiasm for the device wanes. The negative results are reported and industry representatives criticize those reporting the results, citing inexperience of the operator or perhaps inappropriate use of the technology. In this article, the primary surgeon had previously performed 6 cases at another hospital. Most of the cases were done in conjunction with industry representatives and both representative and the surgeon were satisfied with the immediate technical results of the atherectomy. Therefore, regardless of whether one is enthusiastic or not enthusiastic about peripheral atherectomy, the poor results reported here may very well be what an individual surgeon can expect in similar types of patients with similar lesions. The authors' recommendation that this "time-consuming modality should be used more judiciously" seems reasonable.

G. L. Moneta, MD

Iliofemoral Pulsion Endarterectomy
Wall ML, Davies RSM, Sykes TCF, et al (Univ Hosp Birmingham, UK)
Ann Vasc Surg 23:259-263, 2009

We present our experience with a technique of endarterectomy for use in patients with iliofemoral occlusive disease, in which the atheromatous plug is extruded from the intact artery by external manipulation (pulsion). A retrospective review of consecutive patients who underwent surgical iliofemoral pulsion endarterectomy (IFPE) in two vascular surgery units between 1998 and 2006 was performed. Primary and secondary graft patency, limb salvage, and patient survival rates were determined using Kaplan-Meier methods. Fifty-eight IFPEs were carried out successfully on 54 patients (36 men, 18 women, median age 66 years) presenting with critical limb ischemia ($n = 23$), with claudication ($n = 29$), or in conjunction with abdominal aortic aneurysm repair ($n = 6$). Mean (range) follow-up was 17 months (1-69). During this period six patients (all male, mean age 64 years) underwent iliofemoral bypass using a prosthetic graft when the iliac arteries were found unsuitable for endarterectomy because of hypoplasia or heavy calcification. Two-year cumulative primary patency of IFPE was 95%, secondary patency 100%, limb salvage

98.5%, and patient survival 73%. This modification of iliac endarterectomy is a relatively simple and safe technique that eschews prosthetics and offers a durable solution for the majority of patients with extensive iliofemoral occlusive disease (Figs 1 and 2).

▶ There are a number of techniques available for the performance of endarterectomy of the iliac vessels. Through a retroperitoneal incision the artery can be opened directly and open endarterectomy performed and the artery then either closed primarily or with a synthetic or autogenous patch. Alternatively, and

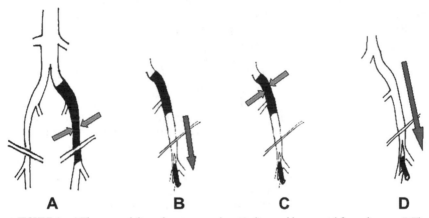

FIGURE 1.—**A** The external iliac atheromatous plaque is disrupted by external finger fracture. **B** The cylinder of atheroma is squeezed distally through the previously endarterectomized femoral artery. **C** The process is repeated proximally up to the pulsating common iliac core. **D** Fragmentation of the common iliac core is often required to squeeze the atheroma downward. (Reprinted from Wall ML, Davies RSM, Sykes TCF, et al. Iliofemoral pulsion endarterectomy. *Ann Vasc Surg.* 2009;23:259-263.)

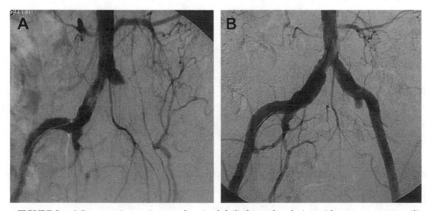

FIGURE 2.—**A** Preoperative angiogram showing left iliofemoral occlusion with a patent common iliac stump. **B** Angiogram performed 6 months after a left IFPE showing a widely patent iliac artery. (Reprinted from Wall ML, Davies RSM, Sykes TCF, et al. Iliofemoral pulsion endarterectomy. *Ann Vasc Surg.* 2009;23:259-263.)

more commonly used, is a technique of eversion endarterectomy in which the iliac artery is divided just above the circumflex iliac vessels, and the plaque everted through an eversion technique of the vessel. The authors describe in this case another method of endarterectomy of the iliofemoral system. In the authors' technique of pulsion endarterectomy, the femoral artery is opened in the groin through a longitudinal arteriotomy. Common femoral and distal external artery endarterectomy is performed in the standard fashion. When inflow is inadequate, the ipsilateral iliac bifurcation is then approached retroperitoneally through an oblique iliac incision. Plaque in the external iliac artery is then palpated and disrupted by external finger fracture techniques. The authors note that a strong pinching action is required and proximal clamping is avoided but intermittent distal clamping is necessary for hemostasis. The technique results in a detached cylinder of atheroma that is squeezed distally and delivered through the previously endarterectomized femoral artery. Once the external iliac artery has been treated in this way, the maneuver is repeated proximally up the pulsating common iliac artery to the aortic level. The authors note that the large plaque of the common iliac artery may be difficult to extrude through the smaller external iliac artery. They suggest extensive fragmentation of the plaque by external digital compression so that it can be extruded distally, avoiding arteriotomy of the proximal external iliac/distal common iliac arteries. If the common iliac plaque cannot be extruded through the distal external iliac artery, a small common iliac arteriotomy can be made to facilitate extraction of the common iliac plaque. Care must be taken around the aortic bifurcation to avoid dislodgement of the atheromatous material down the contralateral limb (Figs 1 and 2).

The technique should be of interest to vascular surgeons wishing to avoid long lengths in the iliac vessels and to those who perform iliac endarterectomy infrequently. It avoids the use of a prosthetic material, whether it be a patch or a stent, and sacrifice of the circumflex iliac vessels that occurs with an eversion technique. Some judgment will be required in avoiding the technique in severely calcified iliac arteries, as these appear to be the ones that are most prone to producing arterial rupture.

G. L. Moneta, MD

Superficial femoral artery autograft reconstruction in the treatment of popliteal artery aneurysm: Long-term outcome

Paraskevas N, Castier Y, Fukui S, et al (Hôpital Saint-Joseph, Paris, France; Hôpital Bichat and Assistance Publique, Hôpitaux, Paris, France)
J Vasc Surg 48:311-316, 2008

Objective.—This prospective, observational study evaluated the safety and efficacy of superficial femoral artery autograft reconstruction in the treatment of popliteal artery aneurysms in the absence of a suitable saphenous vein.

Methods.—From March 1997 to April 2007, data from patients with popliteal artery aneurysms treated by superficial femoral artery reconstruction were prospectively collected in two centers. The procedure was performed through a medial approach. The superficial femoral artery was harvested in the upper third of the thigh and used as the conduit for reconstruction, and the harvested segment was replaced by a polytetrafluoroethylene graft. The patients were observed for survival, limb salvage, and reconstruction patency. The results were calculated by the Kaplan-Meier method.

Results.—During the 10-year study period, 37 popliteal artery aneurysms in 32 patients (all men; median age, 71 years) were treated by reconstruction using the superficial femoral artery. Indications for surgical treatment were symptomatic or complicated aneurysms in 11 (30%). Four (11%) of the 37 popliteal artery aneurysms were thrombosed, and 33 (89%) were patent. At surgery, 35% had a single vessel runoff. Because of acute ischemia, reconstruction was performed as an emergency procedure in three patients (8%). There were no perioperative deaths, early amputations, or early thrombosis. The mean follow-up period was 36 months (range, 7-103 months). Two grafts thrombosed during follow-up. At 3 years, the primary and secondary patency rates were 86% and 96%, and overall limb salvage was 100%. Follow-up duplex ultrasonography did not detect any aneurysmal dilatation of the autograft.

Conclusion.—Our experience shows that superficial femoral arterial reconstruction is a safe and useful treatment option in patients with popliteal artery aneurysms who lack suitable saphenous veins. This reconstruction seems to be a good alternative to prosthetic bypass crossing the knee joint, and our results suggest that this study should be continued.

▶ At first glance this seems like a silly operation. An operation that otherwise would consist of 2 anastomoses is turned into an operation that consists of more extensive dissection and 4 anastomoses. Nevertheless, the idea of placing a piece of autogenous artery across the knee joint makes some sense when there is no good autogenous vein available and the alternative is prosthetic. Patients with aneurysmal disease have less trouble with occlusions of prosthetic grafts compared with those with occlusive disease and, therefore, replacing the proximal superficial femoral artery with polytetrafluroethylene (PTFE) may indeed be associated with a relatively low rate of graft-related complications. Indeed, the authors were able to achieve a 3-year primary patency rate of 86% and a 3-year secondary patency rate of 96%. Although I would not recommend this technique for patients with adequate saphenous vein, it is reasonable to consider in patients with popliteal aneurysm who otherwise would require reconstruction using a deep vein or a prosthetic graft placed either through a standard open operation or an endoluminal procedure.

G. L. Moneta, MD

Through-knee amputation in patients with peripheral arterial disease: A review of 50 cases

Morse BC, Cull DL, Kalbaugh C, et al (Greenville Hosp System Univ Med Ctr, SC)

J Vasc Surg 48:638-643, 2008

Background.—For good rehabilitation candidates, the biomechanical advantages of the end weight-bearing through-knee amputation (TKAmp) compared with the above knee amputation (AKA) are well established. However, the TKAmp has been abandoned by vascular surgeons because of poor wound healing rates related to long tissue flaps and challenges to prosthetic fitting related to the femoral condyles. Since 1998, we have performed the modified "Mazet" technique TKAmp procedure that creates shorter flaps to close the wound and greatly facilitates prosthesis fitting. The purpose of this study is to review our results with TKAmp in patients with peripheral vascular disease who were not candidates for below-knee amputation.

Methods.—The records of all patients who underwent through-knee amputation between 1998 and 2006 were retrospectively reviewed. Mean follow-up was 33 months (range, 38 days to 99 months). Amputations for trauma and malignancy were excluded. Patient survival, maintenance of ambulation, and independent living status were analyzed using Kaplan-Meier survival analysis methods.

Results.—Fifty patients underwent TKAmp using a modified Mazet technique. The mean age was 63 years; 50% were men, and 50% had diabetes mellitus. All patients had peripheral arterial disease. Thirty-five patients (70%) had prior revascularization procedures. Those patients averaged 2.2 revascularization procedures prior to amputation. There were three (6%) perioperative deaths. The ipsilateral common femoral artery was patent in 43/50 (86%) of patients at the time of amputation. Forty patients (80%) had open wounds and three patients (6%) had a failed below-knee amputation at the time of TKAmp. Thirty-eight patients (81%) healed their TKAmp wound. Nine patients failed to heal and were revised to an above knee amputation. The cumulative probability of regular prosthetic usage and maintenance of ambulation was estimated to be 0.56 at 3 years and 0.41 at 5 years. The probability of maintaining independent living status at 3 and 5 years was 0.77 and 0.65, respectively. Survival probabilities for patients in this series were 0.60 at 3 years and 0.44 at 5 years.

Conclusion.—These data show that the TKAmp is associated with an acceptable primary healing rate and satisfactory functional outcomes in patients with peripheral arterial disease. The advantages of TKAmp over AKA make it the preferred alternative for patients with vascular disease who are candidates for prosthetic rehabilitation (Fig 1).

▶ Through-knee amputation has a bit of a checkered history. A theoretic advantage of the through-knee amputation versus an above-knee amputation

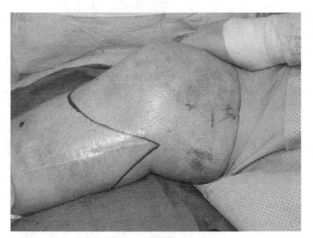

FIGURE 1.—"Fishmouth" incision. (Reprinted from Morse BC, Cull DL, Kalbaugh C, et al. Through-knee amputation in patients with peripheral arterial disease: a review of 50 cases. *J Vasc Surg.* 2008;48:638-643, with permission from the Society for Vascular Surgery.)

in patients who are candidates for rehabilitation would seem to be a longer lever arm with the through-knee amputation than the above-knee amputation. This longer lever arm should provide better balance and control of the prosthesis. However, the procedure with preservation of the femoral condyles can result in a rather bulbous stump that has been traditionally difficult to fit with a prosthesis. In addition, early small series of through-knee amputations suggested a high incidence of wound complications. In this series, with exclusion of patients with aortic iliac occlusive disease, the healing rate for a through-knee amputation was 93%. The authors have modified the traditional technique by using equal flaps rather than a long anterior flap, resecting the femoral condyles, and removing the patella. In the discussion accompanying this article, Dr Cole points out that in the last 40 years, the technology for lower extremity prostheses has improved dramatically. The combination of improved prostheses and improved wound healing using the technique described makes a through-knee amputation a viable alternative in selective patients (Fig 1).

G. L. Moneta, MD

Vascular injury during anterior exposure of the spine
Hamdan AD, Malek JY, Schermerhorn ML, et al (Beth Israel Deaconess Med Ctr, Boston, MA)
J Vasc Surg 48:650-654, 2008

Objectives.—Fusion of the spine is often performed from an anterior approach requiring mobilization of aorta, iliac artery, and vein. This study describes the preferred techniques and incidence of vascular complications at a spine center.

Methods.—Information and operative notes on all consecutive patients undergoing anterior exposure were entered into a database that was retrospectively reviewed. Four hundred eighty-two procedures performed on 480 patients at one spine center between January of 1997 and December of 2002 were analyzed. Demographics, technique, levels of exposure, and history of prior spine surgery were recorded. Primary outcomes measured included intraoperative vascular complications, estimated operative blood loss, and operative mortality. Vascular injury was defined as any case in which a suture was required to control bleeding. Major vascular injuries were defined as those requiring transfusion, vascular reconstruction, or blood loss greater than 300 cc.

Results.—An intraoperative vascular injury occurred in 11% (54/480) of patients. The majority of these (45/54) were minor injuries treated with simple suture repair. Nine (1.9%) major vascular injuries did occur; the majority identified and treated during the exposure and not the spinal fusion. One patient required a return to the operating room 24 hours after the initial procedure for removal of packs placed to control severe bleeding from an avulsed branch of the internal iliac vein. Median estimated blood loss (EBL) was 150 cc and there were no mortalities. Eighty-three percent of overall injuries involved exposure of L4-5, and this was statistically significant odds ratio (OR) 2.73, $P = .005$. The lowest incidence of injury occurred when L5-S1 alone was exposed (5.1% of injuries) OR .34, $P = .01$. Prior spine procedures did not significantly increase the risk of injury, $P = .67$. Other factors that did not significantly increase risk included gender, multiple levels vs single levels and technique of exposure.

Conclusion.—Exposure to the lumbar spine can be readily accomplished via a retroperitoneal approach. Minor vascular injuries during exposure, mostly venous, are not uncommon and are easily repaired. They are increased when L4-5 is part of the exposure and are lowest when L5-S1 alone is exposed. Major injuries occur in less than 2% of patients.

▶ Anterior fusion of the lumbar spine, either alone or in combination with a posterior procedure, is now common. The increasing frequency of this procedure relates to the increasing need to redo spine surgery and the development of artificial discs and bone grafts that require an anterior exposure. When exposing the lumbar spine, mobilization of the iliac artery and veins and/or aorta is required. The extent of exposure is determined by the site of the intended orthopedic procedure. An overwhelming tenant of anterior exposure of the lumbar spine is to provide sufficient access to the anterior disc area and even sometimes the lateral aspect of the involved disc. I think there are several points that can be gleaned from the article. First of all, exposure at the L4-L5 level is the site most frequently associated with vascular injury. This makes sense as exposure at that level requires relatively extensive mobilization of the iliac vessels and their retraction to the right. Because the problems are overwhelmingly at the L4-L5 level, exposure of multiple levels versus a single level does not increase the risk of vascular injury. The authors point out that previous spine surgery also was not a risk factor for vascular injury. However, the large majority of patients undergoing anterior exposure who had previous spine surgery had their previous operation from a posterior approach. It would seem intuitive that the results would be quite different if the previous operations had been via an anterior rather than posterior approach to the spine. Most of the injuries in this series occurred during exposure of the spine and not during the course of the actual implantation of the orthopedic device. Nevertheless, significant injuries can occur during the actual implantation of the artificial disc or bone graft. The instruments used by the orthopedist to implant these devices are not exactly "vascular friendly." Surgeons providing anterior exposure of the spine for their orthopedic colleagues are urged to remain in the operating room and scrubbed during the actual implantation of the orthopedic device.

G. L. Moneta, MD

19 Miscellaneous

Competence assessment of senior vascular trainees using a carotid endarterectomy bench model
Black SA, Harrison RH, Horrocks EJ, et al (St Mary's Hosp, London, UK; Imperial College School of Medicine, London, UK)
Br J Surg 94:1226-1231, 2007

Background.—Competency-based assessment is being introduced to surgical training. The value of bench-top technical skills assessment using a synthetic carotid endarterectomy (CEA) model was evaluated in vascular trainees and consultants.

Methods.—Forty-one surgeons (13 junior trainees, 15 senior trainees and 13 experienced consultants with experience of more than 50 CEAs) performed a three-throw knot-tying exercise on a jig and a CEA on the bench model. A composite score for knot-tying was calculated, incorporating electromagnetic motion analysis. CEA technical skill was assessed using validated rating scales by blinded video analysis.

Results.—Senior trainees performed better than junior trainees in knot-tying ($P = 0.025$) as well as generic ($P < 0.001$) and procedural ($P < 0.001$) skills on CEA model assessment. There was no difference between senior trainees and consultants on any of these measures. The CEA model interobserver reliability was high for all rating scales (generic $\alpha = 0.974$, procedural $\alpha = 0.952$, end-product $\alpha = 0.976$).

Conclusion.—Senior trainees achieved the same score as consultants, suggesting a similar level of basic technical skill and knowledge required to perform CEA, and were significantly better than junior trainees. Performance on the bench model could provide an early assessment for suitability to proceed to operative training in a competency-based training and assessment programme.

▶ There is a growing literature, most of it from Europe, in the use of models to both teach vascular-related technical skills and assess competence in the performance of vascular surgical procedures. As demonstrated in this study, such models (Fig 1 in the original article) can, in association with assessment tools, provide quantitative scores that may differentiate between surgeons of various levels of experience and, therefore, presumably varying levels of technical competence. It remains to be proven whether this can serve as a surrogate for clinical competence, and if the performance on models parallels operating room skill in the performance of vascular surgical procedures. Nevertheless, simulation and the use of models in clinical training is a genie that is not likely to go back in the bottle. The Society for Vascular Surgery recently formed a committee to evaluate vascular surgical training. The committee would be wise to investigate how models may improve the efficiency of vascular surgical training. The days of merely placing bright people in the hospital and having them emerge years later as a trained surgeon are rapidly drawing to a close.

G. L. Moneta, MD

Experienced Endovascular Interventionalists Objectively Improve their Skills by Attending Carotid Artery Stent Training Courses

Van Herzeele I, Aggarwal R, Neequaye S, et al (Surgical Technology, Imperial College, London; et al)
Eur J Vasc Endovasc Surg 35:541-550, 2008

Objective.—Carotid artery stenting (CAS) is an advanced endovascular intervention with a steep learning curve. Virtual reality (VR) simulation has been proposed as a means to train and objectively assess technical performance.

Aim.—To objectively assess psychomotor skills acquisition of experienced interventionalists attending a two-day CAS course, using a VR simulator.

Methods.—Both cognitive and technical skills of 11 interventionalists were trained in a two-day course using didactic sessions, case reviews, supervised VR simulation and live-cases. Pre- and post-course skills were assessed through performance on the same CAS procedure using metrics derived from the simulator.

Results.—Significant differences were noted between pre- and post-course performance for procedure (36 vs. 20 min., $p = 0.005$), X-ray (20 vs. 11 min., $p = 0.016$) and delivery-retrieval time of the embolic protection device (12 vs. 9 min., $p = 0.007$). Advancement of the guiding catheter without a leading wire occurred to a greater extent pre- versus post-course (199 vs. 152 mm., $p = 0.050$) as did spasm of the internal carotid artery (4 vs. 2, $p = 0.049$).

Conclusions.—This study has objectively proven a benefit for experienced interventionalists to attend CAS courses for skills acquisition, measured by a VR simulator. These data can be used to offer participants an insight into their skills and objectively audit course efficacy.

▶ This is another example of virtual reality simulation creeping into vascular surgical training and assessment. In this case, physicians experienced in catheter-based interventions, but not carotid stenting, underwent simulator training in carotid stenting. The results indicated it was possible to greatly improve simulator performance in the procedure with training on the simulator. The participants felt the training was effective. The study highlights the requirements for evaluating new educational techniques in surgical or interventional procedures. There must be a clinically relevant model, pre- and post-performance evaluations, objective measurements of performance, and participant evaluation of the process. The study also highlights the limitations of simulation, in that there is not necessarily a direct translation to improved clinical practice, and the variables evaluated in the model may not be clinically relevant. For example, cutting down the time to perform a carotid stent does not necessarily translate to improved clinical outcome, nor does reducing fluoroscopy time necessarily result in improved clinical outcomes. Everyone is aware of "slow" surgeons who have perfectly satisfactory results and "fast" surgeons whose results may not be as optimal. Simulation training and other techniques of modeling vascular procedures are highly interesting but have a long way to go before they will, can, or should be widely accepted. This is an area of academic inquiry that will expand rapidly in the next 5 to 10 years.

G. L. Moneta, MD

Article Index

Chapter 1: Basic Considerations

Rosuvastatin to Prevent Vascular Events in Men and Women with Elevated
C-Reactive Protein   1

Genetically Elevated C-Reactive Protein and Ischemic Vascular Disease   3

Glucose Control and Vascular Complications in Veterans with Type 2 Diabetes   5

Low-Dose Aspirin for Primary Prevention of Atherosclerotic Events in Patients
With Type 2 Diabetes: A Randomized Controlled Trial   6

The prevention of progression of arterial disease and diabetes (POPADAD) trial:
factorial randomised placebo controlled trial of aspirin and antioxidants in
patients with diabetes and asymptomatic peripheral arterial disease   8

Effect of Statins Alone Versus Statins Plus Ezetimibe on Carotid Atherosclerosis in
Type 2 Diabetes: The SANDS (Stop Atherosclerosis in Native Diabetics Study)
Trial   9

Plasma Levels of Soluble Tie2 and Vascular Endothelial Growth Factor Distinguish
Critical Limb Ischemia From Intermittent Claudication in Patients With Peripheral
Arterial Disease   11

Long-term clinical outcome after intramuscular implantation of bone marrow
mononuclear cells (Therapeutic Angiogenesis by Cell Transplantation [TACT]
trial) in patients with chronic limb ischemia   12

Hepatocyte Growth Factor, but not Vascular Endothelial Growth Factor,
Attenuates Angiotensin II-Induced Endothelial Progenitor Cell Senescence   14

Polydeoxyribonucleotide (PDRN) restores blood flow in an experimental model of
peripheral artery occlusive disease   16

Gene expression analysis of a porcine native abdominal aortic aneurysm model   17

Intra-abdominal fat and metabolic syndrome are associated with larger infrarenal
aortic diameters in patients with clinically evident arterial disease   18

Biomechanical properties of abdominal aortic aneurysms assessed by
simultaneously measured pressure and volume changes in humans   19

Genomewide Association Studies of Stroke   21

Local Delivery of Gene Vectors From Bare-Metal Stents by Use of a Biodegradable
Synthetic Complex Inhibits In-Stent Restenosis in Rat Carotid Arteries   23

Adventitial delivery of platelet-derived endothelial cell growth factor gene
prevented intimal hyperplasia of vein graft   24

Metalloproteinase expression in venous aneurysms   25

Sox18 induces development of the lymphatic vasculature in mice   27

Chapter 2: Coronary Disease

General and Abdominal Adiposity and Risk of Death in Europe   29

Prevalence and extent of dyslipidemia and recommended lipid levels in US adults
with and without cardiovascular comorbidities: The National Health and
Nutrition Examination Survey 2003-2004   30

Telmisartan, Ramipril, or Both in Patients at High Risk for Vascular Events   31

Effect of PCI on Quality of Life in Patients with Stable Coronary Disease   33

Drug-Eluting or Bare-Metal Stents for Acute Myocardial Infarction   34

Chapter 3: Epidemiology

Angina pectoris is a stronger indicator of diffuse vascular atherosclerosis than intermittent claudication: Framingham study   37

Patients with peripheral arterial disease in the CHARISMA trial   38

Symptomatic Peripheral Arterial Disease in Women: Nontraditional Biomarkers of Elevated Risk   40

Von Willebrand Factor, Type 2 Diabetes Mellitus, and Risk of Cardiovascular Disease: The Framingham Offspring Study   41

The Obesity Paradox in Patients With Peripheral Arterial Disease   43

Progression of Peripheral Arterial Disease Predicts Cardiovascular Disease Morbidity and Mortality   44

The epidemiology of abdominal aortic diameter   46

Carotid artery stenting has increased rates of postprocedure stroke, death, and resource utilization than does carotid endarterectomy in the United States, 2005   47

Endovenous laser ablation: Does standard above-knee great saphenous vein ablation provide optimum results in patients with both above- and below-knee reflux? A randomized controlled trial   48

A Predictive Model for Identifying Surgical Patients at Risk of Methicillin-Resistant *Staphylococcus aureus* Carriage on Admission   49

Chapter 4: Vascular Lab and Imaging

Reappraisal of velocity criteria for carotid bulb/internal carotid artery stenosis utilizing high-resolution B-mode ultrasound validated with computed tomography angiography   51

Color Doppler Ultrasonography in Occlusive Diseases of the Brachiocephalic and Proximal Subclavian Arteries   53

Duplex ultrasound velocity criteria for the stented carotid artery   54

Grading Carotid Intrastent Restenosis: A 6-Year Follow-Up Study   55

Validation of a method for determination of the ankle-brachial index in the seated position   56

Duplex ultrasound of the superficial femoral artery is a better screening tool than ankle-brachial index to identify at risk patients with lower extremity atherosclerosis   58

Assessment of the medial head of the gastrocnemius muscle in functional compression of the popliteal artery   60

Duplex criteria for determination of in-stent stenosis after angioplasty and stenting of the superficial femoral artery   61

Efficacy of duplex ultrasound surveillance after infrainguinal vein bypass may be enhanced by identification of characteristics predictive of graft stenosis development 64

Bleeding into the intraluminal thrombus in abdominal aortic aneurysms is associated with rupture 65

Assessment of renal artery stenosis: side-by-side comparison of angiography and duplex ultrasound with pressure gradient measurements 67

Magnetic resonance angiography of collateral blood supply to spinal cord in thoracic and thoracoabdominal aortic aneurysm patients 69

Chapter 5: Perioperative Considerations

Effects of extended-release metoprolol succinate in patients undergoing non-cardiac surgery (POISE trial): a randomised controlled trial 73

Predictors and outcomes of a perioperative myocardial infarction following elective vascular surgery in patients with documented coronary artery disease: Results of the CARP trial 75

Intensive Blood Glucose Control and Vascular Outcomes in Patients with Type 2 Diabetes 76

Effect of Statin Therapy on Mortality in Patients With Peripheral Arterial Disease and Comparison of Those With Versus Without Associated Chronic Obstructive Pulmonary Disease 78

Clinical outcome in patients with peripheral artery disease. Results from a prospective registry (FRENA) 80

Are patients with thrombophilia and previous venous thromboembolism at higher risk to arterial thrombosis? 81

A comparison of recombinant thrombin to bovine thrombin as a hemostatic ancillary in patients undergoing peripheral arterial bypass and arteriovenous graft procedures 82

Femoral vs Jugular Venous Catheterization and Risk of Nosocomial Events in Adults Requiring Acute Renal Replacement Therapy: A Randomized Controlled Trial 83

Oral Vitamin K Versus Placebo to Correct Excessive Anticoagulation in Patients Receiving Warfarin: A Randomized Trial 85

Preoperative Shower Revisited: Can High Topical Antiseptic Levels Be Achieved on the Skin Surface Before Surgical Admission? 86

Five Day Antibiotic Prophylaxis for Major Lower Limb Amputation Reduces Wound Infection Rates and the Length of In-hospital Stay 87

Use of vacuum-assisted closure (VAC) therapy in treating lymphatic complications after vascular procedures: New approach for lymphoceles 88

Rehospitalizations among Patients in the Medicare Fee-for-Service Program 90

Chapter 6: Grafts and Graft Complications

Aortic reconstruction with femoral-popliteal vein: Graft stenosis incidence, risk and reintervention 93

Predictors for Outcome after Vacuum Assisted Closure Therapy of Peri-vascular
Surgical Site Infections in the Groin   94

Chapter 7: Aortic Aneurysm

Abdominal Aortic Aneurysm Development in Men Following a "normal" Aortic
Ultrasound Scan   97

Growth predictors and prognosis of small abdominal aortic aneurysms   98

Analysis of Expansion Patterns in 4-4.9 cm Abdominal Aortic Aneurysms   99

Abdominal aortic aneurysm events in the women's health initiative: cohort study   101

Fit patients with small abdominal aortic aneurysms (AAAs) do not benefit from
early intervention   102

Peak wall stress measurement in elective and acute abdominal aortic aneurysms   103

The Rupture Rate of Large Abdominal Aortic Aneurysms: Is This Modified by
Anatomical Suitability for Endovascular Repair?   105

Anatomic Suitability of Ruptured Abdominal Aortic Aneurysms for Endovascular
Repair   107

National trends in the repair of ruptured abdominal aortic aneurysms   108

Common iliac artery aneurysm: Expansion rate and results of open surgical and
endovascular repair   110

Natural history of common iliac arteries after aorto-aortic graft insertion during
elective open abdominal aortic aneurysm repair: A prospective study   112

Endovascular treatment of thoracoabdominal aortic aneurysms   114

Chapter 8: Abdominal Aortic Endografting

Endovascular vs. Open Repair of Abdominal Aortic Aneurysms in the Medicare
Population   117

Lifeline registry of endovascular aneurysm repair: Open repair surgical controls in
clinical trials   118

Comparison of the effects of open and endovascular aortic aneurysm repair on
long-term renal function using chronic kidney disease staging based on glomerular
filtration rate   119

Zenith abdominal aortic aneurysm endovascular graft   121

The Powerlink system for endovascular abdominal aortic aneurysm repair:
Six-year results   122

What is the clinical utility of a 6-month computed tomography in the follow-up
of endovascular aneurysm repair patients?   123

The trifurcated endograft technique for hypogastric preservation during
endovascular aneurysm repair   124

Branched devices for thoracoabdominal aneurysm repair: Early experience   126

Chapter 9: Visceral and Renal Artery Disease

Renal Stenting for Incidentally Discovered Renal Artery Stenosis: Is There any
Outcome Benefit?   129

Embolic Protection and Platelet Inhibition During Renal Artery Stenting   130

Efficacy of protected renal artery primary stenting in the solitary functioning
kidney   131

Operative mortality for renal artery bypass in the United States: Results from the
National Inpatient Sample   133

Outcomes after endarterectomy for chronic mesenteric ischemia   135

Isolated spontaneous dissection of the splanchnic arteries   136

Epidemiology, risk and prognostic factors in mesenteric venous thrombosis 137

Superficial venous thrombosis: Prevalence of common genetic risk factors and their
role on spreading to deep veins   139

Chapter 10: Thoracic Aorta

Characterization of the inflammatory cells in ascending thoracic aortic aneurysms
in patients with Marfan syndrome, familial thoracic aortic aneurysms, and
sporadic aneurysms   141

Degree of fusiform dilatation of the proximal descending aorta in type B acute
aortic dissection can predict late aortic events   142

Outcomes and Survival in Surgical Treatment of Descending Thoracic Aorta With
Acute Dissection   143

Complicated acute type B aortic dissection: Midterm results of emergency
endovascular stent–grafting   144

Aortic remodeling after endografting of thoracoabdominal aortic dissection 146

Early and midterm results after endovascular stent graft repair of penetrating aortic
ulcers   147

Outcome and Quality of Life After Surgical and Endovascular Treatment of
Descending Aortic Lesions   148

Population-based outcomes of open descending thoracic aortic aneurysm repair 150

Pivotal results of the Medtronic Vascular Talent Thoracic Stent Graft System: The
VALOR Trial   152

Hybrid procedures for thoracoabdominal aortic aneurysms and chronic aortic
dissections – A single center experience in 28 patients   153

Visceral aortic patch aneurysm after thoracoabdominal aortic repair: Conventional
vs hybrid treatment   154

Chapter 11: Leg Ischemia

Incident Physical Disability in People with Lower Extremity Peripheral Arterial
Disease: The Role of Cardiovascular Disease   157

Asymptomatic Peripheral Arterial Disease Is Associated With More Adverse Lower
Extremity Characteristics Than Intermittent Claudication   158

Risk attitudes to treatment among patients with severe intermittent claudication   159

Treadmill Exercise and Resistance Training in Patients With Peripheral Arterial Disease With and Without Intermittent Claudication: A Randomized Controlled Trial   160

Functional assessment at the buttock level of the effect of aortobifemoral bypass surgery   162

Long-term results of a multicenter randomized study on direct versus crossover bypass for unilateral iliac artery occlusive disease   163

The management of severe aortoiliac occlusive disease: Endovascular therapy rivals open reconstruction   165

Female gender and oral anticoagulants are associated with wound complications in lower extremity vein bypass: An analysis of 1404 operations for critical limb ischemia   167

Factors associated with early failure of infrainguinal lower extremity arterial bypass   168

Disparity in Outcomes of Surgical Revascularization for Limb Salvage: Race and Gender are Synergistic Determinants of Vein Graft Failure and Limb Loss   170

Prospective 2-Years Follow-up Quality of Life Study after Infrageniculate Bypass Surgery for Limb Salvage: Lasting Improvements Only in Non-diabetic Patients   171

Major Lower Extremity Amputation after Multiple Revascularizations: Was It Worth It?   172

Preservation for Future use of the Autologous Saphenous Vein during femoro-popliteal Bypass Surgery is Inexpedient   173

Revascularization to an isolated ("blind") popliteal artery segment: A viable procedure for critical limb ischemia   175

Bypass to the Perigeniculate Collateral Arteries: Mid-term Results   176

Angioplasty for Diabetic Patients with Failing Bypass Graft or Residual Critical Ischemia after Bypass Graft   177

The Adjuvant Benefit of Angioplasty in Patients with Mild to Moderate Intermittent Claudication (MIMIC) Managed by Supervised Exercise, Smoking Cessation Advice and Best Medical Therapy: Results from Two Randomised Trials for Stenotic Femoropopliteal and Aortoiliac Arterial Disease   179

Contemporary outcomes after superficial femoral artery angioplasty and stenting: The influence of TASC classification and runoff score   180

Cost-effectiveness of endovascular revascularization compared to supervised hospital-based exercise training in patients with intermittent claudication: A randomized controlled trial   181

Comparison of Results of Subintimal Angioplasty and Percutaneous Transluminal Angioplasty in Superficial Femoral Artery Occlusions   183

Efficacy of Cilostazol After Endovascular Therapy for Femoropopliteal Artery Disease in Patients With Intermittent Claudication   185

Cilostazol reduces restenosis after endovascular therapy in patients with femoropopliteal lesions   187

Local Delivery of Paclitaxel to Inhibit Restenosis during Angioplasty of the Leg   189

Midterm outcome predictors for lower extremity atherectomy procedures   190

Do Current Outcomes Justify More Liberal Use of Revascularization for
Vasculogenic Claudication? A Single Center Experience of 1,000 Consecutively
Treated Limbs   191

Outcomes of Combined Superficial Femoral Endovascular Revascularization and
Popliteal to Distal Bypass for Patients with Tissue Loss   192

Improving limb salvage in critical ischemia with intermittent pneumatic
compression: A controlled study with 18-month follow-up   193

Fifty percent area reduction after 4 weeks of treatment is a reliable indicator for
healing—analysis of a single-center cohort of 704 diabetic patients   195

Outcomes of surgical management for popliteal artery aneurysms: An analysis of
583 cases   196

Chapter 12: Upper Extremity and Dialysis Access

The natural history of vascular access for hemodialysis: A single center study of
2,422 patients   199

Arteriovenous Fistula Formation using Transposed Basilic Vein: Extensive Single
Centre Experience   200

The brachial artery-brachial vein fistula: Expanding the possibilities for
autogenous fistulae   203

Effect of Clopidogrel on Early Failure of Arteriovenous Fistulas for Hemodialysis:
A Randomized Controlled Trial   204

Fistula Elevation Procedure: Experience with 295 Consecutive Cases During
a 7-Year Period   206

Plication as Primary Treatment of Steal Syndrome in Arteriovenous Fistulas   207

Risk of Hemodialysis Graft Thrombosis: Analysis of Monthly Flow Surveillance   209

Secondary Patency of Thrombosed Prosthetic Vascular Access Grafts with
Aggressive Surveillance, Monitoring and Endovascular Management   211

Brachial artery ligation with total graft excision is a safe and effective approach to
prosthetic arteriovenous graft infections   212

Chapter 13: Carotid and Cerebrovascular Disease

The fate of patients with retinal artery occlusion and Hollenhorst plaque   215

Aortic Atherosclerosis, Hypercoagulability, and Stroke. The APRIS (Aortic Plaque
and Risk of Ischemic Stroke) Study   216

The relationship between serum levels of vascular calcification inhibitors and
carotid plaque vulnerability   218

Aspirin and Extended-Release Dipyridamole versus Clopidogrel for Recurrent
Stroke   220

Markers of instability in high-risk carotid plaques are reduced by statins   222

General anaesthesia versus local anaesthesia for carotid surgery (GALA):
a multicentre, randomised controlled trial   224

Factors associated with stroke or death after carotid endarterectomy in Northern
New England   226

Statistical modeling of the volume-outcome effect for carotid endarterectomy for 10 years of a statewide database — 228

Association between minor and major surgical complications after carotid endarterectomy: Results of the New York Carotid Artery Surgery study — 230

Carotid endarterectomy was performed with lower stroke and death rates than carotid artery stenting in the United States in 2003 and 2004 — 231

Significance of postoperative crossed cerebellar hypoperfusion in patients with cerebral hyperperfusion following carotid endarterectomy: SPECT study — 232

Long-Term Results of Carotid Stenting versus Endarterectomy in High-Risk Patients — 234

Alert for increased long-term follow-up after carotid artery stenting: Results of a prospective, randomized, single-center trial of carotid artery stenting vs carotid endarterectomy — 235

Carotid Artery Stenting in High-Risk Patients: Midterm Mortality Analysis — 236

Carotid artery stenting: Identification of risk factors for poor outcomes — 237

A randomized trial of carotid artery stenting with and without cerebral protection — 238

Effects of Age and Symptom Status on Silent Ischemic Lesions after Carotid Stenting with and without the Use of Distal Filter Devices — 239

A risk score to predict ischemic lesions after protected carotid artery stenting — 241

Endovascular treatment for carotid artery stenosis after neck irradiation — 242

Results in a consecutive series of 83 surgical corrections of symptomatic stenotic kinking of the internal carotid artery — 243

Thrombolysis with Alteplase 3 to 4.5 Hours after Acute Ischemic Stroke — 246

Chapter 14: Vascular Trauma

Blunt thoracic aortic injury: Open or stent graft repair? — 249

Endovascular Stenting for Traumatic Aortic Injury: An Emerging New Standard of Care — 250

Endovascular repair of traumatic thoracic aortic disruptions with "stacked" abdominal endograft extension cuffs — 251

Blunt intraabdominal arterial injury in pediatric trauma patients: injury distribution and markers of outcome — 253

Penetrating femoropopliteal injury during modern warfare: Experience of the Balad Vascular Registry — 254

Post-Traumatic Ulnar Artery Thrombosis: Outcome of Arterial Reconstruction Using Reverse Interpositional Vein Grafting at 2 Years Minimum Follow-Up — 255

Chapter 15: Nonatherosclerotic Conditions

Abdominal aortic coarctation: Surgical treatment of 53 patients with a thoracoabdominal bypass, patch aortoplasty, or interposition aortoaortic graft — 259

Complex vascular reconstruction of abdominal aorta and its branches in the pediatric population — 262

Quality of life of patients with Takayasu's arteritis   263

Intermittent claudication in diabetes mellitus due to chronic exertional
compartment syndrome of the leg: An observational study of 17 patients   264

Predictors of Prosthetic Graft Infection after Infrainguinal Bypass   265

Chapter 16: Venous Thrombosis and Pulmonary Embolism

Incidence, clinical characteristics, and long-term prognosis of travel-associated
pulmonary embolism   269

Clinical Predictors for Fatal Pulmonary Embolism in 15 520 Patients With Venous
Thromboembolism: Findings From the Registro Informatizado de la Enfermedad
TromboEmbolica venosa (RIETE) Registry   271

Chronic Kidney Disease Increases Risk for Venous Thromboembolism   272

Activated Partial Thromboplastin Time and Risk of Future Venous
Thromboembolism   273

Etiology and VTE risk factor distribution in patients with inferior vena cava
thrombosis   275

Incidence of deep vein thrombosis related to peripherally inserted central catheters
in children and adolescents   276

A 10-year analysis of venous thromboembolism on the surgical service: The effect
of practice guidelines for prophylaxis   277

Clinical probability assessment and D-dimer determination in patients with
suspected deep vein thrombosis, a prospective multicenter management study   278

Evaluation of Wells score and repeated D-dimer in diagnosing venous
thromboembolism   279

D-dimer and factor VIII are independent risk factors for recurrence after
anticoagulation withdrawal for a first idiopathic deep vein thrombosis   281

Identifying unprovoked thromboembolism patients at low risk for recurrence who
can discontinue anticoagulant therapy   282

Thromboembolic Consequences of Subtherapeutic Anticoagulation in Patients
Stabilized on Warfarin Therapy: The Low INR Study   284

Deep Vein Thrombosis of Lower Extremity: Direct Intraclot Injection of Alteplase
Once Daily with Systemic Anticoagulation—Results of Pilot Study   285

Chapter 17: Chronic Venous and Lymphatic Disease

Determinants and Time Course of the Postthrombotic Syndrome after Acute Deep
Venous Thrombosis   289

A Randomized, Double-Blind Multicentre Clinical Trial Comparing the Efficacy of
Calcium Dobesilate with Placebo in the Treatment of Chronic Venous Disease   290

Comparisons of side effects using air and carbon dioxide foam for endovenous
chemical ablation   291

The importance of deep venous reflux velocity as a determinant of outcome in
patients with combined superficial and deep venous reflux treated with endovenous
saphenous ablation   293

Endovenous laser ablation: Does standard above-knee great saphenous vein ablation provide optimum results in patients with both above- and below-knee reflux? A randomized controlled trial 294

A Prospective Study of Incidence of Saphenous Nerve Injury after Total Great Saphenous Vein Stripping 295

The appropriate length of great saphenous vein stripping should be based on the extent of reflux and not on the intent to avoid saphenous nerve injury 296

A prospective evaluation of the outcome after small saphenous varicose vein surgery with one-year follow-up 298

Iliac vein compression syndrome: Outcome of endovascular treatment with long-term follow-up 299

Ovarian vein incompetence: a potential cause of chronic pelvic pain in women 300

Chapter 18: Technical Notes

EVAR of Aortoiliac Aneurysms with Branched Stent-grafts 303

Successful devascularization of carotid body tumors by covered stent placement in the external carotid artery 304

Repair of complex renal artery aneurysms by laparoscopic nephrectomy with ex vivo repair and autotransplantation 306

Intraoperative Retrograde Mesenteric Angioplasty for Acute Occlusive Mesenteric Ischaemia: A Case Series 308

Midterm Patency following Atherectomy for Infrainguinal Occlusive Disease: A Word of Caution 309

Iliofemoral Pulsion Endarterectomy 310

Superficial femoral artery autograft reconstruction in the treatment of popliteal artery aneurysm: Long-term outcome 312

Through-knee amputation in patients with peripheral arterial disease: A review of 50 cases 314

Vascular injury during anterior exposure of the spine 315

Chapter 19: Miscellaneous

Competence assessment of senior vascular trainees using a carotid endarterectomy bench model 319

Experienced Endovascular Interventionalists Objectively Improve their Skills by Attending Carotid Artery Stent Training Courses 320

Author Index

A

Abraira C, 5
Abularrage CJ, 263
Acher CW, 135
Acosta S, 137
Ades P, 160
Ageno W, 85
Aggarwal R, 320
Albrecht T, 189
Aleksynas N, 183
Alexandrou A, 131
Alferiev I, 23
Alhadad A, 137
Allison MA, 46
Allon M, 204
Altavilla D, 16
Altinel O, 190
Alvarez L, 80
Amberger N, 222
Amoroso S, 300
Antusevas A, 183
Ashton HA, 97
Azuma J, 14

B

Backes WH, 69
Bakay M, 23
Ballard JL, 58
Ballotta E, 112, 175
Bandyk DF, 64, 167
Bannazadeh M, 190
Barbato JE, 123, 238
Baril DT, 61
Beck AW, 93
Beck GJ, 204
Beckert S, 195
Beckman MO, 65
Belch J, 8
Bena JF, 165
Benvenisty A, 192
Bertoglio L, 154
Bianchi C, 236
Bis JC, 21
Bishop V, 236
Bitto A, 16
Black SA, 319
Blankensteijn JD, 173
Bluhmki E, 246
Böckler D, 153
Boeing H, 29
Bosch JL, 181
Bozinovski J, 143

Brabham VW, 293
Brach JS, 157
Brahmanandam S, 167
Breslau PJ, 295
Bronder CM, 206
Brothers TE, 265
Brown LC, 102, 105
Bruijnen H, 171
Burkett AB, 251
Busch MA, 222
Buth J, 19

C

Cacoub PP, 38
Caliò FG, 243
Cambria RP, 121
Campbell I, 8
Caniano DA, 253
Caprini A, 27
Carpenter JP, 122
Castier Y, 312
Chang B, 262
Chang R, 285
Chassin MR, 230
Chaudhuri A, 87
Chavanpun JP, 64
Chen CC, 285
Chigurupati R, 309
Chisci E, 55
Chloros GD, 255
Chung SW, 309
Chuter TAM, 114, 121
Ciaranello AL, 212
Cini M, 281
Ciocca RG, 231
Clark NP, 284
Clerici G, 177
Clerissi J, 177
Clouse WD, 254
Coerper S, 195
Coleman EA, 90
Collier JW, 103
Colyer W, 130
Cook NR, 40
Cooper CJ, 130
Coselli JS, 143
Cosmi B, 281
Criado E, 259
Criado F, 152
Criqui MH, 44
Crowther MA, 85
Cull DL, 206, 314
Cushman M, 272

D

Da Giau G, 112, 175
Davies RSM, 310
Décousus H, 271
Delate T, 284
de Latour B, 176
Delis KT, 193
Dellagrammaticas D, 48, 294
Delvecchio C, 172
Dember LM, 204
den Hoed PT, 181
Desai T, 51
de Virgilio C, 207
DeZee KJ, 168
Di Stasi C, 300
DiTomasso D, 46
Di Tullio MR, 216
Dias NV, 303
Dick F, 148
Diener H-C, 220
Dillavou E, 238
Dirven M, 173
Doughman T, 200
Drieghe B, 67
Druce PS, 97
Dubois J, 276
Duckworth W, 5
Duncan AA, 110
Dunlap AB, 215
Duong ST, 119, 180
Duprey A, 176, 242
Duscha BD, 11

E

Edmiston CE Jr, 86
Edmundsson D, 264
Egorova N, 108
Elf JL, 278
Eliason JL, 254, 259
Elliott BM, 265
Engelhardt M, 171
English SJ, 237
Ernemann U, 241
Estallo L, 99
Evans JC, 37

F

Fagan MJ, 103
Faglia E, 177
Fairman RM, 152, 237
Farber M, 152

Favre J-P, 242
Fayad P, 234
Ferreira M, 126
Ferrucci L, 158
Findley CM, 11
Fishbein I, 23
Flanigan DP, 58
Fleg JL, 9
Flu HC, 295
Forsberg C, 159
François M, 27
Frankel DS, 41
Fukui S, 312

G

Galal W, 43
Gallagher KA, 306
Gammie JS, 250
Garcia B, 56
Garcia D, 85
Garel L, 276
Garg P, 34
Geisbüsch P, 147, 153
Gerasimidis T, 218
Ghandehari H, 30
Giacovelli JK, 108
Gich I, 290
Giglia JS, 172
Giles KA, 150
Gloviczki P, 110
Go MR, 123
Goldenberg S, 17
Golemati S, 218
Gómez R, 99
Goncalves I, 200
Goodney PP, 226
Gornik HL, 56
Gorter PM, 18
Gröschel K, 239, 241
Granke K, 82
Greenberg JI, 129, 203
Greenberg RK, 118, 121
Greenhalgh RM, 102, 105
Greenstein AJ, 230
Greindl M, 235
Groner JI, 253
Gruppo M, 112, 175
Guo D-C, 141
Guralnik JM, 158, 160
Gurm HS, 234

H

Haagensen M, 60
Hacke W, 246

Haddad GK, 211
Haddad JA, 211
Hafez H, 97
Haller ST, 130
Hamdan AD, 150, 315
Hamed O, 88
Hamming JF, 295
Hamner CE, 253
Handa M, 24
Harbarth S, 49
Harper SJF, 200
Harris EJ, 107
Harrison RH, 319
Hayes PD, 87
He R, 141
Healy MG, 191
Heng MS, 103
Hevelone N, 170
Hill JS, 231
Hinder D, 148
Hiramoto JS, 114
Hobson RW II, 54
Hoch JR, 135, 249
Hocking JA, 93
Hoeks SE, 43, 78
Hoffmann K, 29
Homma S, 216
Horowitz MB, 238
Horrocks EJ, 319
Hosking B, 27
Howard BV, 9
Huang Y, 110
Hynecek RL, 17

I

Ihnat DM, 180
Iida O, 187
Ikram MA, 21
Illuminati G, 243
Imhoff L, 129
Immer FF, 148
Ioannou CV, 296
Irwin C, 25

J

Jackson BM, 237
Jaquinandi V, 162
Jencks SF, 90
Jensen JS, 3
Jensen M, 192
Jhaveri A, 117
Jin Z, 216

Johnson ON III, 196
Julian JA, 289

K

Kadoglou NPE, 218
Kahn SR, 282, 289
Kakkos SK, 211
Kalbaugh CA, 191
Kalbaugh C, 314
Kam A, 285
Kamal-Bahl S, 30
Kannel WB, 37
Karr SB, 304
Kashyap VS, 165, 215
Kaste M, 246
Kastrup A, 239
Katsargyris A, 131
Kaupas RS, 183
Kavros SJ, 193
Kawasaki T, 185
Kaye AJ, 262
Kim J, 61
Klonaris C, 131
Kobayashi M, 232
Kölbel T, 94
Kolm P, 33
Kosmorsky GS, 215
Kostas TT, 296
Kotelis D, 147, 153
Koyama T, 142
Kraiss L, 25
Krepel CJ, 86
Kunte H, 222
Küper MA, 195
Kuper SG, 206
Kwan K, 46

L

Labruto F, 65
Lal BK, 54
Lantis J, 192
Lanziotti L, 126
Laporte S, 271
Larson JC, 101
Lederle FA, 101
Lee JT, 107
Legnani C, 281
Lehmann R, 269
Leon LR Jr, 119
Letterstål A, 159
Leus M, 269
Levien LJ, 60

Lew W, 82
Li W, 24
Li Z, 255
Linnemann B, 81, 275
Ljungqvist M, 279
Lucas L, 146
Lucas RM, 255
Lustgarten JJ, 304

M

MacCuish A, 8
Macsata RA, 196
Madaric J, 67
Malek JY, 315
Margolis KL, 101
Marone EM, 154
Marston WA, 293
Martínez-Zapata MJ, 290
Marui A, 142
Massaro JM, 41
Matoba S, 12
Mauri L, 34
Mavor AID, 48, 294
May S, 203
McCarter DHA, 308
McDermott MM, 158, 160
McFalls EO, 75
McPhee JT, 47, 231
Meigs JB, 41
Mell MW, 135
Mendes R, 293
Merkx M, 19
Mess WH, 69
Messina LM, 47
Mete M, 9
Milio G, 139
Miller DC, 144
Mills JL Sr, 119
Minà C, 139
Minion DJ, 124
Mismetti P, 271
Mitchell RG, 11
Miyata T, 136
Moainie SL, 250
Mochizuki T, 142
Modrall JG, 133
Moll FL, 18
Monreal M, 80
Monsen C, 94
Monteiro M, 126
Moreno RM, 290
Morioka K, 24
Moritz P, 279
Moritz T, 5

Moritz TE, 75
Morrison N, 291
Morse BC, 314
Moyes LH, 308
Muck PE, 88
Mureebe L, 108
Murphy EH, 93

N

Nägele T, 239
Nanto S, 187
Nassar R, 209
Naydeck BL, 157
Nazarian SM, 228
Neequaye S, 320
Neschis DG, 250
Neuhardt DL, 291
Nguyen LL, 167, 170
Nijenhuis RJ, 69
Nilsson C, 278
Ninomiya JK, 44
Nourissat A, 242
Nourissat G, 176

O

Ogasawara K, 232
Ogawa H, 6
Oguzkurt L, 299
O'Hare JL, 298
Ohira T, 273
Olofsson P, 159
Olsen DM, 146
O'Malley AJ, 117
Ou HW, 236
Ozkan U, 299

P

Papagiannis A, 199
Papanikolaou V, 199
Paraskevas N, 312
Parienti J-J, 83
Patel A, 76
Pavkov ML, 165
Pfister K, 235
Phelan MW, 306
Picquet J, 162
Pillai J, 60
Piper S, 37
Pischon T, 29
Pogue J, 31

Polito F, 16
Powell JT, 105
Pradhan AD, 40
Probst H, 163

R

Ram SJ, 209
Rapp JH, 114
Reed AB, 172
Resch TA, 303
Rhee RY, 61, 123
Ricco J-B, 163, 243
Ridker PM, 1
Robinson D, 58
Robison JG, 265
Rodger MA, 282
Rodriguez JA, 146
Rogers CR, 291
Rogers FB, 277
Rogers SO, 170
Rosenthal D, 251
Rosero EB, 133
Roy J, 65
Rypens F, 276

S

Sacco RL, 220
Sadat U, 87
Sadek M, 17
Sanada F, 14
Sarac TP, 190
Sarno G, 67
Saumet J-L, 162
Sax H, 49
Scanlon JM, 304
Schanzer A, 47, 212
Schanzer H, 212
Scharmer C, 171
Scharn DM, 173
Schermerhorn ML, 117, 150, 315
Schindewolf M, 81, 275
Schlösser FJV, 98
Schmidt H, 275
Schnaudigel S, 241
Seabrook GR, 86
Seshadri S, 21
Setacci C, 55
Setacci F, 55
Shaalan WE, 51
Shackford SR, 277
Sharafuddin MJ, 309

Shirakawa M, 136
Shrier I, 289
Shrivastava S, 40
Sidawy AN, 118, 168, 263
Silbaugh TS, 34
Sin DD, 78
Singh N, 168
Siragusa S, 139
Slater BJ, 107
Slemp AE, 262
Slidell MB, 196, 263
Smith JM, 88
Smith ST, 133
Soga Y, 185
Söderberg M, 279
Solomon C, 157
Sonesson B, 303
Sorial E, 124
Spertus JA, 33
Spronk S, 181
Stanley JC, 259
Stehman-Breen C, 272
Steinbauer MGM, 235
Stern T, 306
Strandberg K, 278
Suess C, 269
Suga Y, 232
Suliman A, 129, 203
Sun W, 141
Svensson O, 264
Svensson P, 137
Svensson S, 94
Sykes TCF, 310
Synn A, 25
Sze D, 144

T

Takayama T, 136
Tangelder MJD, 98
Taniyama Y, 14
Taylor SM, 191
Taylor ZC, 180
Tefera G, 249

Teo KK, 31
Tepe G, 189
Tercan F, 299
Terrien CM, 277
Theivacumar NS, 48, 294
Thompson RE, 228
Thompson SG, 102
Tinder CN, 64
Tofighi B, 54
Tola M, 53
Toolanen G, 264
Tropeano G, 300
Tshomba Y, 154
Turner NS, 193
Tybjærg-Hansen A, 3

U

Uckay I, 49
Uematsu M, 187
Uslu OS, 53

V

Vandenbroeck CP, 298
van Gestel YRBM, 43, 78
Van Herzeele I, 320
van 't Veer M, 19
Vass DG, 308
Vega de Céniga M, 99
Veligrantakis M, 296
Verhagen HJM, 98
Verhoye JP, 144
Vilaseca B, 80
Visseren FLJ, 18
Vrochides D, 199

W

Wahlgren CM, 51
Wall ML, 310
Wang GJ, 122

Wang J, 230
Ward HB, 75
Wattanakit K, 272
Weaver FA, 82
Weber TF, 147
Weintraub WS, 33
Wellons ED, 251
Wells PS, 282
White R, 273
Whitman B, 298
Williams MV, 90
Wingard DL, 44
Witt DM, 284
Wolski K, 56
Wong ND, 30
Woodward EB, 254
Work J, 209

X

Xenos E, 124

Y

Yadav JS, 234
Yaghoubian A, 207
Yamane BH, 249
Yenokyan G, 228
Yokoi H, 185
Yurdakul M, 53
Yusuf S, 31, 220

Z

Zacho J, 3
Zakai NA, 273
Zeller T, 189
Zgouras D, 81
Zwolak RM, 118